David Låg Tomasi

Medical Philosophy

A Philosophical Analysis of Patient Self-Perception in Diagnostics and Therapy

STUDIES IN MEDICAL PHILOSOPHY

Edited by Alexander Gungov and Friedrich Luft

ISSN 2367-4377

David Låg Tomasi

MEDICAL PHILOSOPHY

A Philosophical Analysis of Patient Self-Perception in Diagnostics and Therapy

ibidem-Verlag

Stuttgart

Bibliographic information published by the Deutsche Nationalbibliothek
Die Deutsche Nationalbibliothek lists this publication in the Deutsche Nationalbibliografie; detailed bibliographic data are available in the Internet at http://dnb.d-nb.de.

Bibliografische Information der Deutschen Nationalbibliothek
Die Deutsche Nationalbibliothek verzeichnet diese Publikation in der Deutschen Nationalbibliografie; detaillierte bibliografische Daten sind im Internet über http://dnb.d-nb.de abrufbar.

Cover picture: © David Låg Tomasi, 2016.

ISSN: 2367-4377

ISBN-13: 978-3-8382-0975-3

© *ibidem*-Verlag / *ibidem* Press

Stuttgart, Germany 2016

Acknowledgments

Making sure to list all the people without whom this book would not have been possible is indeed a very difficult task. It is my hope that my memory will not fail me and that all the great experiences I cherish in my heart and my mind will leave a mark, at least in part, in the writing for this thesis.

Firstly, I would like to acknowledge all the professors and academic staff at the University of Sofia "St. Kliment Ohridski" and the Bulgarian Academy of Sciences for all the great conversations and learning opportunities through the years: Prof. Maria Dimitrova, Prof. Valeri Dinev, Prof. Julia Vaseva-Dikova, Prof. Asen Dimitrov, Prof. Aneta Karageorgieva, Prof. Plamen Makariev, Prof. Nedyalka Videva, Dr. Elena Tsenkova, Ms. Deyana Andonova, Ms. Irena Cheresharova, and Ms. Sasha Nikolova-Livsey. I also want to thank all the participants, the patients, the multidisciplinary treatment team and all the staff on the Inpatient Psychiatry Unit, Shepardson 3 and Shepardson 6, as well as all the staff at the University of Vermont Medical Center and College of Medicine. I am especially grateful to Dr. William Tobey Horn and Prof. Lou Colasanti for their assistance and supervision, and to Prof. Friedrich Luft as well as Dr. Ilaria Rubbo for their work and contributions. I also want to acknowledge the wonderful example of Dr. Dietfried Schönemann and Ms. Margarethe Wiedenhofer in helping me discover a true passion for medicine.

Furthermore, a big thank you goes to the Inpatient Psychiatry Group Therapists Carol Clawson, John Derivan, Lindsay Enman, Sheri Gates, Kevin Melo, Annie Rapaport, Emily Reyns, Joshua Shupp-Star, Adoria Tudor, and Alixandra West. I want to acknowledge the great support of the University of Vermont College of Medicine, the University of Vermont College of Medicine and the University of Vermont Medical Center, especially Dr. Robert Pierattini, Dr. Alan Rubin, Lauren Tronsgard-Scott, Katharine Monje, Stacey Ward, David Hunt, Denise Quint and Gale Weld. This has been a wonderful journey and I am grateful for all the beautiful people who were very generous in giving up some of their time to take part in our surveys and questionnaires, and the academic, research, and medical professionals who helped me with their knowledge, their insights, and their experiences.

A special *благодаря Ви много* goes to my Professor Dr. Alexander Gungov. He has been an incredible source of academic strength, interesting and passionate debates, and constant encouragement. I am grateful and truly privileged to be receiving the attention of such a noble person and wonderful teacher.

Last but not least I would like to acknowledge the understanding, the support and the encouragement of my family both in Europe and the USA, especially my wife Livija and my son Lucas Andrej.

This study is dedicated to you.

David Låg Tomasi

Table of Contents

List of Figures

List of Tables

Foreword

Does medicine warrant its own philosophy? In antiquity, doctors and philosophers identified the physical body as the space in which life was located and originated. They used the word psyche or soul to refer to forces organizing, inspiring, and energizing the body. Ancient physicians strived to achieve a balance, an aequinimitas in their patients; William Osler strived to achieve the same for the physicians themselves. Probably both patients and physicians need to be in balance. My pathologist friends tell me they have never encountered a soul; what a pity! Of course, by the time they arrive on the scene, the souls are gone. The soul is an octopus, multi-armed, since it organizes growth, development, and the exercise of full-ranged natural capacities.

Medical philosophy includes epistemology, ontology/metaphysics, aesthetics, and ethics of medicine. Perhaps the most notorious discipline is medical ethics, which overlaps with bioethics. Philosophy of medicine can be distinguished from the philosophy of healthcare, which is mostly concerned with ethical, political, and overall economical issues arising from healthcare research and practice. Medical epistemology today includes the genome and all the "omics" disciplines. Necessarily, "evidence-based" medicine (EBM) must also be included. This "buzz" word is an approach to medical practice intended to optimize decision-making by emphasizing the use of evidence from well-designed clinical trials and carefully conducted prospective research. Not only the economic implications are obvious, but also the Hippocratic admonition to "do no harm" arises here. Physicians conducted worthless blood letting for two millennia before the practice was discontinued.

Our author is a psychotherapist; the term "soul doctor" would do his philosophical mission too little justice. Tomasi aims to explore the relationships between medicine and philosophy particularly with regards to neurosciences, psychiatry, and psychology, since these areas of medicine particularly address connections between mind and body. René Descartes concerned himself with this same (more limited of course) issue, termed *Cartesian dualism*. Descartes made ontological space for modern medicine by separating body from mind – "while mind is superior to body as it constitutes the uniqueness of the human soul" (the province of theology), body is inferior to the mind as it is mere matter. Medicine simply investigates the body as a machine, maintain the non-philosophers. Tomasi introduces his material and the numerous chapters that divide his topic. Interestingly, he cites Aulus Cornelius Celsus, whom most physicians will not know. This Roman encyclopedist compiled *De Medicina*, a compendium on diet, pharmacy, surgery, and related fields (25 BC–50 AD). During Celsus' time, medicine was clearly a part of philosophy and evolved, as did philosophy, to include development of the scientific method (Bacon and Descartes) and a steady march of ethical principles from Hippocrates, who moved towards empiricism to Kant who formalized a respect for moral law.

Tomasi briefly reviews the topic of medical philosophy historically. He touches on highlights, including Galen's treatise, *The best physician is also a philosopher*. Galen was very interested in the debate between the rationalist and empiricist medical sects, still a timely topic. Nevertheless, Galen was primarily a scientist (albeit limited) and all of his claims could be supported by scientific evidence related to his time. Relevant to the thesis topic, Galen believed that there is no distinction between the mental and the physical. Tomasi carefully outlines his questions.

Hermeneutics (text interpretations) is a controversial topic that has particular political and economic implications. Interestingly, Tomasi considers the case of Paracelsus who named himself after Celsus and stayed true to his real name that includes Bombastus. Modesty was not one of his virtues. Paracelsus would probably not have survived EBM, even in his own time. His hermetical views that sickness and health in the body rely on the harmony of Man (microcosm) and Nature (macrocosm) come across well today. Indeed, Paracelsus is credited as providing the first clinical/scientific mention of the "subconscious". Tomasi's brief discussion of hermeneutics and suicide is very timely. The topic of "assisted suicide" where physicians act upon patient requests is currently hotly debated. Pythagoras, for example, was against the act, though more on mathematical, rather than moral grounds, believing that there were only a finite number of souls for use in the world, and that the sudden and unexpected departure of one upset a delicate balance.

Hegel would be shocked to encounter neuroscience, perhaps less so phenomenology. Tomasi emphasizes Hegel's *Phänomenologie des Geistes*. Hegel divides consciousness into sense-certainty, perception, and force through understanding. The physicist Ludwig Boltzmann criticized the obscure complexity of Hegel's works, referring to Hegel's writing as an "unclear thoughtless flow of words." Mathematics is extremely important to philosophy, and as far as the reviewer knows, pure mathematics is an *a priori* experience. Tomasi suggests that mathematical modeling is of value. He could not be more correct!

Medicine will drown in systems biology (or systems medicine). The hope here is that by gathering all information on a patient, all clinical data, her/his genomic sequence, all proteins she/he produces or can produce etc., some medical insight will be accrued. The proponents call this approach "Big Data". George Orwell would have used the term "Big Brother". Medical philosophy is desperately needed here.

Is the patient still at the center of the work? Here, Tomasi delves into Aristotle and Kant. Particularly the latter is important here and the reviewer is interested in Kant's doctrine of right and doctrine of virtue. Tomasi provides a helpful table model of physician-patient relationships. Notable is the subheading, "experimental philosophy". Can medical philosophy be subjected to EBM? We shall see!

Wither complementary, alternative, and traditional medicine? The ancients (balance wheels) taught primarily that. Alternative medicine is any practice that is put forward as having the healing effects of medicine, but does not originate from evidence gathered using the scientific method, is not part of biomedicine, nor is contradicted by scientific EBM. This grouping consists of a wide range of health care practices, products and therapies, ranging from being biologically plausible but not well tested, to being directly contradicted by evidence and science, or even harmful or toxic. Despite significant expenditures on testing alternative medicine, including $2.5 billion spent by the United States government, almost none have shown any effectiveness greater than that of false treatments (placebo), and alternative medicine has been criticized by prominent figures in science and medicine as being quackery, nonsense, fraudulent, or unethical.

If we could chide the ancients, we could mention that they concerned themselves with the wealthy and the "worried well". Hippocrates did not serve in the Peloponnesian wars where he might have observed blood, yellow bile, black bile, and phlegm in the flesh of his dying patients. Galen served the wealthy Romans. No evidence is known that he sought out the typhus, malaria, sepsis, worm-ridden, or wounded Roman patients that must have surrounded him everywhere. Earth, Fire, Air, and Water were not the issues because his patients could afford all these attributes. Were these two icons solely "society" doctors? "According to many defenders of the scientific and therapeutic superiority of modern conventional Western biomedicine, the positive results of alternative therapies are entirely due to the placebo effect." These therapies also have rough sledding in EBM, except for influences of political correctness.

Much of philosophy through the ages has concerned God and proving that God exists. Plato believed in the afterlife. Many philosophers developed proofs (scholastics and beyond) and perhaps proofs are not necessary. Spinoza equated God with the material universe. He has therefore been called the "prophet" and "prince" and most eminent expounder of pantheism. More specifically, in a letter to Henry Oldenburg he states, "as to the view of certain people that I identify God with Nature (taken as a kind of mass or corporeal matter), they are quite mistaken". For Spinoza, our universe (cosmos) is a mode under two attributes of "Thought and Extension". God has infinitely many other attributes, which are not present in our world. Einstein stated that he believed in Spinoza's God. Back we move to the soul octopus; could we all meet together on that issue?

Tomasi mentions Rudolf Steiner. Steiner was a 19th-early 20th century phenomenon, who founded "anthroposophism", in central Europe. The movement he founded attempted to find a synthesis between science (about which he knew little) and spiritualism (where he was a self-proclaimed expert). This movement should not be underestimated. In the philosophically oriented phase of his movement, Steiner attempted to find a synthesis between science and spirituality. His philosophical work of these years, which he termed spiritual science, sought to apply the clarity of thinking characteristic of Western philosophy to spiritual questions. Steiner advocated a form of ethical individualism, to which he later brought a more explicitly spiritual approach. Steiner based his epistemology on Johann Wolfgang Goethe's worldview, in which: "Thinking ... is no more and no less an organ of perception than the eye or ear. Just as the eye perceives colors and the ear sounds, so thinking perceives ideas." But then again, Goethe was a pretty good poet, but was he a philosopher (or was Steiner)?

Tomasi also discusses Camus and Sartre. Camus's first significant contribution to philosophy was his idea of the absurd. He saw it as the result of our desire for clarity and meaning within a world and condition that offers neither, which he expressed in The Myth of Sisyphus and incorporated into many of his other works, such as "The Stranger" and "The Plague". Sartre's primary idea is that people, as humans, are "condemned to be free" (lovely idea). Sartre read Martin Heidegger's, "Being and Time", an ontological investigation through the lens and method of Husserlian phenomenology (Edmund Husserl was Heidegger's teacher). Reading *Being and Time* initiated Sartre's own philosophical enquiry. Reviewing Sartre's *Being and Nothingness* we would rely on Gustav Boltzmann's interpretation of Hegel. Nonetheless, Tomasi synthesizes this material well (as well as it can be done). Perhaps in this chapter, Joseph Heller could have appeared. Catch-22 is a paradoxical situation from which an individual cannot escape because of contradictory rules. An example includes: "To apply for this job, you would have to be insane; but if you are insane, you are unacceptable for the job". A mathematical description has been worked out to solve catch-22.

What is meant by *Translational Science?* This clinician is grateful for a philosopher's answer. Take for instance the first public health measures (Avicenna), and the first vaccinations (before and after Jenner). We are continuing to and already have eliminated numerous diseases (small pox, "great" pox, polio, tetanus, diphtheria, pertussis and others) from the planet. Translational research applies findings from basic science to enhance human health and well-being. In a medical research context, it aims to "translate" findings in basic research into medical and nursing practice and meaningful health outcomes. Translational research implements a "bench-to-bedside" approach, from laboratory experiments through clinical trials to point-of-care patient applications, model, harnessing knowledge from basic sciences to produce new drugs, devices, and treatment options for patients. Most clinicians/scientists operate in the opposite direction, namely from patient-to-bench. Politicians call the buzzwords here and unfortunately they are overwhelmingly economic rather than directed at curing or eliminating disease. Clinicians have been performing this mission since Celsus, to Paracelsus as best we can. We need to lean back, breathe in, and read books such as this to rediscover the ground upon which we stand. Albert Einstein is quoted: "When I study philosophical works I feel I am swallowing something which I don't have in my mouth". He managed relativity and we can too. Our author can help us in managing the field.

Friedrich C. Luft, MD
Professor of Medicine

Introduction by William Tobey Horn

In an effort to understand the mechanisms causing individuals' suffering, psychiatrists often focus on neurobiological theories, neuroimaging, and lab values, sometimes obscuring the very patients they are attempting to understand. Absent intention to comprehend the nuances of the human experience, many psychiatrists succumb to materialistic biological reductionism. As a psychiatrist, I have found that to counter the temptation of reductionism it is essential to apply intention to the development of the patient-provider relationship. Establishing quality relationships enables psychiatrists to avoid treating patients as neurobiological abstractions and allows them to instead understand the entirety of a patient's unique experience. Moreover, these relationships are integral to helping a patient heal. Reading Dr. David Låg Tomasi's book, Medical Philosophy: Philosophical Analysis of Patient Self-Perception in Diagnostics and Therapy, and my great fortune of having the opportunity to be his clinical supervisor at the University of Vermont Medical Center reified and expanded this perspective.

On meeting Dr. Tomasi, I was immediately struck by his generosity of spirit, compassionate nature, impressive intellect, and diversity of interests and knowledge. These personal qualities are evident throughout his book and give life and meaning to his philosophical and empirical analysis. Philosophical analysis is critical for psychiatry—and all of medicine—in that it leads us to question and challenge our assumptions. When philosophical analysis is combined with an empirical study, as Dr. Tomasi accomplished in this book, it grounds the analysis in something more translatable to non-philosophers. As a result, the work can have a more significant impact helping those in the medical profession better understand how to help patients heal.

In his book, Dr. Tomasi defines the diverse underpinnings of Medical Philosophy and elaborates on how these underpinnings inform the field's role in academics and society. A bold and visionary thinker, his analysis of diverse topics—such as patient self-perception, the mind-brain problem, the limitations of evidence-based medicine, the role of complementary and alternative medicine, and the impact of patients' faith and/or connection to a higher purpose on healing—demonstrates how Medical Philosophy can help to shape our understanding of medicine, psychiatry, psychology, and neuroscience. Moreover, he explains how Medical Philosophy can help these fields focus on individuals and their humanity. His own work achieves this aim.

Dr. Tomasi's book highlighted what I have observed in academic psychiatry, that many psychiatrists are dismissive of interventions outside of the sphere of evidence-based pharmacological and therapeutic approaches, for example rejecting treatments from the world of complementary and alternative medicine. Yet, our patients are turning to these interventions in ever-increasing numbers. Moreover, interventions such as mindfulness and meditation that were once considered "alternative" have research to support their effectiveness. This is not to say that all "alternative" modalities of treatment are simply awaiting anointment as the next evidence-based treatment. Rather, patients might perceive benefit from treatment that conventional medicine has not yet recognized—and might never recognize—as effective. Most importantly, to best help the patient heal, the provider needs to listen openly to the patient's experience and not dismiss outright that which the provider does not understand or agree with. Working with Dr. Tomasi in person, I was influenced by his compassion and openness with patients. Reading his book reaffirmed this humanistic orientation to patient-provider relationships for me, as I expect it will for most readers.

Dr. Tomasi was beloved by patients on the Inpatient Psychiatry Unit at the University of Vermont Medical Center. Frequently, patients with whom I had a difficult time connecting opened up to Dr. Tomasi—often through discussions of spirituality. Dr. Tomasi's work highlights that many patients benefit from a spiritual orientation, one that gives their lives and their healing process meaning. Dr. Tomasi's work taught me that exploring patients' own spirituality and higher purpose in the context of the patient-provider relationship can be integral to recovery and growth.

Dr. Tomasi's book deepened my awareness of the shortcomings of medicine and of psychiatry. His work also offered and inspired potential solutions to overcome these shortcomings. Most importantly, his work enhanced my understanding of the patient experience and, in doing so, my understanding of what it means to be human. I believe that most readers will share this experience.

William Tobey Horn, MD
Assistant Professor of Psychiatry
University of Vermont Medical Center

Introduction

Philosophy is the mother of all sciences.

Exploring the relationship between medicine and philosophy is somewhat akin to exploring the connection between philosophy and science as a whole. Where do the interdisciplinary fields of theoretical medicine, medical philosophy, cognitive neuroscience, and neuropsychology intertwine? Why is there a need to address questions such as the ones usually found in medical science within the framework of a philosophical analysis and/or debate?

This study intends to analyze the various philosophical perspectives within medical science, with a particular focus on those disciplines, such as neuroscience, psychiatry, and psychology, dealing with the direct connection between mind/brain and the rest of (human) body. More specifically, it tries to address issues related to the above listed topics taking in consideration the perspective of the patient, in terms of perception and self-perception, within the framework of diagnosis and therapy. Furthermore, this investigation follows the specific structures and methods of the theoretical approach with a specific epistemological analysis of comparative empirical research. The ultimate purpose is to open up the discussion and generate new questions, inferring information from the data examined as well as the reasoning process. Furthermore, the aim of this research is directed at a deeper understanding of human nature, examining the links and mutual influence between perception, beliefs, sense of meaning and purpose, and the healing process. We divided this study into seven main areas of investigation, corresponding to seven chapters. The first chapter discusses general aspects of Medical Philosophy, including a broad overview of its history, defined questions and applicability of results, and the relation between the epistemology of medicine and some elements of the comparison (also in causal terms) between self-image and the healing process. In chapter two we analyze the language, the reasoning and cognitive processes, and the methods of several philosophical perspectives. We also compare them with the methodologies used in modern medicine, thus drawing important considerations as to why the analysis of psychology and psychiatry is especially important and useful in our analysis. The third chapter discusses a specific set of philosophical considerations, starting with Hegel and Merleau-Ponty but without forgetting the classics and the postmodernists (and making sure not to ig-

23

nore terms often associated with philosophy of mind), in search of the best way to address fundamental questions such as the mind-brain and embodied cognition problems, and suggesting a model. A further explanation of the goal of the study is also included in this section. With chapter 4 we literally put the patient "at the center of therapy", discussing the core issues of perception and self-perception, experimentation, and therapeutic implications. The fifth chapter represents one of the possible applications of Medical Philosophy in clinical settings. The debate around Integrative Medicine is at the center of modern scientific investigation and public policy, and we attempt to examine claims, theories, and practices under the lenses of logic, culture and identity following again a multifaceted examination of what it means to be human. For chapter six and seven we present a possible connection on a deeper level; the first addressing transcendental elements, the second translational elements. Chapter six discusses all those consideration that "lie between worlds" and represent the connection between the individuality of human beings and a sense of (higher) purpose and meaning. Chapter seven instead uses the broad range of topics covered in the first part of this writing and re-morphs them into a discussion on research method and scope, social implications, and epistemological suggestions without solution of continuity. The Appendix at the end of this volume represents part 8 of our analysis. It presents the empirical research conducted at the University of Vermont Medical Center, Inpatient psychiatry Unit, through the *Focus Group Questionnaire*, and the *Health Perception Survey*.

The debate between an Evidence-based medicine (EBM) and a patient-centered medicine (PCM) is a logical outcome originating in these considerations, and the practical application of one perspective versus the other will certainly impact not only the theoretical premises of such science, but the very effect of clinical approaches, from the relationship between patient and health care provider, to the structuralization and scientific base of the definition of (a specific) illness or disease, its diagnosis, prognosis, and treatment, thus the whole medical-therapeutic spectrum. Medical Philosophy has been with us from a very long time; in fact we could argue that the name itself represents an alternative synonymical version of "Philosophy of medicine" or "Iatrophilosophy", thus comprising a vast spectrum of subfields such as theoretical medicine, epistemology, medical and bio- ethics, ontology and metaphysics. At the same time, Medical Philosophy represents the theoretical base for disciplines like metaethics, philosophy of healthcare, public health (policy) and healthcare practice. From this perspective, Medical Philosophy could possibly include, or at least be strongly interconnected with, the modern field of translational science, and even move beyond it. The interaction between medicine and philosophy was a fact since the very beginnings of our civilization, especially within the geographical and cultural apparatus of what is now considered the European (sphere of) influence, in particular in ancient Greece.

The roots of the Apollonian *philosophia divina* are translated into the *medicus* who, not only observes, examines, discusses, diagnoses, treats but also understands, knows, comprehends and "measures" or "expresses, talks about, gives voice to, pronounces" a "measure"[1]. In this sense, Medical Philosophy is a synthesis of this interaction, which once more connects the terms *Doctor* and *Medicus* in a broader and deeper sense, which ultimately impacts the translational aspects of such science. According to Aulus Cornelius Celsus,

> "At the beginning medical science thought of itself as part of philosophy, because both the treatment (cure) of diseases and the analysis (contemplation) of natural things are known due to the work of the same authors, especially given that the ones who resorted to medicine were the ones who weakened their body in the quietness of meditations and in the night vigils. Thus, we know that we can find many learned philosophers in this science: among them the celebrated Pythagoras, Empedocles, and Democritus. Hippocrates, whom some believe to be Democritus' disciple, was in fact the first one, among all those we should mention, to separate this discipline [medicine] from philosophy."[2]

---

[1]   See the Latin verb *mèdeor*, from *med-mað*, related to the Sansc. *Medhâ* (mind, knowledge), connected to the Zend.-Aves *madhas* (science, or therapeutic knowledge) and *mah-ayā -mi* (as in "I teach"). The term is further linked to the Gr. Μῆτις (wisdom, skill, art and craft or "know how"), Gr. (and arch. Lat.) *Manth-àno*, to the It. *mente, meditare, rimedio, maestro*. Linguistically and conceptually, the word is connected to the Old Germ. *munter* "awake, lively, alert" (Old H. Germ. *Magan*, basis for *mögen*, and Old Irish/Norse *mega*), Old Ch. Slav. *madru* "wise, sage," (as well as components of мочь / мо̌hu / мо̌га and other languages from Old Ch. Slav. *moumu*) Lithuanian *mandras* "wide-awake". It has also been postulated, that the Avestan root might be connected with *Mazdā-* (nom. *Mazdå*) reflecting Proto-Iranian *Mazdāh*, as in *Ahura Mazda*.

[2]   Celsus, A. Cornelius 1985 (tr.) *De Medicina*, Book I, Introduction, translated by Angiolo del Lungo, editor Dino Pieraccioni, Florence: Sansoni Editore.

Chapter 1
A brief history of Medical Philosophy

1.1 General Aspects

In recent times, especially between the mid to the late twentieth century, the debate around Medical Philosophy addressed the problematic aspect of separating philosophy of medicine from either philosophy or medicine, thus creating a separate discipline. In order to better understand what Medical Philosophy is, studies, relates to, provides in terms of scientific research etc., we must be clear on the meaning and definition of the concept. As *Theoretical Medicine* or *Scientific Medicine* we identify a specific part or branch of medicine interested in the analysis and debate of theoretical, scientific, epistemological, ontological, methodological, conceptual and linguistic aspects of the discipline and its related research and practice. In fact, from a purely academic perspective, the study of medicine presents in this modern day and age a vast array of definitions, titles and degrees, such as MBBS, MFM, MD, ND, Dr.rer.med., Dr.med.scient., PhD, ScD/Dsc, DClinPract, DClinRes, etc. In practice, the fields of philosophy and medicine are deeply intertwined as shown through the analysis of main questions pertaining to both fields, as well as by simply examining what practitioners and researchers do in their everyday clinical and scientific work. Certainly, in the analysis of conceptual and methodological issues raised by the current scientific (especially medical) research, we understand how Medical Philosophy overlaps with fields such as bioethics or public health policy, not to mention translational science. Why is there a need to address the existence of this separate discipline?

Specifically, the ontology of general medical science and its analysis of the conceptual terms used in medical research and practice arise from the philosophical aspects of the ontological revolution. This dramatic shift in logical definitions due to a new perspective on reality, from an omnicomprehensive organismic viewpoint to a more materialistic, definitely mechanistic one, is arguably connected with the Cartesian dualism in theoretical and applied science. At the same time, important theoretical discoveries in the field of medicine contributed to this new paradigm. A giant of theoretical medicine, histology and microscopical anatomy, the Italian physician and scientist Marcello Malpighi, stated that the body was indeed a machine. Another champion of iatromechanics, William Harvey (who also studied in Italy at the University of Padua) also worked beyond the Hippocratic-Aristotelian-Galenic methodological framework, by presenting an explanation of (human and animal in general) physiological phenomena in mechanical terms. A similar worldview was the one of Giovanni Alfonso Borelli, widely considered the Father of biomechanics (as well as teacher and mentor of Malpighi). From this perspective, their scientific method could arguably be included in a radical reductionistic sphere, as opposed to a vitalistic one, and as base for the modern scientific method in medicine. Furthermore, we could argue that these premises are to be considered the necessary conditions for a further development, starting from the XIX century on, of a scientific method whose epistemological analysis is rational (and, according to some, rationalist), realist and methodologically skeptical, and whose philosophical viewpoint and ontological nature is materialist (or, again, materialistic) and systemic (which is not *dia*stemic, we should note).

These factors have had a direct impact in the noseological classification of illness, as defined by an evidence-observative-etiological base toward a monogenic conception of disease. But this epistemological debate is right understood only if we still want to consider the association between philosophy and medicine, from the ultra (in terms of qualitative overcoming) identification of Galen in his treatise *That the Best Physician is also a Philosopher*. To be sure, Galen also followed Hippocrates in warning medicine against a certain type of philosophy, namely some of the considerations of the Pythagoreans and more generally the pre-Socratics. In fact, his modality of direct observation constituted an *in medio* standpoint, between rationalism and empiricism. Historically speaking, parallels between medicine and philosophy are at the center of the fundamental works by Avicenna, Averroes, Al Farabi, and Maimonides.

The beginnings of medical science and of the scientific worldview in general are deeply rooted in the continuous historic change which ultimately led to the social and cultural movements of the Renaissance, all the way to the Age of Enlightenment. We do not know precisely the specific features of the human worldview in ancient times, and from this perspective the fields of archaeology and anthropology do represent a fundamental support of any kind of knowledge on the subject of medicine, and of science in general. We postulate, based on the current comparative knowledge, that archaic sciences were based on a complex collection of magic, mystical, spiritual, divine, and perhaps obscure forces, although we cannot assert for sure that all these forces were necessarily embodied in quasi-human form, as it is often depicted with good and evil spirits, demons, gods and goddesses, tricksters, angels, and similia. We also know that some cultures used rocks, bones, and symbolic signs like divinized alphabets letters to predict a specific medical or social/personal outcome, for instance in the case of the Runes or the work of the *Augures*. In this sense, we understand how the process of healing was believed to happen through the help of special contacts and connections with higher (or lower) spheres of reality. What is important to notice though, is that in ancient times, and from a certain point of view this reflects also in contemporary tribal autochthonous cultures such as the aboriginal and east/west African, diseases and related therapies and possible cures present a social dimension. Thus, the healing process, although led by a superior, and in some cases mysterious, power was ultimately connected to the patient's own culture, ethnic environment or (family, tribe, village, etc.) society. We could argue that this would fit into a dualistic worldview, with a material(istic) elements such as plants, flowers, potions, amulets, rocks, etc., and spiritual(istic) connections (as explanation) such as spirit guides and gods, all tied together by a combination of spiritual-materialistic practices and rituals. In these practices we recognize the healer's (and, in some cases, the patient's) altered state of consciousness, the meta-communication with a different realm of reality or astrological investigations. We could also argue that other practices, some still present in current times also in the Western society, especially in complementary and alternative medicine, present a layered interpretative structure of explanation, function, and purpose of medical treatments. Please note that we use the term *Western* throughout this volume in a broader, and yet translated sense. There are certainly plentiful elements within Western culture which could and should rightfully be considered the philosophical, cultural, and scientific basis for many integrative, complementary and alternative approaches, as we will see in the concept of "Central Medicine". In this sense, "Western" indicates a culture that is generally intended to be derived from a European/Indoeuropean (or related through cultural exchange, as well as precursors) substratum, specifically originating from [in alphabetical order] an Arabic, Baltic, Celtic, Germanic, Hellenic, Jewish, Latin, Slavic, Turkic, Ugro-Finnic, Basque, etc. cultural heritage). However, due to the very historical nature of the evolution of Western culture, some of the aforementioned approaches are not considered "conventional" and "standard" in modern times. This especially true from a *non-continental* (in the philosophical sense) perspective and especially in regard to the development of Western culture in the USA and the Commonwealth areas. We argue that part of the reason for this situation is again historically connected, and more specifically related to the cultural and philosophical "split" between a shared, traditional, folk, ethnic (etc.) background which (in the case of Europe) "naturally" (which is not to say "without struggle") evolved into modernity (e.g. in the case of rational thought and scientific method), and was instead "uprooted" and "separated" from its (this) origin (in the case of USA & Commonwealth), so that in the latter case, the very history of (medical) science dates to the time of European expanding (and colonizing) abroad, especially since the XIX century[3]. This is precisely why in this study we propose and defend the position according to which a more comprehensive view in medicine, especially from the patient-provider relationship standpoint, is very much needed. It is a work of reconnecting, even recollecting. We find this heritage in the case of practices such as iridology, homeopathy, chirology, (according to some) chiropractic, osteopathy etc., all the way to ayurvedic, anthroposophic and general herbal medicine which is arguably connected with the European *doctrine of signatures* from Dioscurides and Galen, to Paracelsus, William Cole, Giambattista della Porta (not to mention Giuseppe Giovanni Battista Vincenzo Pietro Antonio Matteo Balsamo, best known as *Conte di Cagliostro*), to Samuel Hahnemann and Rudolf Steiner. A good example of this practice (using the concept of resemblance to some extent directly derived from a Neo-Platonic macrocosm and microcosm schema) is the claimed positive properties of the walnut, which, due to its physical similarity to the human brain, is used in the treatment of neurological disorders. This allegorical component is described by the following words by Michel Foucault:

---

[3]   This is especially important from a social and ethical, as well as political standpoint, especially in regard to the side effects of bad policy making practices, such as overmedication or chemical/artificial approaches versus traditional/folk remedies: "One doctor in Latin America who was also a statesman did try to stem the pharmaceutical invasion rather than just enlist physicians to make it look more respectable. During his short tenure as president of Chile, Dr. Salvador Allende quite successfully mobilized the poor to identify their own health needs and much less successfully compelled the medical profession to serve basic rather than profitable needs. He proposed to ban drugs unless they had been tried on paying clients in North America or Europe for as long as the patent protection would run. He revived a program aimed at reducing the national pharmacopoeia to a few dozen items, more or less the same as those carried by the Chinese barefoot doctor in his black wicker box. Notably, within one week after the Chilean military junta took power on September 11, 1973, many of the most outspoken proponents of a Chilean medicine based on community action rather than on drug imports and drug consumption had been murdered." Illich, I. 1976. *Limits to Medicine; Medical Nemesis: The Expropriation of Health*. London, UK: Marion Boyars Publishers, pp. 68–69.

"Up to the end of the sixteenth century, resemblance played a constructive role in the knowledge of Western culture. It was resemblance that largely guided exegesis and the interpretation of texts; it was resemblance that organized the play of symbols, made possible knowledge of things visible and invisible, and controlled the art of representing them."[4]

From this perspective, this doctrine is not exclusively European, being extensively used also (for example) in Traditional Chinese Medicine with a series of basic components (natural elements, human senses and body organ, plant's taste, smell and color, time of the day and of the year) used to analyze and quantify their combination within the idea of body/spirit equilibrium. Thus, similarly to what happens in Ayurvedic medicine, disease and illnesses originate in the imbalance between bodily systems.

This viewpoint is shared by the importance given to arithmetic structure across cultures. In the case of the Chinese (medical) science and philosophy we have the number 2 (*Yin* and *Yang* of Taoism), the 3 (*Vayu, Pitta, Kapha*) for the Indian tradition, the 4 humors for the (Greek) hippocratic method (Blood-air; Yellow bile-fire; Black bile-earth; Phlegm-water)[5]; the 6 (3+3 opposites) for the Jewish *kabbalah*, the Mesopotamian 7, etc. The very conceptual background behind this point of view needs further analysis, especially when we realize that the vast majority of the above mentioned assumptions, scientific, and more generally philosophical in nature, are deeply embedded in a substratum (which is also a *supra*stratum and *intra*stratum) of culture and history, often addressed by Medical Anthropology, which we will be discussing in Chapter 2. In particular, we need to agree on the prominent impact and influence of the historical data on the very perception of medicine as a science, thus a Medical Philosophy which would not take in consideration history of medicine and more in general history of culture, is doomed to become shallow and imprecise. The analysis of the philosophical components of medicine can benefit from the Heideggerian view on perception and circumspection from the perspective of objectivity, a necessary premise in the approach and clinical application of modern medicine. In this sense we also reenter concepts such as *Vorhandenheit* and *Zuhandenheit*. In the attempt to understand the patient, his

---

[4]   Foucault, M. 1966. *The Order of Things: An Archaeology of the Human Sciences*, (Les Mots et les choses: Une archéologie des sciences humaines) New York: Pantheon Books, p. 17.

[5]   It is interesting here to note that the number four does not enjoy such a high conceptual (and spiritual) degree in TCM, or in Chinese culture in general. In fact, in the Southeast Asian regions such as China, Japan, Korea, Malaysia, Singapore, Taiwan, and Vietnam we can identify practices linked to the so-called (within the Western culture addressed and defined superstitions) *tetraphobia*.

singularity and individuality, both in cultural and diagnostic terms, we could argue that this circumspection is in part based on a form of pre-reflective understanding, in the hermeneutic tradition, of the patient 1) as a whole, and 2) as an individual. This alternating form of path to knowledge, from the medical perspective, is appropriately identified by Tucker:

> "We all know this but over the ages this art/science ratio has undergone a dramatic change. The medical pendulum is swinging from the art to the science side. However, in my opinion, the best clinician is one who armed with this scientific knowledge, practices using excellent clinical judgment (which of course is his art). Compassion and understanding are a large part of this art."[6]

Certainly, the decision-making apparatus that every physician needs to possess in order to accurate diagnose and treat a specific illness or disease is a necessary *conditio-sine-qua-non* of advanced, empirical, rational, experimental modern medicine. In this sense there is nothing "magical" about the physician ability to link the individual *quadro clinico* to the pathology of the case. The problem indeed is how to contextualize the situation within the parameters of observable data and patient's history. The physician here is required to follow the rules of the most recent, cutting-edge biomedical research, in particular the combination, appropriately addressed by philosophers such as Bluhm and Bunge, of Randomized Control Trials and theoretical approach to investigate mechanisms of action. How does Medical Philosophy address the issues related on the very approach, attitude and education in the field of medical science? Further help can come to use from the words by Mark Wrathall in discussing Hegel's position on technology:

> "So, for example, education is increasingly aimed at providing students with 'skills' for critical thinking, writing and study, rather than at teaching students facts or training them in disciplines. This is because skills, unlike disciplines, will let students adapt to any conceivable work situation. This is driven by the need for an economy that can flexibly reconfigure itself and shift its human resources into whatever role happens to be necessary at the moment"[7]

[6]   Tucker NH. 1999. *Presidential message Art vs Science* Jacksonville Medicine, 50(12).
[7]   Wrathall, M. 2006. *How to Read Heidegger*, New York: W. W. Norton, p. 100.

1.2 Application and epistemological considerations

a) Defining the questions

In this sense we also understand the methodological component of medicine as addressed by Medical Philosophy, a discipline that is interested in addressing questions such as:

- How can we understand the specifics of scientific method within medicine from the perspectives of ontological revolution and (Cartesian) dualism[8], especially in the context of the mind-body or mind-brain problem?
- Is a disease or illness a mere list of clinical signs and/or related biomarkers?
- Are clinical data, albeit valid in terms of quantity and quality, sufficient (although here we should not forget the parameters of 'necessary' or 'required') to describe a disease and provide a correct diagnosis?
- Is contemporary medicine a combination of Evidence-Based Medicine and Theoretical Medicine?
- Does the Hierarchy of Evidence need re-examination in its order, content and concept?
- Are Randomized Control Trials necessary and sufficient to validate a therapeutic intervention?
- To what extent the positivistic aspects of the lack of hypothesizing and mechanism-seeking are still part of medical science and practice?
- How do we define things, in ontological and epistemological terms, which we do not perceive with the commonly accepted array of scientific methods and technologies?
- Is medicine a form of natural philosophy, a (hard) science or craft, technology, art?
- Is it possible to integrate the above form and definitions of medicine, also in relation to the steadily growing aspect of medical and scientific technology?
- What is the room for each of these aspects in medical curriculum, education and academia?

---

[8] In this regard, we should also mention the Ontology of General Medical Science (OGMS), which includes a list of definitions of very general terms, generally applied to human population, that are used across medical disciplines, from 'disease', 'disorder', and 'disease course', to 'diagnosis', and 'patient'. Furthermore, it is important to note that the Ontology of General Medical Science provides a theoretical analysis of disease, further elaborated by specific ontologies of disease such as the Infectious Disease Ontology (IDO) and the Mental Disease Ontology (MDO).

- Why is it necessary to define forms of complementary, alternative, traditional, non-traditional, school-, and scientific medicine?
- How do we define the above mentioned forms of medicine, and should these be included in medicine as a therapeutic science?
- How do we define placebos, their biological effects, and their clinical and medical efficacy?
- Are there universal biomedical truths or do we have to include and/or control for individual, culture, ethnicity, society, personal beliefs, spirituality and religion in addressing this question?
- To what extent is modern academic, pharmacological and biomedical research affected, or even controlled, by commercial interests?
- Do philosophy, philosophical debate and positions contribute to the advance of medicine as a science and therapeutic practice?
- Furthermore, is it necessary to select/exclude specific philosophies and/or philosophical methods from the paradigm of Medical Philosophy?

The last question in particular addresses a key problem in defining what Medical Philosophy is, does and ought to/should do, and if is essentially and structurally different from Philosophy of medicine. James Marcum gives us his definition:

> "I opt for the philosophy of medicine relationship, which I hold to be a sub-discipline of philosophy. The relationship between the two disciplines is more than simply philosophy and medicine in that they share more than common problems and is more than philosophy in medicine in that philosophers use medicine not just to do philosophy but to understand the nature of medicine itself. I define philosophy of medicine specifically as the metaphysical and ontological, the epistemological, and the axiological and ethical analyses of different models for medical knowledge and practice. Such a definition is rooted in a standard topology for philosophical analysis. The aim of this analysis is to unpack the nature of medicine itself as articulated in the question: What is medicine? This question is at the center of the quality-of-care crisis facing modern western medicine and represents the primary issue for my philosophy of medicine"[9].

Beside what medicine is, in this study on Medical Philosophy we are asking ourselves what medicine does and ought to do, especially from the perspective of patient-provider relationship. In particular, the very existence of patients and disorder are questioned by some[10] in their ontological and epistemological

---

[9]   Marcum, J.A. 2008. *An introductory philosophy of medicine: humanizing modern medicine.* New York: Springer, p. 8.

[10]   To quote Mario Bunge: "The physicians who disbelieve the independent existence of their patients won't treat or charge them. Thus anti-realism is an obstacle to medical practice and

existence and justification. This is especially true in the fields of psychiatry, psychology and mental health[11]. In fact, even from the perspective of scientific application and therapeutic effectiveness, these fields are subject to an enormous and fast paced change, although they are far from the success of other branches of medicine[12]. This lack of success is to an important extent, due to the very nature of the problems related to mental health, which are not only biological, but also philosophical, and spiritual. Certainly this is not to say that philosophy alone or biology alone will be able, in reasonable time, to completely solve all these problems. However, we argue that the most effective way to understand the complexity of human beings in relation to psychological issues is to combine all the aforementioned perspectives in a solid theoretical discussion[13]. However, there are also difficulties in achieving this goal, ultimately because of the great differences between philosophical positions, which

---

public health". Bunge, M. 2013. *Medical Philosophy. Conceptual Issues in Medicine*, Singapore: World Scientific Publishing, p. 223.

[11]   Ibid., "Some postmodern authors have denied that diseases are real. In particular, the antipsychiatry movement was based on the opinion that what pass for mental disorders are only social dysfunctions (see Shorter 1997). But of course, the brain can get sick, just like any other organ, whereas society cannot, except metaphorically. It is also obvious that, if all mental disorders were imaginary, anyone could feel and behave sanely or insanely at will." Aside from the hard criticism throughout his book, it is interesting to note that Bunge talks here about the anti-psychiatry movement is a (reductive) past tense, although this position, albeit not entirely coded in a well-recognizable movement, is alive and well, like in the work of Peter Breggin, Sandy Steingard and Robert Whitaker. See also http://www.mad inamerica.com/ and the work of Mario Beauregard at the University of Arizona.

[12]   "[Thomas R. Insel, MD, director of the National Institute of Mental Health] believes the diagnosis and treatment of mental illness is today where cardiology was 100 years ago. And like cardiology of yesteryear, the field is poised for dramatic transformation, he says. "We are really at the cusp of a revolution in the way we think about the brain and behavior, partly because of technological breakthroughs. We're finally able to answer some of the fundamental questions." Weir, K. 2012. *The roots of mental illness. How much of mental illness can the biology of the brain explain?*. Monitor on Psychology, Vol 43, No. 6, Washington, DC.: American Psychological Association, p. 32.

[13]   "Decades of effort to understand the biology of mental disorders have uncovered clues, but those clues haven't translated to improvements in diagnosis or treatment, he believes." We've thrown tens of billions of dollars into trying to identify biomarkers and biological substrates for mental disorders". [Jerome Wakefield, professor of social work and psychiatry at NYU] says. "The fact is we've gotten very little out of all of that. [...] You can think of the brain as a computer, he adds. The brain circuitry is equivalent to the hardware. But we also have the human equivalent of software. "Namely, we have mental processing of mental representations, meanings, conditioning, a whole level of processing that has to do with these psychological capacities," he says. Just as software bugs are often the cause of our computer problems, our mental motherboards can be done in by our psychological processing, even when the underlying circuitry is working as designed. "If we focus only at the brain level, we are likely to miss a lot of what's going on in mental disorders." Ibid., p. 33.

do not all follow the same pattern, target or method. For instance, Mario Bunge is especially critical of a vast array of philosophical positions, originating in Aristotelian, Pre-Socratic, Continental and Postmodern philosophy and beyond:

> "The ancient Greeks made much of the difference between *episteme* or science and *doxa* or opinion. The postmoderns deny this difference, but the rest of us have kept it because we care for truth and well-grounded action"[14].

> "[...] physicalism and chemism were primitive but perhaps unavoidable phases of materialist philosophy, biology, and medicine"[15]

> "In short, in medicine, as elsewhere, we must distinguish peel from pulp. This distinction, inherent in scientific realism, is denied by the anti-realist philosophies, such as objectivism, phenomenalism, fictionism, and conventionalism"[16]

> "The history of anatomy confutes Karl Popper's thesis (1963) that scientific advances are not born either from observations or from experiments, but from myths and criticism of the latter"[17]

> "[The] combination of rationality with materialism and with the realistic principle of the autonomous existence, lawfulness, and intelligibility of the universe was unique and it was modern *avant la lettre*. This may also have been the main contribution of pre-Socratic philosophy. It was indeed a new way of looking at things and exploring them, that overcame confusions, obscurities, fantasies, and irrational fears. What a contrast to the obscurantism and pessimism of the self-styled postmoderns, in particular the radical skeptics and the constructivist-relativists! These philosophers inhibit the search for truth because they deny that it is possible and desirable; they suspect that scientific research is a political conspiracy and attempt to pass off obscurity for profundity"[18]

It is interesting to note, that Bunge speaks of "Psychiatry [as] the only branch of medicine where symptomatic diagnosis still prevails – a clear sign of its backwardness"[19]. We must certainly agree that the lack of further scientific (biomedical, empirical, as well as theoretical) basis to the definitions and claims of modern psychiatry represent a lack of the discipline. At the same time, we would argue that this scientific handicap could perhaps lead to a new

---

[14]   Bunge, M. 2013. *Medical Philosophy. Conceptual Issues in Medicine*, Singapore: World Scientific Publishing, p. 102. As a comment to this quotation, we might ask the author whether this case is probabilistic or frequency-related.
[15]   Ibid., p. 35.
[16]   Ibid., p. 162.
[17]   Ibid., p. 32.
[18]   Ibid., pp. 11–12.
[19]   Ibid., p. 79.

way to look at psychiatry, and medicine as a whole. Does that mean that medical practice should just focus on personal impression, or even intuition? Bunge continues:

> "The so-called clinical eye is a kind of intuition, or pre-analytic and fast thinking. We indulge in it when pressed for time or lacking in information. But only the intuitionist philosophers, like Henri Bergson, George E. Moore, and Edmund Husserl, have claimed that intuitions are infallible"[20]

Is it therefore absolutely no room for pre (perhaps non-) analytic thinking and/or intuition in medical practice? Trosseau argues:

> "The worst man of science is he who is never an artist, and the worst artist is he who is never a man of science. In early times, medicine was an art, which took its place at the side of poetry and painting; today they try to make a science of it, placing it beside mathematics, astronomy, and physics"[21].

Perhaps we should investigate a little more not just the concept of intuition, but certainly the relationship it has with more psychological, and generally neurological models such as short-, mid-, and long-term memory. Many have in fact argued for the imprecision of human intuitive powers, when these can be linked with memory-related phenomena such as *source misattribution* and *confabulation*. For instance, we could refer to *perceptual blindness* and *inattentional blindness*, as relatively recently presented in *the Invisibile Gorilla* and the related "Gorilla experiment" by Chabris and Simons[22]. In fact, the authors refer to their experiment and describe some of their methods as

> "[using] a wide assortment of stories and counterintuitive scientific findings to reveal an important truth: Our minds don't work the way we think they do. We think we see ourselves and the world as they really are, but we're actually missing a whole lot. [...] Again and again, we think we experience and understand the world as it is, but our thoughts are beset by everyday illusions. [...] The Invisible Gorilla reveals the numerous ways that our intuitions can deceive us."[23]

---

[20]   Ibid., p. 94.

[21]   Trosseau A. 1869 *Lectures on clinical medicine,* The New Sydenham Society, 1869 Submitted by AL Wyman: Filler. Medicine: art or science; 2(320): 1322.

[22]   Chabris, C., and Simons, D. 2011 *The Invisible Gorilla.* New York, NY: Crown Publishing Group.

[23]   Ibid. See *Introduction,* as well as the general overview at http://www.theinvisibleg orilla.com/.

Without examining all the specific characteristics of such models, we have the duty to investigate what me mean here, in a scientific and clinical setting (especially when medical decision making processes are involved), by "counterintuitive", "our minds", "deceiving" and the very relation between "illusion" and "intuition". In fact, "many researchers have commented on the complexity and possibly elusive character of medical reasoning"[24]. To be sure, when discussing clinical decision-making, we cannot put educated and experienced physicians as well as other medical practitioners in the same category as the general public, and for this very reason we should not apply the same discourse and expectations. However, if it is true that by "us" the authors here intend human beings in general, regardless of their titles or academic experiences, we should really ask ourselves (this time all of us, or at least the ones interested in these themes[25]) whether this lack of "intuitive infallibility" affects medical diagnosis and prognosis in important ways, in terms of quantity and quality. This is certainly another central theme addressed by Medical Philosophy. Therefore, we must at least go back to the most commonly accepted definition of intuition within the philosophical debate, or a form of *a priori* knowledge characterized by its immediacy. This can also be applied, in a more translated way, to experiential (some even argue, existential) (form of) (personal) belief. A certain confusion arises when, especially in analytic philosophy, which to some extend sees itself (and it is seen) as a *corollarium* to rational and empirical science, philosophers often call on intuitive perspectives when addressing methodologies used to test and verify claims. In particular, we could refer to the platonic "Justified True Belief"[26] and its further analysis, such as the "Gettier Problem", or the works by Martin Cohen, Fred Detske, Alvin Goldman, Richard Kirkham, Bertrand Russell, Alvin Plantinga, Nicla Vassallo, and others[27]. Beyond Intuitionism (in the sense proposed by Luitzen Egbertus Jan Brouwer) and conceptual intuition, proposing a particular definition of knowledge and

---

[24]   Hammrick, H., & Garfunkel, M. 1991. *Editor's Column-Clinical decisions: How much analysis and how much judgment?* Journal of Pediatrics, 118, 67, as discussed in: Fleming, M.H. 1991. *Clinical Reasoning in Medicine Compared With Clinical Reasoning in Occupational Therapy.* American Journal of Occupational Therapy, November 1991, Vol. 45, 988–996, p. 992.

[25]   Although we could argue that, since we are talking about (human) health in general, this definitely affect us all.

[26]   A concept generally accredited to Plato, and closely linked to the cognitive and epistemological debate around the term Belief.

[27]   See related bibliographical references, as well as the following link at the University of California San Diego http://philosophyfaculty.ucsd.edu/faculty/rarneson/Courses/gettierphilreading.pdf.

constructing a hypothetical case and possibly rejecting it, the core problems is the definition and distinction between the connection "state of mind" and judgment, and whether this judgment is the same as belief and/or a spontaneous manifestation, or even the (therefore postulated) necessary truth.

If we need to apply the discourse on intuition within the framework of Medical Philosophy, and linking it to the requirements and characteristics of clinical practice, we certainly must understand if the methods of philosophy, analytical, continental (and/or?) beyond are indeed valid and if they are (considering the skeptical paradigm in the process), if we can separate them from the fields of natural, social, mathematical sciences or even "common sense" (if this last concept makes sense at all, given the above listed premises of human intuition). Analytic philosophers tend to identify as "rational" those intuitions which are necessary, such as mathematical truths in calculus, as a way to differentiate them from (general) beliefs. This position concentrates on the possibility of holding beliefs which are not "intuitive", or having intuitions for statements (or, in a more analytical way, prepositions) which we can (cognitively) declare false. Another positions is simply considering intuitions as a form of experiential/experienced belief, which differs according to the personality of the individual, the cultural and social (sub) structures, beliefs (often intended as the same as intuition), religion, tradition, etc.

Furthermore, we need to remember the "basic sensory information" as found by Kant in the "cognitive faculty of sensibility", a position which is somewhat linked to the neurological concept of perception and proprioception (thus in a more physical form), since our mind, in the Kantian description, produces and morphs our intuitions within (in the form of) space, versus what happen with our internal intuitions, which (our) mind casts in the form of time. The above mentioned mathematical truths are according to Kant forms of "knowledge of the pure form of intuition", thus not empirical/experimental; a position further elaborated by Brouwer, Heyting, and in part by constructivists in general, with the special characterization rejection of the *principium tertii exclusi* and the use of the *reductio ad absurdum* to prove the existence of something. Should we then assume that there are different levels of intuition beyond what is scientifically acceptable? And if that is the case, how do we judge different subfield in science, from a theoretical and empirical standpoint? Bunge rightfully argues that "the weight assigned to an empirical datum relevant to a given hypothesis depends on the latter's theoretical status"[28], thus reclaiming the very importance of Medical Philosophy in the scientific medical research and practice. However, the author steers the analysis of the theoretical aspects within this philosophical subfield toward a specific set of scientific levels:

> "[...] in the immature sciences, it is advisable to adopt the *refutationist* strategy recommended by Popper (1935), in opposition to the *confirmationism* or *inductivism* preached by the positivists such as Rudolf Carnap, Hans Reichenbach, and at one time Bertrand Russell as well."[29]

> "Certainly, philosophers such as Anaxagoras, Democritus, Epicurus, Empedocles and many other pre-Socratic scholars presented a worldview in which the rational element of reason was taken in (high) consideration, promoting a strong scientific foundation from philosophy."[30]

Due to the very nature of psychiatry and neurosciences at this stage of scientific development, it is definitely appropriate to maintain an epistemological approach such as critical rationalism[31]. In fact, we can argue that the subjective element, both from the perspective of the patient and the one of the doctor, plays a fundamental role, especially when it comes to empirical generalizations lacking a strong theoretical background, basis, and support. In this sense, criti-

---

[28]   Bunge, M. 2013. *Medical Philosophy. Conceptual Issues in Medicine*, Singapore: World Scientific Publishing, p. 132.

[29]   Ibid. Furthermore, we should look at the problem from the perspective of falsifiability, which is the core of modern evidence-based science. For instance, William Whewell's focus on hypothesis' generation within science helps us frame the inductive method in terms of a specific conceptual-philosophical framework that not only addresses the collection of data (also in terms of possible confirmation bias) but also guides their interpretation. This point of view is strictly related to Whewell's analysis of the inductive method, which happens through the selection of the (fundamental) idea, such as space, number, cause, or resemblance/likeness; the formation of the conception, or more special modification of those ideas, as a circle, a uniform force, etc.; and finally the determination of magnitudes. Karl Popper is well understood in this context through his "all swans are white" hypothesis, in which he focused on the principle of falsifiability, namely by proposing the null hypothesis idea in which one attempts to disprove or falsify a hypothesis, contrary to the "No non-white swans will ever be found", which is, indeed, falsifiable.

[30]   Ibid. In this regard, Bunge seems to contradict himself, criticizing pre-Socratic philosophy throughout Chapter 1 and supporting the claim that this philosophy contributed indeed to the development of modern (medical) science on p. 11 and following.

[31]   For a special focus on Popper's metaphysics and "Objective Knowledge", especially in regard to the connection with the Cartesian Dualism and the „Drei-Welten-Theorie", see Brianese, G. (Editor) 1998. *"Congetture e confutazioni" di Popper e il dibattito epistemologico post-popperiano* (Popper's Conjectures and Refutations and the post-Popper epistemological debate). I ed. – XIII, Turin: Paravia.

cal rationalisms holds scientific theories "accountable", in the sense that they should be rationally criticized, and even be subjected to tests (in the case of empirical science) which may falsify them, following the principle of falsifiability. To be sure, if such claims cannot be subjected to this principle, they are not necessarily "wrong", but they are not empirical, in the epistemological sense. Furthermore, we also need to be aware of the complexity of life perspectives and worldviews on the ontological and, by extension, diagnostic aspects of psychiatry. This discipline is in fact one of the closest, among medical practices, to the connections to and between patient's and clinician's perception. The reason, once more, is the level of complexity of (human) brain and being human in general. Furthermore, one of the key concepts linking Medical philosophy and psychiatry is the focus on symptomatic evidence as foundation for the mental health diagnostic apparatus, by far inferior (if here we decide to only focus on empirical, evidence-based research) to the characteristics of other branches of medicine. From this perspective, psychiatry is not too far away from the unsolved problems of ancient medicine, namely the (perceived) absence of a well-structured cause-effect relation.

Throughout history, we can identify a vast array of philosophical systems upon which medicine structured its own scientific view and method. In particular, the symbolic, transcendental, spiritual, and/or magic worldview was the basis of the connection between human life and activities, including medical practice, with the hope and expectation of a positive outcome as result of a healing process linked to the divine element. In various forms and characters, God or the Gods intervened and/or assisted human in their path toward health/salvation (*Salus*). Philosophically speaking, illness and disease have always been complicated, even mysterious concepts, at least until the revolution of post-Cartesian dualistic evidence-based medicine, daughter of the Age of Enlightenment. There was certainly an active search of possible cause-effect relations as grounding element of disease, whether suffering and pain might have come from internal and/or external environmental factors, such as natural phenomena. From this perspective, an empirical, material attitude always permeated the science of medicine. This is especially true for herbal medicine, but can be certainly applied to a broader analysis of Medical Philosophy. Before Cartesian dualism, the scientific monism did not take away anything from the empirical model. On the contrary, this type of medicine was actively seeking *supra*natural (even supernatural, or, in complete fairness we should say *intra*natural) element attached, embedded, permeating the natural elements.

b) Medicine as art, science, and technology

Another very important focus of Medical Philosophy is the analysis of Healthcare and Healthcare Systems, in particular:

- Is healthcare a fundamental right of all people, regardless of age, race, creed, color, sex, national origin, religion, sexual orientation, gender identity, disability, marital status or socioeconomic status, etc.?
- Who is the target population who benefits from, has access to, and deserves healthcare? How can we identify it?
- How can we turn observations in the laboratory, clinical/medical settings and community into interventions that improve the health of individuals and the public (translational process)?
- More specifically, how can we go from diagnostics and therapeutics to medical procedures and behavioral changes (thus involving Behavioral Medicine)?
- How can we investigate and understand the scientific and operational principles underlying each step of the translational process (Translational Science)?
- Costs/Benefits, part 1: How can healthcare be administered to the greatest number of people in the best possible way?
- Costs/Benefits, part 2: What should be the basis for calculating the cost of treatments, hospital stays, drugs, etc.?
- Costs/Benefits, part 3: What are the necessary parameters for clinical trials, patient's rights and quality assurance?
- Who/what, if anybody/anything, can decide when a patient is in need of "advanced care plan" and "comfort measures" (end of life process, euthanasia)?

How can we address all the above listed questions, with a solid scientific method, with an analysis which is factual and yet not reductionist/reductivist, objective and yet epistemologically and ethically respectful of the individual subjectivity? Does this require a specific subset of Medical Philosophy or is generally understood as been part of medicine as science and practice? If the latter is the correct hypothesis, how do we understand medicine as combination of science, art, technique/technology and philosophy? According to Patel, Arocha, and Zhang:

> "The practice of medicine requires art as well as science. The latter argues for a deeper understanding of the mechanisms underlying disease processes and use of scientific evidence in making patient care decisions. The study of medical reasoning and thinking underlies much of medical cognition and has been the focus of research in cognitive science and arti-

ficial intelligence in medicine. Expertise and medical knowledge, organization, the directionality of reasoning, and the nature of medical errors are intricately tied to thinking and decision-making processes in medicine. With the recent advancement of technology in medicine, technology-mediated reasoning and reasoning support systems will be a focus for future research."[32]

Certainly, it is not easy to define medicine without taking in consideration art, science, and technology, especially given that medical cognition mainly focuses on research analysis of "everyday", "real", "actual" clinical tasks in order to foster more effective medical practices, methods and interventions. Medical Philosophy helps understand which elements, and to what extent, are present in every day clinical practice, in hypothesis making and diagnostics, as well as in therapeutic intervention and decision making in the laboratory. We could rightfully argue that medicine is a form of art based on science. However, we would encounter issues of order, structure and perhaps ethical/practical value of defining these terms as linked in a superior-inferior, or origin-evolution type of dichotomy. Furthermore, we might also get caught in a superficial, perhaps even incorrect application of this relation, especially when we decide to completely separate the realms of art and science, thus discarding the technological sub-element within the Aristotelian view on episteme, techne and phronesis.

To be sure, we would also need to discuss whether medical science is a pure, "hard" science, or should be considered a form of applied science. Moreover, as we previously discussed, the uncertainty of specific medical subfields is part of what medicine is, as commonly accepted within the realm of science, a constantly changing, always challenging method which discards practices and perspectives in the light of newer evidence. Medical Philosophy investigates these problems, and also contributes to a better understanding of the personal, subjective, and even emotional aspects of medical practice. To be sure, here we refer not only to the general aspects of doctor-patient relationship, but also on the results and clinical outcomes of clinician's and patient's behavior under conditions of pressure and stress[33], especially when dealing with diffi-

---

[32]   Patel, V.L., Arocha, J.F., Zhang, J. 2012. *Thinking and reasoning in medicine*. In: Holyoak, K., Morrison, R.G. 2012. *The Oxford Handbook of Thinking and Reasoning*. Oxford Library of Psychology. Oxford, UK: Oxford University Press.

[33]   Which ultimately affect the whole biopsychosocial aspects, considering that stress itself is cause for genetic changes at the level of the DNA, with particular regard to the structure and functions of telomeres, which can ultimately be negatively affected (in the sense that the cell either is subjected to inflammation processes or cease to exist) by high levels of cortisol, due to (chronic) stress.

cult decision-making processes, such as in the case of chronic disease, palliative care, and advance care planning.

Needless to say, the need for a better inclusion of medical humanities within modern medicine is not only ethically required, but absolutely mandatory in the light of the most recent research of clinical outcomes affected by doctor-patient relationship. When we address issues related to decision-making aspects in medicine, we are working within the debate of medical reasoning, thus examining the cognitive processes at the base of patient/doctor perception, understanding and comprehension, clinical decisions and problem solving in general. This perspective also addresses scientific approaches, medical curricula, academic environment as well as the philosophical debate over cognitive and neuroscience, as well as human and artificial intelligence. What is important to note here is that Medical Philosophy helps us shed some clarity on the very big confusion, especially in the Western, post-industrial society, between science and technology. Certainly, effective (from the therapeutic point of view) medical decision-making involves a skilled understanding and ability to use technology, first and foremost to understand, monitor, examine, and treat disease from the analysis of symptoms to therapy, thus covering diagnosis and prognosis. Therefore, the medical community generally divides medical reasoning into two main, interconnected, and mutually dependent subareas: clinical reasoning and biomedical reasoning. At the same time, we need to remember that even the most advanced and sophisticated medical technology does not, alone, provide absolute(ly) correct results 100% of the time.

First of all, the complexity of medical diagnosis, especially in field related to the human brain, contributes to the difficulty of monitoring neurological data. Second, however precise our technologies might be, medical reasoning and decision-making works only with a solid, yet open, theoretical basis. In this regard, we could go back to the words by Thomas Huxley, as quoted by Sanders:

> "Applied science is nothing but the application of pure science to particular classes of problems. No one can safely make these deductions unless he or she has a firm grasp of the principles. Yet the idea of the practice of clinical medicine as an art persists."[34]

---

[34]   Saunders J. 2000. *The practice of clinical medicine as an art and as a science.* Medical Humanities. 26: 18–22. For further reference, please see: http://www.w3.org/1999/xlink" xlink:href="http://mhbmjjournalscom/cgi/content/ full/26/01/18.

We could argue that modern medicine is comprised of scientific analysis and "artistic" practice. Thus, medicine is science and art together, helped by technology and supported by theory. At the same time, the historical perspective (also in Hegelian terms) is fundamental to understand the impact of culture and civilization on science as a whole, and therefore on the relationship, in terms of percentage of applicability but also in terms of ethical and moral value, between science, art, and technology in medicine. Moreover, medical science and practice differed through time and space, thus across geographic, ethnic, racial, and cultural areas. Therefore, this analysis of medical reasoning covers perspective on history, space, cognition, semantics (and specific medical ontologies), and methodological strategies, for instance when addressing elements from clinical and translational science, such as study design, decision support systems, and public policy.

In analyzing clinical reasoning, Medical Philosophy generally focuses on the decision-analytic approach (investigating with a structured quantitative model) on one side, and on the information-processing approach (using the methods of cognitive science in monitoring reason), also liked to perspectives of more general problem-solving, on the other. More specifically, the decision-analytic approach applies a mathematical model to the clinician's performance, in order to capture possible mistakes in the process of making decisions. The information-processing approach relies instead on pure empirical observation and protocol analysis, similarly to developmental/cognitive psychology patters. The whole goal is obviously a better medical performance within the relationship doctor-patient, especially within the perspectives of a social contract, in the sense that the physician is responsible for the individual patient and his/her individual diagnosis, and to the society at large:

> "A medicine that cares or cures, helps or heals has an even greater consequence for humanity than that of merely mending, tending, patching or preventing the various ailments that are the result of being alive. [...] Practicing the art of medicine one can mend the aches and pains of fellow human beings. The act of giving service with a humane touch—in the form of medicine, is the purest gesture of peace and communication; or we can say, manifestation of medicine in an art form."[35]

c) Self-Image, Academic Achievement, Healing Process

Medical Philosophy has a clear message: modern medicine needs to focus on both the individual and humanity as a whole. From the viewpoint of cognitive

---

[35]   Achtenberg J. 1996. What is medicine. Alternative therapy. May; 2(3): 58–61.

science, the human information processing research has focused, at least in general and within an analytical approach, on the individual, to infer more generalizable considerations linked to personal, rational, intellectual, academic performance. How can we understand concepts such as experience, knowledge, and again, performance, within the realms of academic, scientific, and clinical medicine, especially in those realms that are closely related to the analysis of brain functioning and mental health? Let us make sure we understand this point: the physician's strength lies in scientific research and technical (clinical) skills. However, what is also very important in diagnostics and therapy is the physician's capacity for clinical judgment. In this sense, "clinical medicine remains an interpretive practice"[36], based on practical reasoning, or *phronesis*. Aristotle states in the theory of rhetoric, that phronesis is one of three essential qualities that a speaker must possess along with two others, goodwill (*Eunoia*, or ευνοια from the Greek *eu* = good and *voια* = intelligence, possible translation of "benevolence") and virtue (from the Greek αρετή, *are-te*)[37]. The philosopher also thinks that the acquisition of phronesis, translated as "wisdom", is:

> "Also about the details, which become known based on experience, while the young are not experienced: in fact, is the length of time that produces the experience. You could ask the reason: why can someone be a mathematician, but not a wise or a physicist? You should probably answer that the objects of mathematics are derived by abstraction, while the principles of wisdom and of physics are derived from experience."[38]

How can we relate to the sum of our experiences? According to Michel Foucault, a method is developed by actually applying it, not by talking about it.[39] Bent Flyvbjerg explains this concept in terms of a movement from explanation (why/theory) to narrative (how/analysis)[40]. This concept is also analyzed by

---

[36]   Montgomery, K. 2006. *How doctors think: clinical judgment and the practice of medicine*. New York, NY: Oxford University Press, p. 5.

[37]   Sievke, Franz G., *Aristoteles: Rhetorik. Übersetzt mit einer Bibliographie, mit Erläuterungen und einem Nachwort*, (the Rhetoric by Aristotle, translation and commentary), 5. Auflage, München (5 edition, Munich), 1985

[38]   Aristotle, *Nicomachean Ethics*, 1142a in: Abbagnano N., and Fornero G. 1992. *Filosofi e filosofie nella. storia*, (Philosophers and Philosophies in history), Torino: Paravia, Torino.

[39]   Urbanski S. 2011. *The Identity Game: Michel Foucault's Discourse-Mediated Identity as an Effective Tool for Achieving a Narrative-Based Ethic*, The Open Ethics Journal, 2011 -5, pp. 3–9.

[40]   Flyvbjerg, B. 1993. *Aristotle, Foucault and Progressive Phronesis: Outline of an Applied Ethics for Sustainable Development*; in: Winkler, Earl R. & Coombs Jerold R., *Applied Ethics*, Cambridge: Blackwell Publishers, p. 18–19

David S. Yeager, primarily through randomized experiments in school settings[41]. This empirical approach allows, in his opinion, to "better understand
the system of forces affecting behavior and development through active participation and work by the student, as an individual as well as a vital member of
the community"[42]. In a recent lecture at the Community College of Vermont[43],
he showed the statistical data related to the concept of "academic success"
linked to the college-level student performance in the United States (randomized 500 students took part in the survey). His study further explained how
cognitive factors interact with structural and physiological influences to create
positive or negative trajectories for youth. These components are not only used
from a statistical data research point of view, but they serve the purpose of
designing new experiments. This in turn leads to specific interventions who are
created by the researchers and by the students themselves, focusing on cognitive aspects of perception and self-perception. In particular, the focus on the
relationship between self-image[44] and academic success gives the whole process a new framework of analysis, completely based on the student's experience. Therefore, this constitutes a combination of meta-analysis, experiment,
and longitudinal intervention guided by social scientific methodology. Yeager
believes that this approach may be useful for addressing important problems
facing society.

In this sense we can understand how this kind of wisdom, filtered through
personal experience, has indeed a practical application for a study of social
issues. For this reason, phronesis is often translated as "practical wisdom", and
sometimes as "prudence", from the Latin term *prudentia*. In modern times, this
word came to signify positive concepts such as "ability to value or evaluate",
"caution", "carefulness", but also perceived-negative terms such as "reluctance
to take risks", even "procrastination". The latter seems to represent an oxymo-

---

[41]   Yeager, D.S., Walton, G., & Cohen, G.L. 2013. *Addressing achievement gaps with
psychological interventions*, New York, NY: Phi Delta Kappan, p. 62–65.

[42]   Yeager, D.S. & Dweck, C.S. 2012. *Mindsets that promote resilience: When students believe
that personal characteristics can be developed*, Educational Psychologist, 47, p. 1–13.

[43]   Yeager, D.S. *Productive Persistence: A Practical Theory of Student Success*, lecture at the
CCV – Community College of Vermont Summer Institute, Lake Morey, VT, June 21st,
2013.

[44]   It is important to distinguish, and yet understand the connection between self-perception and
self-image. In the following chapter we will discuss more in depth the philosophical component of scientific research of neural basis, such as the mirror-neuron discovery. For further
reference, see Little, A.C., Jones, B.C., DeBruine, L.M. 2014. *Primacy in the Effects of Face
Exposure: Perception Is Influenced More by Faces That Are Seen First*. Archives of Scientific Psychology, Washington, DC: APA, American Psychological Association, pp. 43–47.

ron, considering that the Latin meaning covers a broad spectrum of terms, from "knowledge", "acquaintance", "discretion", all the way to "foresight" and even "sagacity". Aristotle makes indeed a distinction between two intellectual (dianoetic) virtues, *sophia* and *phronesis*[45]. Sophia (which is also usually translated as "wisdom") is the ability-capacity to think well about the nature of the world, to understand why the world is as it is in terms of universal truths; a viewpoint directly linked to *episteme*. The Phronesis, however, is the ability to see what is the right way to achieve a goal, not in the epistemological sense of universal, unchanged/unchangeable/stable truth, but with a specific focus on what is good and what is bad; *id est* what is desirable for man and society[46]. It is therefore an action, or a series of actions, carried out according to a specific criterion. Aristotle specifies, however, that phronesis is not simply the ability to decide how to achieve a particular goal but it is also the ability to reflect and decide what should be the *end* on the base of experience: "We must therefore keep in mind that a person can possess phronesis, for example, may know the righteous principles of a particular action. However, to apply it in the real world, in a concrete way, in unexpected situations, requires experience"[47]. Plato distinguishes humans in *Politeia* three faculties of the soul: desire, emotion and reason. These are the virtues associated with the prudence (σωφροσύνη, sophrosyne), bravery (ανδρεία, andreia) and wisdom (σοφία, sophía)[48]. Based on this analysis, how can we define phronesis in ethical terms, as an evaluation of good and bad? Aristotle considers ethics as the human behavior focused on achieving good from a concrete (practical) perspective:

> "We must achieve *this* good for its own sake; because of its inner value. This good does not have to be a tool necessary to achieve further goods. It must be the supreme good, what we call *eudaimonia,* the happiness that cannot be, for example, in physical pleasure, as this would degrade the man by putting him in the same realm as animals, nor in wealth since this is not the ultimate good but the means to achieve other goods, nor in the political honors because they do not depend on us but by those who give them to us and are not ends but means to feel gratified."[49]

---

[45] Giannantoni, G., a cura di (editor), 1973. *Aristotele: Opere*, (Aristotle: Works) IV Vol.., Roma-Bari: Laterza, p.67.

[46] Mazzarelli, C., a cura di (editors). 1979 *Etica Nicomachea*, Book VII, Milano: Rusconi, p. 15. Of note, some argue that the sense is indeed *absolute*, given the ethical generalizability model it encompasses.

[47] Ibid., p. 23.

[48] Luckner, A. 2005 : *Klugheit*, De Gruyter, Berlin u.a., p. 87–95.

[49] Mazzarelli, C., a cura di (editors). 1979 *Etica Nicomachea*, Book VII, Milano: Rusconi, p. 28.

In this sense we can interpret the relationship between self-image and academic achievement. According to Yaeger and Walton, randomized experiments have found that seemingly "small" social-psychological interventions in education can lead to large gains in student achievement and sharply reduce achievement gaps even months and years later[50]. These interventions are based on brief exercises that target students' thoughts, feelings, and beliefs, focusing on the way they perceive themselves, school, and academic success. This is very important in our analysis of what is desirable in terms of higher good, as well as happiness. Furthermore, a well-thought analysis of Medical Philosophy should include a discussion on the above mentioned perceptual concepts, both in relation to patient-physician and student-professor interaction. Thus, philosophical reasoning is the preferred path to provide not only a better understanding of these relationships, but also deepen and broaden scientific perspectives and interpretations, core concepts in medical fields. In psychology in particular we agree with Christopher, Wendt, Marecek and Goodman:

> "[...] interdisciplinary training is an important way to provide psychology students with a robust and sophisticated knowledge of culture. A genuinely liberal arts education provides conceptual tools to think about alternative systems of meanings, as well as the perspective to engage in disciplinary reflexivity regarding psychology. [...] psychologists who wish to study people in culture would do best to incorporate empirical methods that move outside traditional laboratory experiments and quantitative measures."[51]

Certainly, the very definition of "liberal arts" in some areas of modern, Western, especially US-American cultural circles is somewhat misleading, and disconnected from the *liberalia studia* of Roman antiquity. In fact, the term has unfortunately quite often been used to describe academic subjects which, from a capitalistic, market-oriented worldview, "don't count as much". Furthermore, we could also argue that far too often the same viewpoint confuses technological innovation with real progress in culture, education, intelligence, capacity for understanding and applying knowledge. This is especially important in the realms of medicine and academia. Thus, we should be careful in addressing students' (in medicine or other fields) ability based on an ill-defined concept of

---

[50]   Yaeger, D.S., and Walton, C.S. 2011. *Social-Psychological Interventions in Education: They're Not Magic*, Stanford, CA: Stanford University.

[51]   Christopher, J.C., Wendt, D.C., Marecek, J., D.C., Goodman, D.M. 2014. *Critical Cultural Awareness. Contributions to a Globalizing Psychology*. In *American Psychologist*. Vol. 69, Num. 7: 645–655 Washington, DC: APA, American Psychological Association, pp. 652–653.

"success", of which the credit system is one of the most apparent symptoms. A sign of a system in which even universities are expected to work like banks.

However, if our scope is to improve academic success, the considerations on a progressive phronesis approach are in this sense directly applied on practical work with the students. It is important to remember, that these interventions do not teach students academic content but instead target students' psychology, such as their beliefs that they have the potential to improve their intelligence or that they belong in school and they are valued for what they do and what they are. Is it really true? How much can we achieve, in terms of academic performance, as well as from the perspective of inner satisfaction, happiness and self-esteem? According to Jürgen Habermas, intersubjective dialogue is indispensable. Habermas further discusses this statement through a comparative analysis of Taylor's position:

> "(1) Morality is tailored to interactive relations between subjects capable of action and not to goods – that is, things in the world that can acquire value and importance for individual agents. In this way morality is set apart from the beginning as a social phenomenon and is delimited from individual aspirations to happiness, existential problems, and sensuous needs. 2) Morality relates to interactions regulated by norms [...]. 3) Morality is understood as a peaceful alternative to violent resolution of action conflicts for which there is no equivalent. [...] In this way morality is secured against all purely naturalistic interpretations. 4) From this assumption there follows, where recourse to collectively binding religious or metaphysical worldviews is no longer available, the more far-reaching assumption that a consensual justification of rights and duties can be generated only through argument, that is, through the cogency of good reasons."[52]

Habermas also defines intersubjective dialogue within the scope of "communicative ethics of need interpretation"[53]. Thus, we should be able to improve, both within ourselves as well as within the community (academic, in this case) through dialogue; which also means comparison, shared information, viewpoints, opinions, attitude, bias etc. Is that how we can create an image of ourselves? The problem lies in what we think defines not only "ourselves"[54], but

---

[52]   Habermas, J. 1993. *Remarks on Discourse Ethics*, in: *Justification and Application*, Cambridge, MA: MIT Press, p. 70–71.

[53]   Jaggar, A. 1993. Taking Consent seriously: Feminist Practical Ethics and Actual Moral Dialogue, in: Winkler, E.R., Coombs J.R., *Applied Ethics,* Cambridge: Blackwell Publishers, p. 83.

[54]   We should note that the assumption of the syntactical as well as cognitive conception of a plural selves versus self leads to the acknowledgment of a bigger problem, *id est* the definition and awareness of society as a plurality, a combination of more personalities, or selves. In this regard, the impact of these considerations on the public sphere is further analyzed by Langdon Winner, especially in regard to "the lack of any coherent identity for

also the ways our *selves* work. Does our self change? Do *we* change? And if we do, what are the benefits of this change? How can we decide what is good or bad, or even what is beneficial and desirable just for ourselves (and our selves), since we are focusing on what we (again, our *selves*?) think is good, regardless of (but we just mentioned that intersubjective dialogue is fundamental) what other people think?

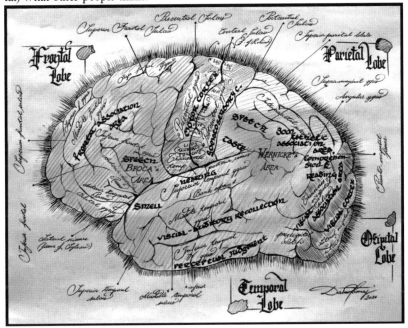

Figure 1. – New and important elements of analysis of cognition and perception come from the analysis of our thought processes under the lenses of neuroscience, especially descriptive neuroanatomy, through investigative methods such as TMS, tDCS, EEG, PET and MRI. (Image by David Låg Tomasi)

In order to answer all these questions a great help comes from the scientific research, in the sense of empirical, epistemological, verifiable (universal?)

the 'public' creates futile rituals of expert advice and disagreement(s) on what is morally justified (and justifiable)." For reference, see Winner, Langdon, *Citizen Virtues in a Technological Order*, in: Winkler, Earl R. & Coombs Jerold R., *Applied Ethics*, Blackwell Publishers, Cambridge 1993, p. 56, 57 and 58.

knowledge[55]. The contribution comes from neuroscience, in particular from the studies on *neuroplasticity*. Brain plasticity refers to the ability of the brain to change its structure and its functionality in terms of pathways and synapses, depending on the activity of their neurons; for instance a neuronal activity related to stimuli received from the external environment. These changes can also happen in reaction to traumatic injury or pathological changes. This capability, which is expressed in degrees and in different ways throughout the nervous system, is based on neuronal plasticity. The results are visible through Magnetic resonance imaging technologies (*MRIs* and *fMRIs*), showing an increase in the size of certain brain regions following their repeated use. Neuronal cells have increased activity and consequently form more synapses between them in enriched environments, especially during learning, and in case of cerebral reorganization. This is very important for the definition of a "self" which takes in consideration the possibility that *today's self* could be different from *yesterday's self*. The implication of this reasoning leads to a new awareness in terms of self-esteem and self-judgment. For example, could a student who always thought of himself as an "art person" discover new parts of himself which might lead to a new understanding of himself as a "math person"? Up to a certain age the neurons have greater capacity for learning. However, there are critical periods that distinguish the possibility of acquisition of a given skill, which is why we as teachers, researchers, scientists, policy-makers and society in general have the moral duty to "leave all the doors open" for personal, cultural and academic discovery. We, as society, are responsible for feeding, protecting and promoting the curiosity of every human being. When this type of social-psychological interventions has lasting effects, it can seem surprising and even "magical", leading people either to think of them as quick fixes to complicated problems or to consider them unworthy of serious consideration[56]. We have to understand that psychological interventions are very powerful but context-dependent.

This means that we have to take in consideration all possible inputs and influences on a definition of self and its relative impact (or ability, which is also *perme*ability) on this type of interventions. In particular, we have to think

[55]   If science research is indeed universal, is there a need to re-verify results and outcome over time? Can science change? If the answer to this question is positive, we could argue that this kind of science is no longer *episteme*.

[56]   See Yeager, D.S., Bundick, M.J. & Johnson, B. 2012. *The role of future work goal motives in adolescent identity development: A longitudinal mixed-methods investigation*, Contemporary Educational Psychology, Vol. 37, p. 206–217.

of context as environment; and environment as historical/chronological/hierarchical (also in terms of student's age and level/grade), cultural, ethnic, geographical, personal, individual, linguistic, cognitive, and psychological-developmental. The other question would be: what are we trying to achieve by looking at this psychosocial interventions form a perspective of progressive phronesis? According to Flyvbjerg, we are living in a "post-era, especially post-immortal; since humanity has finally achieved the ability to effectively destroy itself (...). For more than two centuries instrumental rationality has dominated value rationality."[57] That is where we desperately need phronesis in studying social issues and academic problems, more so if we already have an instrumental goal, which is to increase the academic performance of a certain student or of a college community. We have to combine empirical/practical activity with theoretical work, whether the first is the most important of the two (Aristotle) or the second dominates (Socrates, Plato).

The problem of Giddens' *Double Hermeneutic* is also a very important factor in this type of intervention, but it could carry many positive elements influencing several outcomes. The statement "What counts as a relevant fact or feature is dependent on the interpretation of both researchers and people being studied"[58] is a key to help students succeed, where success is the value-based outcome and the value is defined exactly by our progressive phronesis. Therefore, success is at the same time a specific result following a praxis (the exercise, the dialogue, the problem, the socio-psychological intervention) and the base for future praxis, interpreted as (analytic) combination of different kinds of techne an different kinds of power. Thus, we put into practice Foucault's lesson, which wants us to link techne to goal (outcome, success, academic achievement) instead of linking episteme to techne (an applied epistemic science)[59]. In discussing these approaches, we better understand the definition of social science as "public philosophy" and we put into practice the main characteristics of Aristotelian methodology: the focus on what is context-dependent, concrete and particular and the power of specific and practical example. Certainly, from this perspective, Medical Philosophy is also a social science, as a

---

[57]   Flyvbjerg, B. 1993. *Aristotle, Foucault and Progressive Phronesis: Outline of an Applied Ethics for Sustainable Development*; in: Winkler, Earl R. & Coombs Jerold R., *Applied Ethics*, Cambridge: Blackwell Publishers, pp. 12, 13, 14.
[58]   Ibid., p. 15.
[59]   Ibid., p. 19.

form of patient advocacy "by means of human faculty,"[60] since in this case the role of science has to be necessarily subordinated (in a sociological perspective) to the "humane art of listening."[61]

Thus, since medicine is also a form of applied science, and its practice is a (human) art, the ultimate purpose of medicine is, beyond the scientific enquiry and thirst for knowledge, the sake of the patient. To be sure, excessive biologism in medicine is doomed to fail for these precise reasons, because human behavior, both the physician's and the patient's, is subject not only to the laws of nature, but also to ethical, moral, social, cultural, and certainly theoretical rules. According to Bunge, there are ten major ethical concerns in addressing medicine: amoralism, immoralism or nihilism, radical individualism, holism, negative utilitarianism, religious ethics, deontology, contractualism, utilitarianism, and humanism or agathonism[62]. The latter in particular is defined by Bunge as "egotuism, or a combination of egoism with altruism [whose] top principle [is] *Enjoy life and help live.*"[63] In this regard, we should perhaps discuss whether *alter* and *tu* are interchangeable terms, also in a Levinasian sense.

[60]   Goldman, L., and Ausiello, D.. 2004. *Cecil Textbook of Medicine*, Philadelphia, PA: Saunders, p. 73.
[61]   Ibid.
[62]   Bunge, M. 2013. *Medical Philosophy. Conceptual Issues in Medicine*, Singapore: World Scientific Publishing, pp. 194–196.
[63]   Bunge, M. 1989. *Treatise on Basic Philosophy*, Vol. 8: Ethics: The Good and the Right. Dordrecht & Boston: Reidel.

Chapter 2
Philosophy as basic approach to Medicine

2.1 Hermeneutics and Evidence-Based Medicine

Not surprisingly, the best help in becoming more aware of these conditions in our study comes from Hermeneutics. In fact, since among the main research areas covered by Medical Philosophy, the epistemological debate on the nature and application of Evidence-based Medicine plays a fundamental role, we need to address the problem of evidence and experience first. We could reasonably argue that Hermeneutics is both theory and practice of interpretation,[64] in that culture is contemplated as a whole set of meanings at the base of human existence and, *thus* (empirically speaking), experience. Culture in this sense –which is also shared, *common* sense– contains structure and orientation, in a layered series of perceptions, assumptions which are pre-reflective although not specifically aprioristic, often hidden from the generalized view, and yet providing a solid ground to this shared (moral, ethical, therefore guiding) standpoint. Thus, we could argue that in the hermeneutical analysis (a term used loosely in this case) the very core of scientific method in science, the randomizing aspect of the clinical trial at the center of Evidence-based Medicine is indeed *put on trial*. Furthermore, we could infer that at the base of this criticism lies the very debate between rationalism and empiricism[65] in medical science as a whole, but especially in the most recent, cutting-edge discoveries in neuroscience and neurobiology. To quote Robyn Bluhm, "Neuroimaging looks like rationalism, but is empiricism – just observation, without explanation."[66] In Bluhm's view,

---

[64] Especially because in our analysis we must keep in mind that, in terms of medical scientific analysis, we are always moving from induction to deduction: "induction as a reasoning method on its own is not without problems. It depends upon unbiased observations, and it can be argued that these do not exist. Some observations must be preferred over others and judged as being significant in some way. In hermeneutic terms we cannot avoid bringing our prejudices (or prejudgments) to bear on the observations we make." In: Loftus, S.F. 2006. *Language in clinical reasoning: using and learning the language of collective clinical decision making.* Sydney, AUS: Faculty of Health Sciences, School of Physiotherapy, University of Sydney, p. 33.

[65] Terms, we should not forget, used differently in Medicine and Philosophy, and often considered antithetical, for instance in Newton's analysis of medical science.

[66] Bluhm, R 2014. *Why Evidence-Based Medicine is Bad for Biological Psychiatry*, Psychiatry Grand Rounds lecture at the University of Vermont College of Medicine, Burlington, VT.

Medical Science requires a strong philosophical interpretation to shed light on the weaknesses of EBM as practiced in today's medicine.[67] In fact, to obtain not only reliable results in terms of collecting data, but also to interpret this data as useful and appropriate information to use in clinical settings, medicine needs are to be found in rationalism, with the search of mechanisms and causes, and empiricism, by incorporating prognosis and treatment. More specifically, Bluhm defines modern EBM as "shallow empiricism" in that it completely ignores the specificity of the individual, by focusing on the "Average of the Averages"[68] to infer about a specific (randomized, as it is) patient by the standards of the Hierarchy of Evidence as described in the *User's Guide on Evidence*[69]. In particular, if by rationalism we are willing to embrace a concept that stretches onto a medical realism (thus including anatomical, biological, as well as mechanical aspects), we could look at the very *clinical manifestation* of a disease, instead of a lower level of speculative realism involving the (sub)division of ill-defined symptoms. In fact, to refer once more to Bluhm's work,[70] one of the weakest points of the Feighner Criteria[71] is the *atheoretical* aspect of this psychiatric diagnostic criteria developed at Washington University, with no mention of causes and focus only on description. At the same time, the contemporary debate between the Biological sphere of psychiatry (rationalism) and the mere descriptive analysis of the DSM (empiricism) is a false debate, since the critics to the DSM, can be also applied to the *Research Domain Criteria* (RDoC), also guilty of "shallow rationalism."

---

[67]   In this sense, we should also remember that at the center of the philosophical perspective and scientific method of empiricism, we find figures such as John Locke who not only worked on stating that (empirical, by definition) knowledge comes only or primarily from sensory experience, but also had a direct (clinical) experience in the field of medicine. In particular, he worked with philosophers (and medical scientist) such as Robert Boyle, Robert Hooke, Richard Lower and Thomas Willis, and also obtained a Bachelor in Medicine while studying at Oxford.

[68]   For further discussion, please refer to the Cochrane Collaboration, Oxford, UK – www.cochrane.org.

[69]   Guyatt G., Rennie D., Meade M.O., and Cook D.J., 2014. *Users' Guides to the Medical Literature: A Manual for Evidence-Based Clinical Practice*, 2nd Edition: JAMA & Archives Journals, American Medical Association, New York: McGraw-Hill.

[70]   Bluhm, R 2014. *Teaching Critical Appraisal – of Critical Appraisal*, UVM College of Medicine Faculty Development Workshop, University of Vermont College of Medicine, Burlington, VT.

[71]   Feighner J.P., Robins E., Guze S.B., Woodruff R.A., Winokur G., Munoz R. 1972. *Diagnostic criteria for use in psychiatric research*, Archives of General Psychiatry. 26: 57–66.

How should we address the problem of collecting and presenting data following an appropriate method, which prevented this rationalism to be shallow? Is the mathematical model appropriate for (this, in terms of its intrinsic validity) clinical setting? "How reliable are the diagnoses and prognoses of experts who only use their experience and intuition, or who use objective data but "combine them in the head" instead of feeding them into an algorithm?"[72] We should certainly ask ourselves to what extent the theoretical (here, and only here, in the sense of mathematical) translation (plug-in) matches reality in its complexity. To be sure, we should draw parallels of examination between models. James Marcum writes:

> "Although the humanistic or humane models share many epistemological features with the biomedical model, they also rely on a practitioner's emotions and intuitions. Emotions and intuitions are not necessarily impediments to sound medical judgment and practice; but when judiciously utilized and constrained by the epistemic and empirical boundaries of the biomedical model, they enable a physician to access information about a patient's illness that may exceed quantified data, e.g. laboratory test results."[73]

Marcum here defends a balanced clinical intervention from diagnosis to therapy, while Bunge argues that "[…] forecasts made exclusively on the basis of statistical data and "mechanical" rules are far more successful, and therefore more reliable, than the subjective or intuitive ones made by experts."[74] First of all, we should define whom we mean by "experts". Second, Bunge quotes here the work of Paul Meehl as a valid proof, within Philosophy of Science, of the validity of his claim. Are we sure that a mathematical (algorithmic) translation (plug-in) of data will match reality of the single (individual) patient? Don't we need to discuss again the relationship between particular and general, under the lens (or perhaps, above it) of medical and scientific enquiry, with the help of psychological science and theoretical medicine?[75] Wittgenstein writes that

---

[72]   Bunge, M. 2013. *Medical Philosophy. Conceptual Issues in Medicine*, Singapore: World Scientific Publishing, p. 95.

[73]   Marcum, J.A. 2008. *An introductory philosophy of medicine: humanizing modern medicine*. New York: Springer, p. 12.

[74]   Ibid.

[75]   The theoretical approach is a core concept in social sciences, especially in psychology. However, there are still misunderstandings and imprecise generalization on what psychology actually does. The debate on psychology's need and striving to be admitted in the realm of exact/empirical/"exact"/"hard" science will be discussed in further chapters, but for now let us cite the interesting contribution by Robiner, Dixon, Miner, and Hong: "[…] The National Science Foundation and the U.S. Congress Joint Economic Committee consider psychology a non-STEM discipline. Nevertheless, psychology and medicine are two of the seven "hub

"[...] In psychology there is experimental method and conceptual confusion. [...] The existence of the experimental method makes us think that we have the means of solving the problems which trouble us; though problem and method pass one another by."[76] Certainly, we need to be careful in addressing the components of the kind of rationalism we could (and should) consider "valid." In the view of Heidegger, addressed to a broader field of scientific enquiry, with a special focus on natural sciences, the problem is "[...] one of obtaining and securing the primary way of access to what are supposedly the objects of this science. The relativity theory of *physics* arises from the tendency to exhibit the interconnectedness of Nature as it is 'in itself.'"[77] Furthermore, we also need to be aware of the context in terms of historicity of scientific analysis, especially in psychology and psychiatry, as we previously discussed in Hegelian terms.

---

sciences" that exert substantial influence over other scientific disciplines, according to scientometric and bibliometric analyses (Cacioppo, 2007). As such, the two disciplines are inextricably intertwined, as evidenced by their strong ties (Boyack, Klavans, & Börner, 2005). This interconnectedness provides a foundation for interdisciplinary research, an increasing focus in medical schools, potentially driving growing demand for doctoral psychology faculty. Further, the recent focus on interdisciplinary and translational research by the National Institutes of Health (NIH) has created fertile opportunities for PhD faculty. As Schweitzer and Eells (2008) noted, "Ph.D.s may complement physicians in enhancing a biopsychosocial perspective on treatment and education, while helping meet increasing needs for technical expertise in clinical practice and research" (p. 7). Psychologists' academic training in research is more extensive than that of most health care providers and mental health professionals. Their research skills are applied to diverse biopsychosocial phenomena, spanning basic and applied investigations. [...] Whereas the research contributions of MD faculty trended downward, presumably due to an increased focus on productivity and clinical expectations, the contributions from PhD faculty (i.e., not just psychologists) increased, both in terms of the percentage of PhD faculty serving as principal investigators and in terms of contributions to the total NIH funding pool (Fang & Meyer, 2003). [...] Psychologists are uniquely qualified to play diverse roles in medical education, such as teaching behavioral medicine and professionalism courses, addressing psychological and social aspects of health care and mental health, and supporting evidence-based approaches to practice. See Robiner, W.N, Dixon, K.E., Miner, J.L., and Hong, B.A. *Psychologists in Medical Schools and Academic Medical Centers. Over 100 Years of Growth, Influence, and Partnership*. In: *American Psychologist*. Vol. 69, Num. 3: 217–315 Washington, DC: APA, American Psychological Association, pp. 235–237. In this context, we should also remember the differences, in terms of academic titles and professional v. clinical background, between a US-American "MD" (professional doctorate) and a European, especially UK-British "MD".

[76]   Wittgenstein, L. 1958. *Preliminary Studies for the "Philosophical Investigations", Generally known as The Blue and Brown Books*. Hoboken, NJ: Blackwell Publishers Ltd., Aphorism N. 14.

[77]   Kearney, R. and Rainwater M. 1996. *The Continental Philosophy Reader*, London & New York: Routledge, p. 31.

Steven Behnke[78] discusses several aspects from the cultural perspective within psychological science and therapy, paying particular attention to the importance of language (such in the case of word choices, as in the concept of "termination"), and concludes: "The point is not that there is a "correct" or "incorrect" way to read the APA Ethics Code, but rather – as the SIP commentary emphasizes throughout – *every* reading of the code brings a cultural perspective."[79] Furthermore, the focus on the correctness of interpretation might risk missing the point of what psychology, especially from the perspective of native, traditional and folk psychology is, does and ought to be and do.[80] In

---

[78] Behnke, S.H. 2014. *Always a cultural perspective. The Society of Indian Psychologists comments on the APA Ethics Code*. In *Ethically Speaking*, Monitor on Psychology, Vol. 45, N.10, Washington, DC.: American Psychological Association, p. 37. In the 2014 American Psychological Association Annual Convention, Dr. Melinda Garcia and Dr. Carolyn Morris from the Society of Indian Psychologists (SIP), as well as Dr. Carolyn Barcus from Utah State University addressed issues related to the ethical component of cultural and ethnic substructures in science, from the perspectives of American Indian and Alaska Native psychologists. In particular, Garcia suggested that "We had to go beyond the linear, abstract, Cartesian logic of our European colonizers. In order to do that, we had to embrace who we are and communicate in the language of stories. Stories bring the abstract to life. Stories communicate across cultures." In fact, oftentimes science has consciously or unconsciously avoided broader perspectives which could take into account ethic and cultural differences of such type. In the same article, Stephen Behnke quotes the Society of Indian Psychologists' commentary on the Ethical Standard 8.07 in the American Psychological Association Ethics Code – deception: "Psychologists need to keep in mind the damaging past and current research being done in Native communities. Deceptive resulting in hypersensitivity to ANY research in Native communities. Deceptive research would compound this problem and add to the belief about research doing harm to communities. [emphasis in original] . The author then continues by quoting APA Ethics Code, focusing on the theme of community and on "Reporting Research Results (Ethical Standard 8.10): "Psychological researchers have a duty to consult with community stakeholders about the appropriate ways to share and disseminate the findings with the community being investigated. Psychologists have a further duty to report results effectively, concisely, clearly to the community in a way easily understood by community members. Respecting the dignity and sovereignty of the community dictates that a community member should be included in the writing process and subsequent publication as a community expert in interpreting research outcomes.

[79] Ibid., p. 69.

[80] Critics of these perspectives and approaches have debated the validity and (therapeutic) effectiveness of folk psychology, especially from an empirical point of view. Knobe and Prinz write: "This grand vision says that folk psychology should be understood, most fundamentally, as a tool for predicting and explaining behavior. Researchers who subscribe to this vision often suggest that folk psychology is in many ways similar to a scientific theory. Just as a scientist might posit unobservable entities in order to predict and explain the behavior of the observables, so too the folk psychologist posits unobservable mental states as a way of predicting and explaining human behavior. The key claim here is that we will be able to understand why people ascribe mental states in precisely the way they do if we reflect on the ways in which these ascriptions facilitate the activities of prediction and explanation.

this regard, the hermeneutic analysis of psychological science comes in hand in defining those terms from a much broader perspective. The prereflective understanding of Hermeneutics is also a *para*reflective understanding in the sense given to this field by proponents of this multilayered view of a human being, for instance in the case of Paracelsus. The focus on, and the very first scientific mention of the term in a clinical setting of the term "unconscious" is part of his legacy, together with the five main influences/origins of medical illnesses, diseases and disorders: *Ens Astrorum* or *Ens Astrale* (or the influx and influence of the stars), *Ens Veneni* (through the poison absorbed, inhaled by the body), *Ens Naturale* (the natural predisposition and constitution), *Ens Spirituale* (the influx and influence of the spirit-s), *Ens Dei* (influx and influence of God). Certainly the figure of Paracelsus has been accepted with praise as well as contempt in the history of science and medicine, especially in Germany. For example, Bunge defines Paracelsus "[…] a contemporary of Martin Luther's and a bridge between medieval quackery and modern medicine."[81] Although the above definition of the Swiss German scientist, philosopher, occultist, botanist, physician, alchemist and astrologer is very reductive, the conceptual weight of his contributions is especially important in the fields of psychiatry and psychology.

Starting from this grand vision, it is only a short step to the view that folk psychology must be functionalist. After all, if the vision is correct, it seems that the only properties of mental states that could play a role in folk psychology are those properties that might contribute to prediction and explanation – and the only properties that could be helpful in prediction and explanation are those that have something to do with the state's causes and effects. This chain of reasoning strikes us as a powerful and compelling one. Yet the results reported here have moved us to accept a theory that does not fit well with the functionalist view. On this theory, certain mental state ascriptions are based on the classification of particular entities as 'experiencers,' and this classification is based in turn on a complex system of non-functionalist principles. It is hard to see how a psychological mechanism like this one could be best understood as a tool for predicting and explaining behavior. To bring out the problem here, it might be helpful to emphasize that we seem to be uncovering a mechanism that specifically blocks the ascription of certain mental states even in cases where ascriptions of those mental states would facilitate prediction and explanation. Thus, suppose we find that we can do a better job of predicting and explaining the behavior of a given entity if we sometimes ascribe to it feelings of depression. If the entity in question has the wrong type of physical make-up – e.g., if it is a group agent – a special type of psychological mechanism will kick in and block the ascription of depression to the entity." See Knobe, J. and Prinz, J. 2008. *Intuitions about Consciousness: Experimental Studies.* In: Phenomenology and Cognitive Science. University of North Carolina, Chapel Hill, p. 14.

[81]   Bunge, M. 2013. *Medical Philosophy. Conceptual Issues in Medicine*, Singapore: World Scientific Publishing, p. 166.

Beyond the analysis by C.G. Jung in *Mysterium Coniunctionis*[82] and its more recent critics, we could argue that these fields are fertile ground for complementary, alternative, natural, folk, integrative methodologies. In a positive way, due to the complexity of neurological disorders, therapy and assessment, and for the same reason in a perhaps more negative way, also because of the closeness of yet inexplicable phenomena (certainly symptoms and even more potential treatments) with the lenses of evidence-based medicine. In this sense we understand the position of Christopher, Wendt, Marecek and Goodman:

> "The term folk psychology is often invoked as a pejorative to connote superstitious, old-fashioned, irrational, or prejudicial ideas about human behavior; its antithesis is thought to be "scientific" psychology. By contrast, in the hermeneutic view, folk psychologies entail inescapable presuppositions about self and social relations that orient people in life and enable them to function. [...] Moreover, folk psychology forms the largely unacknowledged substrate of expert psychological knowledge (including scientific psychological knowledge). Any understanding of behavior (e.g., extraversion), emotion (e.g., anger), cognition (e.g., schemas), psychopathology (e.g., delusions or depression), or complex social practices (e.g., courtship or racism) rests on a folk psychology concerning what a person is and what a person is expected to do or experience in a particular situation"[83]

The problem of interpretation in understanding the human mind and brain (leaving aside the dichotomy for a moment) is fundamental not only in psychology, but also in the progressively extensively developed field of medical humanities, especially in Narrative Medicine, as well described by Tricia Greenhalgh and Brian Hurwitz:

> "In the diagnostic encounter, narratives:
> Are the phenomenal forms in which patients experience ill health
> Encourage empathy and promote understanding between clinician and patient
> Allow for the construction of meaning
> May supply useful analytical clues and categories
> In the therapeutic process, narratives:
> Encourage a holistic approach to management
> Are intrinsically therapeutic or palliative
> May suggest or precipitate additional therapeutic options
> In the education of patients and health professionals, narratives:
> Are often memorable

---

[82]   Jung, C.G. 1963 (1990 ed.), *Mysterium Coniunctionis. Untersuchungen über die Trennung und Zusammensetzung der seelischen Gegensätze in der Alchemie*, Olten und Freiburg im Breisgau: Walter-Verlag.

[83]   Christopher, J.C., Wendt, D.C., Marecek, J., D.C., Goodman, D.M. 2014. *Critical Cultural Awareness. Contributions to a Globalizing Psychology*. In *American Psychologist*. Vol. 69, Num. 7: 645–655 Washington, DC: APA, American Psychological Association, p. 648.

Are grounded in experience
Encourage reflection
In research, narratives:
Help to set a patient centered agenda
May challenge received wisdom
May generate new hypotheses"[84]

The search and understanding of meaning from the perspective of the clinician, doctor, therapist and or physician are indeed the central scope of medical hermeneutics. From the abstract of "Clinical interpretation: The hermeneutics of medicine" by Drew Leder:

> "I argue that clinical medicine can best be understood not as a purified science but as a hermeneutical enterprise: that is, as involved with the interpretation of texts. The literary critic reading a novel, the judge asked to apply a law, must arrive at a coherent reading of their respective texts. Similarly, the physician interprets the 'text' of the ill person: clinical signs and symptoms are read to ferret out their meaning, the underlying disease. However, I suggest that the hermeneutics of medicine is rendered uniquely complex by its wide variety of textual forms. I discuss four in turn: the "experiential text" of illness as lived out by the patient; the "narrative text" constituted during history-taking; the "physical text" of the patient's body as objectively examined; the "instrumental text" constructed by diagnostic technologies. I further suggest that certain flaws in modern medicine arise from its refusal of a hermeneutic self-understanding. In seeking to escape all interpretive subjectivity, medicine has threatened to expunge its primary subject — the living, experiencing patient"[85].

From this perspective, illnesses, diseases and disorders are to be interpreted following a multilayered path based on a series of interactions: patient-provider, provider-medical science/knowledge, and also a *quid*, which goes deeper and beyond these relationships. It is the case, for instance, of the placebo/nocebo effect. According to Plato, illnesses originate in metaphysical ignorance, with a special connection to (human) soul. More specifically, in the *Timaeus* we learn how *anoia* and *novs* play a very important role. Both *Mania* and *Amathia* derive from anoia, and generate an imbalance in the soul, thus depriving it from its virtues, especially in connection with essence and consistence in Being, in the (ultimate, absolute, universal) Truth, and finally in the Divine. In this sense, the soul of human beings is in constant motion toward

---

[84]   Greenhalgh T, Hurwitz B. 1999. *Narrative based medicine: why study narrative?* US National Library of Medicine, National Institutes of Health, PubMed BMJ. Jan 2, 1999; 318(7175): 48–50.

[85]   Leder, D. 1990. *Clinical interpretation: The hermeneutics of medicine.* In: Theoretical Medicine March 1990, Volume 11, Issue 1, Dordrecht, the Netherlands: Kluwer Academic Publishers, pp. 9–24.

becoming more rational, this rationality helping the human being to reach higher levels of wholeness and perfection. Thus, education (in a broader sense) helps human beings overcome diseases. There is a constant battle of the soul against the influence of evil which ultimately causes physical and psychical (mental) disorders. The notion of evil is especially important in medicine, in obvious connection with disease, suffering and malpractice. This is exactly where Medical Philosophy can help us improve the science of medicine:

> "[...] philosophy of science has too long ignored the applied branches of science that could breathe new life into stale answers to questions like theory development or evolution. Philosophy of medicine could assist in this endeavor. Second, a robust philosophy of medicine is sorely needed for bioethics. Finally, philosophy of medicine could contribute to the development of medicine itself in terms of clinical trial design or explicating notions of pain and suffering."[86]

To continue in our analysis of Plato, the aforementioned disorders are the root of moral as well as behavioral, vices and general lack of strength. This condition also leads to the corruption of the vital spirit(s), and the following corruption of the humors, connecting the mental and moral sphere to the physical realm, therefore causing the body to get sick. To use a very popular term in modern *new age* circles, this is a *holistic* approach, in the sense that the ultimate cure is not medicine, but regimen. Thus, according to Plato medicine is interpretation, art, and science, and is therefore subordinate or part of philosophy similarly to what taught by Aristotle, Hippocrates, and Celsus. The latter in particular proposed a view in which at the origins of human life, human beings were not affected by moral corruption to the extent that more modern (Celsus' contemporary) civilizations have. Human beings' bodies were not yet influenced by the negative effects of passions, that is why there was no separation between science, religion, and philosophy up until around the V century, in the cultural and scientific centers of the ancient world, Rome/Italy and Athens/Greece. In more recent times, this moral corruption increased both the psychical and the physical *malady* in mankind. This is the time when, according to Celsus, the external part of medicine (the physical) became progressively more separated from the internal part of medicine (the psychical, but also spiritual, in the sense of sacred science). As we will see, this perspective is very similar to the viewpoint of practitioners and proponents of traditional, complementary and alternative medicine, which consider Western modern medicine as overly

---

[86]   Marcum, J.A. 2008. *An introductory philosophy of medicine: humanizing modern medicine*. New York: Springer, p. 5.

focused on the symptomatic exterior physical manifestations of a disorder, instead of focusing on the core of the problem, the bigger picture. The very definition of "alternative" is culture bound, if not even ethno/geocentric in the sense of Western cultural imperialism, considering that traditional medicine is the most common form of medicine in China and India, two of the biggest countries in the world, from a political, cultural, and even capitalistic perspective: together they comprise over one third of the world population, India is the world's biggest Democracy, and China finally became the world's largest economy in December 2014.

A hermeneutic view on medicine is even more important when addressing those issues that by definition are closely connected with the analysis of symptoms, as we previously observed in psychiatry. For example, let us look at the problem of suicide within non-Western cultures:

"In the United States, it is taken as common sense that suicide is a symptom of a serious psychiatric disturbance, typically a mood disorder. [...] On the Indian subcontinent, for example, suicide and suicidal behavior, typically undertaken by individual low in status, often serve as means of redressing grievances or protesting or evading unwelcome or illegitimate demands. The motivation force is anger, not depression, and the intention is to shame the wrongdoer [...]. Suicides in rural China have similarly been linked to familial grievances and the desire to avenge a wrong by publically disgracing the wrongdoer [...]. In fact, the diagnostic manual of the Chinese Society of Psychiatry specifically states that most Chinese individuals who commit suicide do not have mental illnesses [...]. China and India cannot be considered as exotic exceptions to the general rule [...]. With the United States comprising only about 4% of the world's population, one might consider the medicalized view of suicide as the exotic exception."[87]

In the same article, the authors examine the psychological and cultural situation in Taiwan, focusing on a compared analysis of children's upbringing in rural areas, and note that there is "no direct translation of the term "self-esteem' [...] in Mandarin Chinese."[88] Furthermore, the cited study showed that "self-esteem was not a desired developmental outcome but was thought to lead to psychological vulnerabilities such as stubbornness, low frustration tolerance,

---

[87]   Marecek & Senadheera, 2012; Staples, 2012; Widger, 2012; Pearson, Phillips, He, & Ji, 2002; Chinese Medical Association, as cited Pearson et al.; in: Christopher, J.C., Wendt, D.C., Marecek, J., D.C., Goodman, D.M. 2014. *Critical Cultural Awareness. Contributions to a Globalizing Psychology.* In *American Psychologist.* Vol. 69, Num. 7: 645–655 Washington, DC: APA, p. 649.

[88]   Miller, Wang, Sandel, & Cho, 2002 as quoted in: Christopher, J.C., Wendt, D.C., Marecek, J., D.C., Goodman, D.M. 2014. *Critical Cultural Awareness. Contributions to a Globalizing Psychology.* In *American Psychologist.* Vol. 69, Num. 7: 645–655 Washington, DC: APA, pp. 649–650.

and unwillingness to listen to elders."[89] Certainly, this problem of biased judgment affects every field of scientific enquiry, and it is a problem found in many cultures. However, given the self-proclaimed superiority (and, in some cases, the claim of uniqueness in terms of scientific validity) of Western science, this is especially true in the modern Western society. The focus on the individual, the new, and by conceptual translation, the young is a special feature of American society in particular. Thus it is no surprise that US medical and psychological perspectives differ very much in comparison to other geographical and cultural areas. From the perspective of medical philosophy, the above mentioned "unwillingness to listen to elders" is a very good indicator of the intrinsic value of the new-er, the most up-to-date, the latest available element. Within Evidence-based, clinically and empirically-based science and medicine, it is obvious that we should follow whatever the most current research data can provide. However, if we want to dig deeper in the meaning and effectiveness of a therapy, it becomes evident that a medical philosophy taking in consideration hermeneutic perspectives and narrative medicine is more helpful in clinical settings. On the other side of the spectrum, it is also true that sometimes modern medicine, especially in the field of mental health is not well accepted and valued in cultural areas beyond the one associated with "the West"[90]. To be sure, we need to maintain an *internationality* of efforts and scientific research, with a special awareness of strategies, methods, and approaches that are, and ought to be, local and more specialized, in order to provide the best possible care.

---

[89]   Ibid.

[90]   Rebecca Clay of the American Psychological Association recently wrote an article about James E. Maddux, a psychology professor at George Mason University in Fairfax, Virginia, in: Clay, R.A. 2014. *Random Sample. James E. Maddux, PhD*. In: Monitor on Psychology, Vol. 45, N. 11, Washington, DC.: American Psychological Association, p.26: "[...] charged with being an "international ambassador", Maddux has offered workshops on evidence-based treatment in Bulgaria and Romania and given lectures in Lithuania, Poland and Serbia. Eastern European psychologists were alternatively viewed as tools of a repressive state or (in Romania) imprisoned as threats. "Clinical psychology almost came to a standstill in some of these countries", he says. "I Hope I am contributing in some small way to help rebuild clinical psychology in these countries", he says." The definition of "international ambassador" can also be problematic in debates on medical philosophy. First of all, if we want to be open to broader perspectives, thus incorporating a focus on interpretation of medicine, patient-pharmacological and –therapeutic intervention, and patient-provider relationship, we should ask ourselves to what extent one "medical and scientific culture" has a genuine interest of approaching another, or if there are some other interests, sometimes unconscious, sometimes conscious (as in spheres of political influence) at the base of the dialogue.

In regard to the individual-centered approach, which permeates modern American medical scientific and in a broader sense cultural sphere, we need to make sure that we do not confuse this approach with a patient/person-centered perspective, which is still far too distant from modern medicine. In this sense, Western medicine often focuses on the more external layers of what is to be considered the "essence" of a human being, his external, often superficial rights and values.[91] Thus, we come to understand the hierarchy of interests and values of the "modern man." According to Abraham Maslow,[92] human self-actualization happens when a human being ascends the levels of the *hierarchy of needs*, as shown in the following figure. Although the pyramid might suggest a sequential progress in attaining the ultimate goal of each degree, the American psychologist also pointed out that often many needs are present in a person simultaneously. Furthermore, he also revised his approach to reach the conclusion that human self-actualization as defined through the steps of the pyramid was not an automatic outcome of satisfying the other human needs.

[91]   Also in terms of ideation and self (both in direct, as well as indirect object syntax) imagination, especially from the bottom-up or top-down of psychological analysis (as opposed to psychoanalysis), for instance in the interpretation of symbolism, tradition, folklore and dreams in René Guénon.

[92]   Maslow, A.H. 1943. *A Theory of Human Motivation*. Originally published in *Psychological Review*, 1943, Vol. 50 #4, Washington, DC: APA, pp. 370–396.

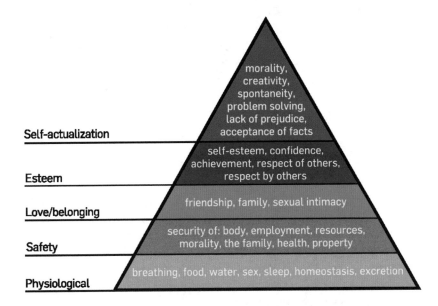

Figure 2. –   Visual summary of Abraham Maslow's hierarchy of needs as presented in "A Theory of Human Motivation" in Psychological Review (1943). In his pyramid, the
more basic needs are represented at the bottom. (Image by Factoryjoe)

Although Maslow's theory is still a very good starting point to examine human
values within a psychological analysis, his perspective has also been criticized
for cultural bias and lack of scientific rigor. How can we investigate the ultimate needs for self-actualization? What are the values at the top of the pyramid? We could definitely argue that concept such as self-sufficiency and self-
determining are integral part of a worldview embedded in modern Western
culture, and related to autonomy and independence; the so-called not-needing-
other-than-itself-in-order-to-be-itself; and ultimately environment-transcen-
dence; separateness/distinction and living by its own (one own's) laws. It becomes apparent how this view is in part rooted in the Cartesian "I", thus connecting the (self) conscious, rational, decisive and deliberative mind to the
very value of one's self as a completely separated entity from the surrounding
element, the environment, the culture, tradition, upbringing of the individual.
This is sharply opposed to a more comprehensive, even omnicomprehensive
hermeneutical perspective on reality. This is one of the missing links in modern medicine; the ability to take into account all the elements of, to use

Heideggerian terms, the *Dasein*. In more recent times, there is a progressively more open approach to traditional forms of medicine. However, as we previously examined, these forms are considered complementary, or integrative to the scientifically acceptable modern Western bio-medicine. If the validity of this approach encounters broad acceptance in medical subfields and specializations such as general surgery, the question is more problematic in psychiatry: "Invariably, the innermost ring is biogenetic, with psychological, interpersonal, societal, and (finally) cultural domains successively layered onto it. Biopsychosocial models usually take this form. The implication is that the outer rings can be peeled off, leaving the core intact: "The bio is the cake; the rest is frosting."[93] The question arising from these considerations is where does our "real" self exist, act, and interact? How and where is our consciousness (located)? As we will discover in the following chapters, an interesting perspective is represented by the Hameroff-Penrose model, but to remain within a purely philosophical debate we could quote Hegel, especially in the accurate interpretation offered by Verene. Through his analysis, we understand how the struggle of consciousness in trying to bring the two moments of *Ansich* together is coded in sense, perception and understanding; the three attempts which failed because these opposites cannot both be apprehended (and comprehended, cognitively understood) as a function of the object. It is the self-consciousness that leads us to the absolute truth, beyond what is illusion. That is where *das Meinen* comes to play –literally *play*– as if it were on the stage of such a representation, its fundamental *role*. It allows consciousness to speak out of itself until it abandons its posts and, in the word of Verene "goes to sleep," before being absorbed into the *verkehrte Welt*. At this point only, language must speak again and forth a new ground,[94] and show that self-consciousness is "the only reality and all reality."[95] The theme of consciousness is further analyzed by Hegel, and reinterpreted by Verene, through the dialectical movement across history *and* philosophy (and therefore, across the history *of* philosophy).

In particular, we see the "truth of self-certainty" associated with the debate on doctrines found in ancient Greece and Rome, in particular through

[93]   Christopher, J.C., Wendt, D.C., Marecek, J., D.C., Goodman, D.M. 2014. *Critical Cultural Awareness. Contributions to a Globalizing Psychology*. In *American Psychologist*. Vol. 69, Num. 7: 645–655 Washington, DC: APA, p. 651

[94]   In this sense we also understand the metaphor of the so-called 'tupsy-turvy world'.

[95]   Marx, Karl, *Early Writings*, trans. And ed. T. B. Bottomore, McGraw-Hill, New York, 1946, pp. 198–199, as quoted in: Donald Phillip Verene, Hegel's Recollection: a Study of Images in the Phenomenology of Spirit (Albany: SUNY Press, 1985), p. 66.

stoicism and skepticism and the figure of Marcus Aurelius, but also Pyrrho-
nism and Sextus Empiricus. The "unhappy consciousness" is instead associated with the religious life of the European Middle Ages. At the same time, we
have to understand that the term *unglücklich* doesn't present a straight forward
parallel with the English term "lucky", since *glücklich, Glücklichkeit* relate to
the Latin term "Fortuna", which is not only Luck, but also a predisposition, a
destiny/destination, etc.[96] Verene writes:

> "In the unhappy consciousness the absolute is turned into a beyond (*Jenseits*). In so doing it
> is misfortune; it experiences an *Unglück*. It is not merely unhappy, for it cannot simply
> change its attitude toward this other and overcome its lack of mastery. Consciousness as
> self-consciousness has mastered the Stoical and Skeptical attitudes of thought. It has thought
> its way through them, but now it becomes unable to think."[97]

What is the role, the mission of Philosophy, from this perspective? Philosophy
exercises its own power in order to focus, to be more specific about the real
data, by giving up its sense of the absolute and freeing itself from this (its)
misfortune. Thus, reason is (becomes, in this interpretation) a deduction from
the stage of self-consciousness. More specifically, "at the end of Self-
consciousness, the self in its unhappy state draws itself forth until it remembers
the fact of its own presence. This is simply an ingenious act on the part of self-
consciousness – it remembers the experience of world reversal at the end of
Consciousness."[98] For the section on Phrenology, Verene decides to analyze
the issue in two ways; first by exploring the section in a general way, in terms
of its implications for psychology and philosophy of mind, and then to bring
out the "general ironic pint" that is hidden in the significance of Hegel's *Phenomenology*. Consciousness focuses on the observation of mind in the stage of
'Observational Reason' which is the first part of a process leading to observational psychology, a stage, element and section before physiognomy (with Lavater) and phrenology (with Gall). This is an action of recording "faculties,
inclinations, and passions."[99] The attempt to connect all these elements together (in the mind), creates a great difficulty, because of the ambiguous meaning
of the world of the individual. Trying to understand the difference between the

---

[96] It would be interesting (and very important, from a cognitive and natural-scientific
perspective) to analyze the etymological components of the term 'glucose' in relation to this
debate.

[97] Donald Phillip Verene, Hegel's Recollection: a Study of Images in the Phenomenology of
Spirit (Albany: SUNY Press, 1985), p.75.

[98] Ibid., p.79.

[99] Ibid., p. 81.

individual and the environment is a hard task, because of the inability to establish this connection "between inner (as the self-consciousness of the individual) and outer (as it *milieu*)."[100] The problem is whether the inner can be reflected in the other, as in the studies by Lavater, and, by comparison an analogy also in behavioral psychology, for instance in the work by Skinner analyzed and quoted in this section by Verene: "What is needed is a technology of behavior.... One difficulty is that almost all of what is called behavioral science continues to trace behavior to states of mind, feelings, traits of character, human nature, and so on."[101] According to Verene, much of this scientific analysis was already contained in Hegel's work and criticism: "We should not be surprised to discover that Skinner has collapsed the inner and the outer."[102] Verene points out that we should all be careful in judging some of these (at least that is how they are referred to in modern times) "pseudosciences," especially considering the great (scientific) admiration Lavater and Gall had in their time. In particular, Hegel says that the science of physiognomy "overlooks the power of the mask."[103] The problem here lies (both ways) in the scientific bias and self-expectation of its ability for analysis. Even Skinner, according to Verene, "believes nothing can hide from the searchlight of scientific experimentation, consciously or unconsciously."[104] He continues:

> "What can Skinner tell us of the psychopath who always wears the mask of sanity? With the question of the face as mask this science encounters in its first attempt at understanding the object, at the end of the section on Consciousness (A.). There consciousness faced the problem in terms of the inner and outer of the object. Here it faces it in terms of the inner and outer of the subject."[105]

Hegel clearly states that a 'science of knowing human beings' is not possible, because the reading of the behavioral signs or deeds of the individual, as well as the physical features of his face are only opinions; there are no laws of char-

---

[100]   Ibid., p. 82.

[101]   B. F. Skinner, *Beyond Freedom and Dignity*, Bantam/Vintage Books, New York, p. 22; cit. in: Verene, D. Ph., 1985. *Hegel's Recollection: a Study of Images in the Phenomenology of Spirit*. Albany, NY: SUNY Press, p. 83.

[102]   Verene, D. Ph., 1985. *Hegel's Recollection: a Study of Images in the Phenomenology of Spirit*. Albany, NY: SUNY Press, p. 83.

[103]   Miller, 318, as cit. in: Verene, D. Ph, 1985. *Hegel's Recollection: a Study of Images in the Phenomenology of Spirit*. Albany, NY: SUNY Press, p. 83.

[104]   Verene, D. Ph., 1985. *Hegel's Recollection: a Study of Images in the Phenomenology of Spirit*. Albany, NY: SUNY Press, p. 84.

[105]   Ibid.

acter.[106] Verene writes that: "Some human beings have a talent for reading meanings in the face, but there are no laws of it. It is a kind of genius, any more than there are laws for the interpretation of aesthetic form."[107] This is the very core of the terms *meaning of mine, meinen, das Meinen, die Meinung*. Furthermore, Verene explains how the transition from physiognomy to phrenology is made by the attempt to locate the *Geist* (again, mind and/or spirit) in an organ. Even though there is a step forward in identifying the abstract sense of self and linking it to the activity of the brain, the mistake of phrenology is the equation mind=brain. Verene goes beyond this consideration, also quoting the dialogue between Hylas and Philonious and demonstrates how the brain, being a sensible thing is a perception of the mind, since sensible things are all immediately perceivable, which is the same as saying they are ideas, which the mind forms of itself: "In principle the brain cannot be equated with the mind, because the mind makes the equation."[108] He continues:

> "If physiognomy is really just behaviorism, then phrenology is what in the tradition of Anglo-American analytic philosophy is called "philosophical psychology" [...] The instinct that philosophical psychology has followed is to get rid of the notion of mind as "inner". It is this search out and destroy mission that it carries out against mind as inner that "philosophical psychology" shares with phrenology."[109]

Psychology does not have a theory of recollection, thus it differs, as a science, from the science of the experience of consciousness. Psychology observes the object, but it cannot comprehend it in terms of a recollection of its own internal being. In this sense, psychology is a "pure" science, not phenomenology: "In the act of recollecting, consciousness is both inside the memory being recalled and outside it as the power of its recall."[110] Verene talked about psychology and behavior, but what about the focus on existence and social life? According to the author, the beautiful soul is the low point of spirit's attempt to have man exist as a social animal: "In the beautiful soul [...] the social animal withdraws into itself."[111] At the same time,

---

[106]   It is certainly interesting, in this context, taking into account Ludwig Eduard Boltzmann's analysis of the "unclear", and "obscure" complexity of Hegel's works.

[107]   Ibid. We could further analyze the relation between the term 'genius' and both the genetic component of the individual, as well as the (neuro)plasticity involved in the environmental effect on (his) being and behavior.

[108]   Ibid., p. 86.

[109]   Ibid. – Verene focuses especially on *The Concept of Mind* by Ryle.

[110]   Ibid., p. 91.

[111]   Ibid., p. 99.

"The beautiful soul can live in the world of the spiritual animal kingdom and the kingdom can easily go on with its activity with the beautiful soul around. Both are sufficiently defective forms of selfhood to be ineffective against each other. In fact, the beautiful soul is in principle understandable to the self of the matter in hand. The beautiful soul is simply activity, but it is purely spiritual activity."[112]

The absolute knowledge, presented in the last chapter of the Phenomenology, is defined through a specific idea, according to which "The content of this picture-thinking [*das Vorstellen*] is absolute Spirit; and all that now remains to be done is to supersede [*das Aufheben*] this mere form of."[113] According to Hegel, through religion, the absolute knowledge presents itself, though not in a conceptual form, proper of the Begriff, but in a pictorial form, as described in and by the Vorstellung.[114] In order to understand what absolute knowledge really is, we should focus on the dual meaning of the term *Aufhebung*, indicating cancellation/annihilation as well as preservation. The latter is the correct interpretation we should use, according to Verene, in describing the shift from religious consciousness and absolute knowing:

"Absolute knowing preserves the content of religion, that to which its scriptural speech refers, and adds to it the proper conceptual form. It replaces the scriptural image with the concretely developed logical category. Now we have the notion of absolute knowing as something in itself—the idea of the thought of thought."[115]

What is even more important, is that absolute knowledge is not the combination of *An sich sein* and *Für sich sein*, but is actually the absolute distance that cannot be reduced between the two terms. Thus, the appropriate philosophical methodology should follow a formal dialectical process, but should engage in

---

[112]   Ibid., p. 103.

[113]   Miller, 788—p. 104, cit. in Ibid., p. 104.

[114]   It is interesting to consider the poetic-imaginative-creative German (almost idiomatic) expression *stell' dir vor*. This pictorial form is essential to comprehend many perspectives and theoretical basis of a quantity, probably the vast majority, of alternative therapies. In part, this is also one of the reasons for the misunderstanding and, in some instances complete rejection, of alternative therapies by modern Western medicine: "[...] it is necessary that all the participants [to the discussion on medical diagnostics, and more generally on the very nature and scope of medicine, N/A] belong to the same medical tradition, as well as to the philosophies according to which reason and evidence trump dogma and intuition. Therefore, the attempts to reconcile scientific medicine with traditional medicine, like those recently sponsored by the World Health Organization, are as pointless as the efforts to reconcile religion with science." (Bunge, M. 2013. *Medical Philosophy. Conceptual Issues in Medicine.* Singapore: World Scientific Publishing, p. 85).

[115]   Verene, D. Ph , 1985. *Hegel's Recollection: a Study of Images in the Phenomenology of Spirit.* Albany, NY: SUNY Press, p. 105.

an "introspective rememorization, recollection" or internal absolute, which brings "to the surface" this memory; a method called *Erinnerung*. Therefore, we understand how, according to Hegel as interpreted by Verene, Revealed Religion is an illusion, for its truth is always something to be represented, not conceptualized, not conceptually understood. In summary, the content of religion is correct, but the form is wrong. This represents a fundamental point in our analysis. In fact the problematic relation between illusion, representation, perception, conceptualization and revelation of metaphysical, spiritual, and religious, especially messianic and/or prophetic type such as premonitions, apocalyptic visions, clairvoyance etc., is at the center of the debate on the ontology and phenomenology of psychiatric events. This is especially true in the translated sense of medical episodes which need to be treated medically versus (spiritual, ghost-like, evil) possessions, which were traditionally addressed by spiritual guides, shamans, gurus, and the most exemplary Christian practice of exorcism.

> "When it has not been trying to disclaim spirituality altogether, psychology has attempted to study religious experience or the experience of spirituality in the same way it has studied mental illness. In general, there has been an underlying denial in the people interested in the areas of spirituality and religion that their very existence is antithetical to psychology as a science. Many people in the fields of religion and psychology, and others with a similar focus, have failed to see how they have needed denial in order to continue trying to do what they do, and this has resulted in a kind of schizophrenia in these fields."[116]

The importance of concepts such as "manifestation" and "epiphany" is particularly relevant in analyzing the cognitive-rational perspective (in term of human thought processes) as preferred method of investigation of such issues. Verene states that "We cannot form the Christ as thought."[117]. Furthermore, the spirit is substance and not subject on the level of religion and consciousness experience is the attempt (or the attempt happens through its experiencing) to unify these two elements, which are also two moments, the Father and the Son. This happens in the identity of a third element, the (Holy / Whole) Spirit, the Ghost (*Geist*). This spirit appears in time as substance, and unsuccessfully tries to unite the elements, which is the same as saying it tries to annihilate (reduce)

---

[116]   Schaef, A.W. 1992. *Beyond Therapy, Beyond Science*. New York, NY: HarperCollins, p. 224.

[117]   Ibid., p. 108—We should also consider the theological implication of the word Χριστός as a translation of "anointed, chosen" in comparison with the Hebrew מָשִׁיחַ instead, for instance to the real—in terms of historical, but also material, biological, human, figure of *Jesus/Issa/Yoshua*.

time. That is exactly why this *Erinnerung* is a denial of time, because "it only annuls time when it accepts the conjunction [and] no longer lives from stage to stage but recollects."[118] Verene also analyzes Kojève perspectives, in particular in opening up new considerations on the ontology and methodology of cognition, which, according to Verene, tries to unify the 'in itself', the known, with the 'in itself for it' or the knower. Thus, cognition always has an object, which is this very process or attempt of unification. Therefore, cognition is "less than absolute knowledge." To move beyond this stage, Hegel identifies the 'beautiful soul' which is both the very intuition of the Divine, as well as the Divine's intuition of itself, the self's own act in contraposition to what was 'content' in religion. This is the reason beyond the divine nature of language (learned at the level of *das Meinen*, since the real cannot be said), of poetry of the very poetic art of intuition, which ultimately leads to philosophy, to a communion with itself.

2.2 Truth in Method

a) Understanding the Language

Alessandro Pagnini's use of Kantian and Aristotelian models to better define structure and limits of medicine as a science is, in this context, very interesting.[119] The same applies to his critical view of claims of "overscientificity" within medicine, and his focus on the importance of the hard/pure scientific method in clinical settings, but also making sure not to blindly follow a reductionist approach in science in general. However, his rejection of pluralistic approaches in medicine, especially narrative medicine and hermeneutics, seems less convincing.[120] In fact, Narrative Medicine is a very appropriate and

---

[118]   Ibid.

[119]   In particular, the author's focus on causal, mechanic explanation versus a teleological and finalistic explanation of reality and mechanisms. See Pagnini A., (Ed.) 2010. *Filosofia della medicina*. Roma: Caroce editore.

[120]   However, we certainly need to distinguish different forms of narrative and different forms of (alternative) practices, since not every therapy that is included in this perspective is equally effective or scientifically proven. In this regard, Illich writes: "Medical procedures turn into sick religion when they are performed as rituals that focus the entire expectation of the sick on science and its functionaries instead of encouraging them to seek a poetic interpretation of their predicament or find an admirable example in some person—long dead or next door—who learned to suffer. Medical procedures multiply disease by moral degradation when they isolate the sick in a professional environment rather than providing society with the motives and disciplines that increase social tolerance for the troubled. Magical havoc, religious injury, and moral degradation generated under the pretext of a biomedical pursuit are

effective approach, especially when dealing with a mental health-related symptomatology which presents a multilayered complexity, both in terms of therapeutic intervention as well as interpretative-diagnostic method.[121] Furthermore,
is also true (scientifically proven) that the very act of learning has positive
impacts on therapy:

> "Not only does memory consolidation lead to [persistent] modifications in synaptic plasticity, but psychotherapy, a form of learning, also produces changes in the permanent storage of information acquired throughout an individual's life and provides new resources to address important psychobiological relationships between affect, attachment, and memory."[122]

In some areas, both geographical as well as cultural an philosophical (in terms
of theoretical basis) of psychology (let us think for instance about Mexico and
Central and South America in general), the ability of the patient to identify
with a customized, and yet archetypal form of personal story/history is fundamental. In terms of expressing oneself as a tool for a better understanding of
psychological analysis, Dougherty thinks that "the best way to induce emotion
is through autobiographical scripts."[123] But again, what is medicine, is it more
of an art or a science, and is it just one form or medicine? Pagnini writes that:

---

all crucial mechanisms contributing to social iatrogenesis." Illich, I. 1976. *Limits to Medicine; Medical Nemesis: The Expropriation of Health*. London, UK: Marion Boyars Publishers, pp. 114–115.

[121] For instance, we can draw elements from the debate on medical reasoning, in particular the focus on forward reasoning: "an epiphenomenon derived from the use of verbal case descriptions and written summaries, where the ambiguity of the original case presentation has been eliminated and the increased certainty of experts is reflected in summaries of reasoning that tend to be organized coherently and linearly from data to solution." In: Norman, G.R., Brooks, L.R., Colle, C.L. and Hatala, R.M. 2010. *The Benefit of Diagnostic Hypotheses in Clinical Reasoning: Experimental Study of an Instructional Intervention for Forward and Backward Reasoning*. In: Cognition and Instruction, 17(4), 433–488, Hamilton, Ontario, CA: Lawrence Erlbaum Associates p. 446.

[122] Tasman, A., Kay, J., Lieberman, J.A. 2003. *Psychiatry. Second Edition. Therapeutics*. Chichester, West Sussex,, UK: John Wiley & Sons, p. 17.

[123] In 1999 the Harvard Medical School associate professor of Psychiatry at Massachusetts General Hospital Dr. Darin Dougherty worked with healthy people with no signs of depression and no history of angry episodes to examine which cerebral regions engage during angry activity. He did his research with the use of positron emission tomography: "The subjects simulated angry moments by recalling the moments in their lives when they felt rage. During angry recollections, the amygdala fired. At the same time, a part of the orbital frontal cortex [...] also engaged, putting the brakes on emotion." Dougherty realized that people with normal, healthy brain function experience anger, but they can suppress it before acting on it. For further reference, see Dougherty, E. 2011. *Anger management. When Emotional Brakes Fail, Depression and anger often go hand in hand*. Scientists probe the nature of wrath in the hope of devising cures. In: Byron, P.B. (Ed.) 2011. The Science of Emotion, Boston, MA: Harvard Medicine, pp. 14–19.

"Medicine is an applied science or a sum of applied sciences that focuses on the health of a single patient [sick person N/A] or of a human population, and that, in order to better achieve this goal, tries, in the systemic observation, in the experimental method and in basic [core N/A] knowledge which are its lifeblood, to increase its own level of scientificity."[124]

The combination of all these elements should therefore help medicine come closer to scientific truth, without falling prey of (pre)assumptions, bias, and general errors. Among the possible medical fallacies we can quote the *post ergo propter hoc*, which we already encountered and will meet over and over again throughout this study, due to the logical component of causal assumptions which need to be constantly verified.[125] This is especially true in areas such as neuroscience/neurology, mind-brain/body problem, and in general dualism versus monism related debates. Certainly, the need to rule out any possible biologically, sociologically, psychologically based comorbidity and correlation without causation is a fundamental step to avoid this type of mistakes. Unfortunately, due to the complexity of human minds, the task can be a very hard one. Furthermore, time is a quite problematic aspect of such a fallacy, considering that, for instance, many diagnoses (as we will see) are doomed to be inaccurate, either in terms of overestimating or (less often, at least from a statistical standpoint) underestimating patients' life expectancy. A good example of correlation might be represented by a chronic problem, which resulted (again, only in chronological, not causational terms) in the death of the subject. Certainly, we will have to rule out every possible *cumcausa* of the issue. Another problem might be the overstated value of a specific definition, especially in diagnostic terms, which can sound "obscure" to anybody who does not have a basic medical, or even linguistic knowledge, in the case of language barrier, or lack of practice with Latin and Greek roots (although this is true for modern evidenced-based medicine in the West, other languages such as Arabic, Urdu and Hindi, Chinese, and Russian have quite an influence on medical terminology as a whole, beside their national value related to the countries in which they are spoken). From the patient's perspective, the difficulties in understanding and/or interpreting information gathered from the physician during a con-

---

[124]   Orig: "La medicina è "una scienza applicata o una somma di scienze applicate" che si occupa della salute del singolo malato o di una popolazione umana, e che, al fine di conseguire al meglio lo scopo, cerca, nell'osservazione sistematica, nel metodo sperimentale e nelle conoscenze di base che ne sono la linfa vitale, di accrescere il proprio livello di scientificità," Pagnini A., (Ed.) 2010. *Filosofia della medicina*. Roma: Caroce editore, pp 15–16.

[125]   Certainly, logical considerations on the standard modi *modus ponens* and *modus tollens*, as well as the principles of including/excluding disjunction have to ba taken into account.

versation have also side-effects in terms of detachment and depersonalization of the healing process: "[...] negligence becomes "random human error" or "system breakdown", callousness becomes "scientific detachment", and incompetence becomes 'a lack of specialized equipment'. The depersonalization of diagnosis and therapy has changed malpractice from an ethical into a technical problem."[126]

Furthermore, the field of psychiatry is especially problematic due to the external/symptomatic-based diagnostic method applied. This is connected to another fallacy, represented by the assumption of correct diagnostic opinion, when shared by many (or the majority) of providers. The best example is perhaps the Rosenhan experiment. Also, there might be a problem related to very memory/recollection of symptomatology from both the patient's and the provider's side. Plus, psychological phenomena such as source misattribution and confabulation play an important role as well, making medical records absolutely necessary, within the limits of personal privacy and limiting possible breach of confidentiality. However, because of the very nature of psychological traumas, disorders, and illnesses, determining possible related disability can be very problematic as well, and requires monitored and constant (re)evaluation, which should be completed by involving the patient whenever possible, as in the Open Dialogue Model. Other fallacies are connected to the treatment itself, for instance in the case of positive or negative outcomes, which are sometimes totally unrelated to the provider's care. The same applies to new and/or alternative therapies, experimental testing, and clinical trials, where standard treatment would possibly (but again, this is where a lot of assumptions and biased views happen) have made a difference. Missed diagnosis fits in the same categories of debate, since it could possibly improve or worsen the therapeutic outcome. Certainly, the patient plays a very important part in maintaining her/his own health, starting from prevention. From a pharmacological intervention standpoint, for each medication, the patient should ask:

a) What is the medicine for? (Although we need to understand the problematic relation with one diagnosis-one problem-one medicine type of assumption, especially in psychiatry)
b) How am I supposed to take it, and for how long?
c) What side effects are involved? What should I do if they occur?

---

[126]   Illich, I. 1976. *Limits to Medicine; Medical Nemesis: The Expropriation of Health*. London, UK: Marion Boyars Publishers, p. 30.

d) Is this medicine safe to take with other medicines and/or dietary supplements I am taking?

e) What food, drink, or activities should I pay particular attention or completely avoid while taking this medicine?

f) Are the medication's label and the provider's prescription, and all the information contained in it, clearly legible and easy to understand?

g) Who is in charge when I am not in (physical, mental, legal, etc.) condition to make decisions?

h) Whom do I contact if I have further question regarding any of the above listed categories?

b) Clinical Reasoning

Philosophy as a basic approach to medicine means concentrating our attention to those procedural cognitive aspects which modulate our understanding of the patient, his/her problem and a possible therapeutic solution in clinical settings and beyond. Generally speaking, there are certain methods and rationales which are used in prognosis and diagnosis. The investigation on the patient's condition follows a specific linear model, starting from the analysis and evaluation of the patient's medical history (which, itself is the result of a prior analysis and evaluation), as well as its interpretation; to the current, illness, disease, disorder; further clinical and empirical observations, laboratory test results, and finally to the generation of hypotheses to identify possible origins and causes of the present patient's condition, in diagnostic terms. Furthermore, modern medical science uses statistical methods as base for this type of investigations, and in general for the analysis of the whole spectrum of medical research, even beyond the therapeutic aspect. For instance, statistical models have been used in biomedical studies as well as in order to address patient-provider communication; patient's and (more often) physician's problem-solving strategies and decision-making abilities (as well as related models); and finally to monitor and quantify specific epidemiological measures such as incidence, rate, prevalence, risk, etc. with respect to the causation. Among the most famous theoretical analysis used to evaluate the evidence of causation (or lack thereof), the model by Austin Bradford Hill, comprising a series of considerations also known as the Bradford Hill criteria[127] is still considered a very useful group of minimal conditions necessary to provide this evidence:

---

[127]   Hill, A. B. (1965). *The Environment and Disease: Association or Causation?*. Proceedings of the Royal Society of Medicine 58 (5): 295–300. See also Phillips, C.V.; and Goodman

1) *Strength*: The concept identifies the size. More specifically, a small association does not mean that a causal effect is not there. However, the larger the association, the more likely that it is causal.
2) *Consistency*: Consistent findings observed by different persons in different places with different samples strengthens the likelihood of an effect.
3) *Specificity*: Causation is likely if a very specific population at a specific site and disease with no other likely explanation. The more specific an association between a factor and an effect is, the bigger the probability of a causal relationship.
4) *Temporality*: Chronological concept according to which a certain effect has to occur after the (its related) cause. Furthermore, if there is an expected delay between the cause and expected effect, then the effect must occur after that delay.
5) *Biological gradient*: Greater exposure should generally lead to greater incidence of the effect, though, in some cases, the mere presence of the factor can trigger the effect. In other cases, an inverse proportion is observed: greater exposure leads to lower incidence.
6) *Plausibility*: A plausible mechanism between cause and effect is helpful.
7) *Coherence*: Coherence between epidemiological and laboratory findings increases the likelihood of an effect.
8) *Experiment*: "Occasionally it is possible to appeal to experimental evidence"[128].
9) *Analogy*: The effect of similar factors may be considered.

Hill observed that, in regard to the discovery of mechanisms, our current medical ability depends on its *historicity*,[129] namely to the amount of knowledge, technical and theoretical, achieved up to a point in time. He notably added that, as a result, "None of my nine viewpoints can bring indisputable evidence for or against the cause-and-effect hypothesis and none can be required sine qua

---

K.J. 2004. *The missed lessons of Sir Austin Bradford Hill*. Epidemiologic Perspectives and Innovations 1 (3): 3. doi: 10.1186/1742-5573-1-3.

[128] Hill, A. B. (1965). *The Environment and Disease: Association or Causation?*. Proceedings of the Royal Society of Medicine 58 (5): 295–300.

[129] In regard to the historical component, not just in terms of history of medical science but even more in depth, at the level of patient's personal/medical history, Fleming noted that "Because the occupational therapist does not make a definitive diagnosis as a part of his or her task, history is not as critical a piece of the puzzle as it is for the physician". Fleming, M.H. 1991. *Clinical Reasoning in Medicine Compared With Clinical Reasoning in Occupational Therapy*. American Journal of Occupational Therapy, November 1991, Vol. 45, 988–996, p. 993.

non."[130] Furthermore, he also made sure to *evidence* that "[...] lack of such [laboratory] evidence cannot nullify the epidemiological effect on associations."[131] Thus, statistical and epidemiological analysis can and it is commonly used by healthcare providers in order to better understand their own clinical reasoning process and improve decision-making abilities in regard to prognosis, diagnosis and therapeutic intervention, and improvement of the latter, which is the ultimate goal of clinical reasoning in medicine. At the same time, in a very interesting article by Maureen Hayes Fleming,[132] researchers have found that, although both physicians and occupational therapists use recognition, hypothesis testing and heuristic search[133] in clinical reasoning, they use those strategies in a different way, especially when it comes to a linear process versus an alternating, continuous examination of the patient's condition.[134] In fact, this is at the base of both propositional reasoning (in the case of Occupational Therapists) and open dialogue (in the case of Psychotherapists). There is therefore a constant movement from prognosis to diagnosis, or better defined, evaluation filtered through the patient's own feedback, in their reasoning frequency. This perspective is also a core concept in the ideas exposed in Medical Philosophy, as established by the analysis of the importance of patient perception and self perception in diagnostics and therapy. Furthermore, the physician tends to follow the standard medical procedure, thus focusing on the statistical analysis, e.g. the generalizability of the diagnosis and related therapy, regardless of the subjective individuality of the patient. The occupational therapist tends to take into account the useful elements (again, in terms of diagnosis and possible therapeutic intervention) of the specific history, condition, presentation, perception and other factors affecting the patient's life. From this point of view we could argue that, based on the research, occupational therapists tend to have a more omnicomprehensive, holistic approach to medicine, similarly to what happens in the realm of complementary and alternative therapies, as we will see in Chapter 5. The same applies to the connection between heuristic and intuitive approaches, used by every healthcare practitioner, but in slightly

---

[130]   Ibid.
[131]   Ibid.
[132]   Fleming, M.H. 1991. *Clinical Reasoning in Medicine Compared With Clinical Reasoning in Occupational Therapy*. American Journal of Occupational Therapy, November 1991, Vol. 45, 988–996.
[133]   As outlined in Newell, A., & Simon, H. 1972. *Human problem solving*. Englewood Cliffs, NJ: Prentice Hall.
[134]   Especially in regard to *pattern recognition*.

different ways.[135] For instance, in the article by Fleming the cited studies have shown that the use of statistics to support therapeutic interventions varies on the base of the aforementioned medical perspectives. Therapists certainly value, understand and employ the "hard data" collected by scientific/medical research, but they use them as a general background in which the individual element (the patient) plays the biggest role, instead of being the variation, the exception to the rule.[136] In fact, these considerations underlie the connection between the variety of research traditions in clinical reasoning to the philosophical background of psychological consideration in medicine,[137] in particular humanistic and positive psychology, as we will see in the next paragraph.

c) Medicine and Psychology: philosophical background and scientific method

Generally speaking, among these traditions we find core viewpoints associated with psychological perspective such as the learning perspective of behaviorism[138] (as well as the various branches of modern behavioral medicine); the

---

[135]   More in detail, "simply shifting from one line of inquiry to the other, [engaging] in conversation as an equal, not as a professional to a patient." Fleming, M.H. 1991. *Clinical Reasoning in Medicine Compared With Clinical Reasoning in Occupational Therapy*. American Journal of Occupational Therapy, November 1991, Vol. 45, 988–996, p. 991.

[136]   "Individualization refers to the tailoring of treatment to the particular skills, needs, and interests of each patient. This interest in the individual would naturally lead therapists away from the medical decision making approach, in which the norm and statistical probabilities are central and individual variations are peripheral." Fleming, M.H. 1991. *Clinical Reasoning in Medicine Compared With Clinical Reasoning in Occupational Therapy*. American Journal of Occupational Therapy, November 1991, Vol. 45, 988–996, p. 994.

[137]   In particular, the evolution from inaccurate research methods as part of phrenology and physiognomy, to the more scientific (in the modern sense) approaches of functionalism (William James in primis), to the psychoanalysis of Freud, and the philosophically related (and often opposed) research by Otto Rank, Carl Gustav Jung, and Wilhelm Reich.

[138]   From its origin with Edward Thorndike, John Broadus Watson, Burrhus Frederic (B.F.) Skinner, and Ivan Petrovich Pavlov (more specifically his research on classical/respondent and operative conditioning) in Psychological Behaviorism, to the development of psychosomatic medicine and health psychology into the behavioral medicine perspective of Anne H. Berman, Lee Birk, John Paul Brady, Kevin S. Masters, Giuseppe Dominic Matarazzo, Ovide F. Pomerleau, William Schofield, Sakari Suominen, and William Steward Agras. "Some research into clinical reasoning has been conducted within the behaviourist paradigm. Rimoldi (1988) tested diagnostic skills of medical practitioners and students in the 1950s and 60s, showing that as expertise increased so the numbers of questions asked and the time taken to solve diagnostic problems decreased. Taylor (1985) argued that this approach was an oversimplification of the kind that occurs when the humanities are studied along the same lines as the natural sciences. The truly interesting questions are avoided, or the research ends up stating the obvious and being irrelevant. Rimoldi's method was an early attempt at simulating clinical problems. However, it can be argued that simulation ap-

biological perspective, in particular the one related to (evolutionary) biopsychology; the cognitive perspective of cognitivism, situated cognition and cognitive science, the socio-cultural perspective, the analysis on elaboration and contrastive (expert/novice[139]) method, and the hypothesis-based (deductive versus inductive) reasoning method.[140] With regard to humanistic and positive psychology, we note that the first tends to orient itself to the psychological tradition of existentialism and phenomenology, as well as to more broad references to theological debate, and even hermeneutics. Thus, the sources for a humanistic approach can be found for example in Camus, Husserl, Merleau-Ponty, Sartre, while positive psychologists often refer to the Classical tradition (especially Aristotle) and the Hellenic, eudaemonist background, as well as in Kierkegaard, Nietzsche, and Tillich; all the way from the medieval tradition of Christian philosophers, to Stuart Mill (especially in regard to the inductive approach and the five methods), Russell, Popper, and Fromm.[141] Certainly the core values shared by positive and humanistic psychology (by some considered either linked by conceptual evolution, or separated by methodological background) are the founding concepts generally discussed in medical ethics. The debate around decision making capacity, ability, capability, personal responsibility, personal freedom and free will, autonomy and agency, determinism and voluntariness are still at the center of modern medical investigation, and should be always taken into consideration by Medical Philosophy. This is

---

proaches are probably better suited for assessment rather than research." In: Loftus, S.F. 2006. *Language in clinical reasoning: using and learning the language of collective clinical decision making*. Sydney, AUS: Faculty of Health Sciences, School of Physiotherapy, University of Sydney, p. 27.

[139] As we previously discussed with regard to the methodological, philosophical, ad clinical differences between physicians and occupational therapists, as well as within medical reasoning in general, in particular the debate on the forward and backward reasoning strategies, which is ultimately based on the literature on the same type of differences in fields such as applied sciences, physics, and even the analysis of possible solutions to chess problems, especially in the case of Elstein.

[140] Although we must distinguish between the Baconian Method, which is definitely empirical and inductive and the Cartesian Method, which operates *following* deduction. For Francis Bacon states in the *Novum Organum* that "Our only hope, then is in genuine Induction. [...] There is the same degree of licentiousness and error in forming Axioms, as in abstracting Notions: and that in the first principles, which depend in common induction. Still more is this the case in Axioms and inferior propositions derived from Syllogisms." (See: *Novum Organum* (English), Fowler, T. (ed., notes, comments) 1878. Oxford, UK: McMillan and Co., Clarendon Press, Oxford, public domain.

[141] See Waterman, A.S. 2013. *The Humanistic Psychology-Positive Psychology Divide. Contrasts in Philosophical Foundations*. In *American Psychologist*. Vol. 68, Num. 3: 123–196 Washington, DC: APA, pp. 124–133.

one of the main reasons why this study focuses on psychological (and psychiatric) method(s) and theoretical basis, not in the sense of a justificationist approach or in terms of higher value in comparison to other branches of medicine, but because the difficulties, in terms of prognosis, diagnosis, and general theoretical and therapeutic understanding encountered in psychology and psychiatry serve as a monitor for every other consideration pertaining human nature and the related attempts to provide health. A good example of the useful interaction is the biopsychosocial approach, as explored in the various subfields of Health Psychology and Behavioral Medicine. Beside the principle of contiguity (namely, that medical/clinical feedback find better response when administrated immediately) and contingency, behaviorism brought to medicine and medical education the very focus on human behavior in terms of measurable outcomes and predictability, including continuous progressive testing. The strengths of cognitivism are linked to disciplines as varied as classical cognitive psychology and neuropsychology, neuroscience and cognitive science,[142] all the way to neurophilosophy (in this sense a bridge to evolutionary biopsychology), by adding the investigation on patterns, structures and processes such as information and memory processing,[143] as well as metacognition, a cognitive form of self-perception, which represents the departure from behaviorism.[144] Furthermore, the psychological debate around cognitive structures is theoretical and truly philosophical in nature, considering the debate around structures, categories, prototypes, cognitive/representational concepts, semantic networks, scripts and schemata.[145] As we previously discussed, the hypoth-

---

[142]   As well as the development of Situated cognition, for instance with Engeström's analysis of the linearisation strategy in medicine. See Engeström, Y., and Middleton, D. (Eds.) 1996. *Cognition and communication at work*. New York, NY: Cambridge University Press; and Robinson, P. and Ellis N.C. (Eds.) 2008. *Handbook of Cognitive Linguistics and Second Language Acquisition*. London, UK: Routledge.

[143]   Including Short-, Mid-, and Long-Term Memory and the neurologically related Long Term Potentiation process (LTP) based on neuronal synchronicity, medical issues such as demyelination, as well as the investigation of phenomena such as confabulation and source misattribution.

[144]   In the sense that "In behaviourism the assumption is that behaviour is what is learned, whereas in cognitivism the assumption is that behaviour is the outcome of what is learned (Stevenson, 1983, as discussed in Loftus, S.F. 2006. *Language in clinical reasoning: using and learning the language of collective clinical decision making*. Sydney, AUS: Faculty of Health Sciences, School of Physiotherapy, University of Sydney, p. 29).

[145]   Certainly, this perspective opens up a further discussion on the relationship between natural (human) and artificial (computer/digital) intelligence, which is beyond the scope of this study. Certainly, we must acknowledge that in the cognitivistic perspective at least, cognition *means* computation. According to Loftus, "Prototypes can be thought of as the "best

esis-based model draws implications from the deductive/inductive approach, in particular from the debate on reasoning processes and principle of falsifiability in Popper, Bradley, Mill, Hume, Whewell, Elstein, and Medawar, while the comparative and contrastive method originates in the work by Robert Lado in connection to behaviorist and structuralist debate, as well as in the cultural-historical psychology[146] of Lev Semyonovich Vygotsky, whose legacy represents a very important philosophical background for our comparison of reasoning processes in medicine and psychology, especially in relation (and contrast) to a phenomenological approach:

---

example" of something (Gruppen & Frohna, 2002). The concept allows for variation around a family resemblance. Bordage and Zacks (1984) claimed that prototypes are consistent with the knowledge organisation of doctors and students. A problem with the prototype in that milieu is that it does not reflect the fact that context has been shown to influence knowledge retrieval (Brooks, Norman, & Allen, 1991). [...]According to the theory of instances, knowledge organisation occurs around individual instances rather than as an abstract based on several cases. However, instance theories leave open questions of how specific instances can be grouped together, and of how instances are extracted from experience. The assumption is that the selection and grouping of instances is a key stage, but it is not clear how this comes about. Schema theory is an attempt to deal with this weakness [and has] featured prominently as knowledge structures in much clinical reasoning literature. They are conceived as higher order structures providing broad abstract frameworks onto which exemplars can be mapped. [...] Scripts are presented as a specialised version of schemas, in an attempt to resolve the perceived generality of schemas. [...] Semantic networks have been proposed as a more dynamic and sophisticated way of representing knowledge. The construct arose from research into artificial intelligence and is essentially a graphic way of representing entities and the relationships between them using nodes and links between the nodes. [...] The cognitive structures mentioned above are believed to be similar to data structures in a computer program". Ibid., pp. 30–31. In regard to the implication of metacognition, two authors, Custers and Boshuizen, are mentioned both my Loftus and Lloyd: "[...] Learning is viewed as an active, constructive process: central aspects of learning are mental activities of the learner, including the active selection of stimuli, organization of the material, construction of responses, and the use of learning strategies. In addition learning is viewed as largely under the control of the learner; learners use the knowledge of how they learn and other factors that influence their learning... (e.g. by planning and monitoring), a phenomenon that is called metacognition – thinking about thinking." Custer & Boshuizen, 2002, in Norman, van der Vleuten, & Newble, p. 172., and quoted by Lloyd, S.H. *An Exploratory Study of the Relationship Between In-Training Examination percentiles of anesthesiology residents and the Vermunt Inventory of Learning Styles.* Manhattan, KS: Department of Educational Leadership, College of Education, Kansas State University, p. 43.

[146] Interestingly, the influence of Thought and Language can be felt even in the very definition of his legacy, to which a broad range of definitions have been attributed, from "the school of Vygotsky", to terms such as sociocultural psychology, socio-historical psychology, cultural psychology, as well as activity theory, cultural historical activity theory, and social development theory.

"We could not describe this new significance of the whole operation otherwise than by saying that it is mastery of one's own process of behavior. It is surprising to us that traditional psychology has completely failed to notice this phenomenon which we can call mastering one's own reactions. In attempts to explain this fact of 'will' this psychology resorted to a miracle, to the intervention of a spiritual factor in the operation of nervous processes, and thus tried to explain the action by the line of most resistance, as did, for example, James in developing his theory of the creative character of the will [...] Reflection is the transfer of argumentation within."[147]

Vygotsky attentively examined the philosophical, structural and methodological crisis of psychology, using a dialectical-integrated approach, and his attempt to combine the objectivist (naturalist) elements of scientific psychology with the Marxist philosophical tradition is still beneficial to Medical Philosophy, in the sense that it helps us (beside the well-known application in medicine through the application of cultural historical activity theory to patient-provider consultation),[148] first understand and compare mechanistic and holistic approaches, and then investigate a possible combination.

We believe that a combination of different approaches is absolutely essential for therapeutic effectiveness, especially in those areas of medicine that closely investigate human nature. However, since we are talking about human medicine, it is hard to imagine a single medical area absolutely and completely not affected by a comorbidity of causes, as well as by a multitude e of effectors, with the purely biological realm, to the social and personal environment, to the very beliefs of the single patient, which is why we decided to investigate patient's view on a variety of topics, including sense of self, sense of meaning and purpose in life. To be sure, as Waterman[149] attentively discussed in regard to psychology, there are important differences between a humanistic and a positive approach. Generally speaking, humanistic psychology is often associated (by the Society of Humanistic Psychology in the first place)[150] with phenomenology, hermeneutic, constructivism, postmodernism, transpersonalism and existentialism, and follows a more qualitative approach in research, often focusing on the individual, singular, subjective and on perspectives similar to

---

[147]   Vygotsky, L.S. 1966. *Development of higher mental functions*. In Leontyev, A.N., Luria, A.R., and Smirnov, A. (Eds.) *Psychological Research in the USSR*. Moscow: Progress Publishers. pp. 33–41

[148]   Staring with Vygotsky, but also in relation the work on general Activity Theory by Alexej Leont'ev and Sergej Rubinstein.

[149]   Waterman, A.S. 2013. *The Humanistic Psychology-Positive Psychology Divide. Contrasts in Philosophical Foundations*. In *American Psychologist*. Vol. 68, Num. 3: 123–196 Washington, DC: APA, pp. 124–133

[150]   Ibid., p. 126.

the ones found in Narrative Medicine. Positive psychology instead, tends to be empirical, pragmatic, and quantitative in nature, with ample size research samples and therapeutic focus on exercises and action-taking. Waterman does not seem convinced in the possibility of an ultimate reconciliation of these two approaches, due to their incompatibility on (of) philosophical grounds.[151] However, he also points out that in terms of therapeutic applicability, both schools present very important messages, with special regard to those areas of scientific enquiry which are still wide open to interpretation, especially in terms of their practical (therapeutic) applicability: "[...] Although therapy techniques are indeed teachable, as with research methodologies, there are also important elements of talent required to be effective using any given therapy."[152] This viewpoint is extremely important in our analysis, since we are indeed proposing a combination of a multitude of techniques and methods, in order to better understand human nature, with the ultimate purpose of playing a part (whether as providers, philosophers or, as it is/should be often the case, both) in improving the healing process. To be sure, we do not want to simply combine *any* random philosophical perspective as background and foundation for this or that psychological theory. In fact, there are some philosophers who advocate for a return to the origins in philosophical method and goals, similarly to what Waterman proposes in terms of shared foundation by positive and humanistic psychology: "Know thyself" seems to be one of these keys of interpretation. This approach is intended to reconnect philosophy to a specific tradition (or set of traditions) which Verene identifies as the great Greco-Roman heritage, in particular Socratic humanism, all the way to the Renaissance era and the Cartesian revolution, which (together with Locke, and therefore combining in his critic both analytic/Anglo-Saxon, as well as Continental philosophy) is guilty of eliminating the complexity, the mystery, and the transcendental elements from the equation "genius-folly",[153] and which represent

---

[151]   Ibid., pp. 129–131.

[152]   Ibid., p. 130. Waterman also provides a broad analysis of various psychological perspective, from the hermeneutical-existential point of view, through client-centered therapy [a term, *client*, which we consider even less appropriate than *patient*, both from a ethical, as well as medico-scientifico-philosophical viewpoint], Gestalt therapy, existential psychotherapy, existentialist-integrative psychotherapy, including the focus of meaning (including meaninglessness and the absurd, but also the process of meaning-making), and the author's *eudaimonic identity theory*.

[153]   An equation which is at the center of the practices of art therapy and outsider art (an expanded version would be *artist = genius = insane*), as we will see in Chapter 5. In particular, Verene refers the old paradigm modern philosophy needs to rediscover in scholars such

the very center of our discussion in terms of patient's perception within a psychiatric/psychological field of action and interpretation. This is especially important in understanding the impact of a translated interpretation and possible alternative cognitive methodology (in the very sense of method of knowing) through art, myth, poetry, rhetoric and eloquence as base of this philosophical method. These elements should serve not only as a theoretical framework for a psychological investigation of the healing process (which is also our goal), but more generally as a guide of human action, including phronesis.[154]

Human action, and decision are also core concepts in the analysis offered by Gadamer,[155] more specifically in the comparison between a (passive) equilibrium brought to us humans by nature (and kept, controlled, monitored by nature itself) versus an opposite (active) equilibrium, entirely depending on our actions. To be sure, disease is a concept linked to time, in the sense that it is a moment(-um) of human choice or decision. When human beings feel[156] that they do not meet the needs of everyday life, health problems arise, and illnesses are created.[157] Thus, health and disease are philosophical (more specifically phenomenological) concepts, and need therefore to be analyzed under the theoretical lenses of (Medical) Philosophy. In fact, health is a phenomenon, an epiphany, a manifestation of (human) existence,[158] structured on a philosophical level of social, ethical, and moral responsibility, toward nature, mankind and values. We agree with this point of view in the sense that we propose and investigate (both through philosophical analysis as well as empirical research) a deeper connection between levels of (human) existence: from an external, phenomenal and in part phenomenological ground, to an experiential (thus

---

as Erasmus van Rotterdam. See Verene, D.P. 1997. *Philosophy and the Return to Self-Knowledge.* New Haven, CT: Yale University Press.

[154] Certainly, we cannot avoid the Aristotelian perspective, but more specifically, here we find closeness to the positions of Cicero, Quintilian, Isocrates, Pico della Mirandola, and Giambattista Vico. To be sure, Verene proposes a philosophical method (and structure) as a *form of memory* based on rhetoric and poetry, both necessary to reach the ultimate goal (which is again the core concept in this study) of accomplishing self-knowledge.

[155] Gadamer, H.-G. 1993. *Über die Verborgenheit der Gesundheit.* Frankfurt a. M., D: Suhrkamp.

[156] This is one of the main reasons why, once again, a qualitative research is a necessary partner of quantitative studies to really dig deeper into the core of the problem, namely the impact of perception (and self-knowledge) in (onto) the healing process.

[157] To be sure, when the *wholeness* of man-nature-reality-existence is broken, diseases appear, and health is the opposite of disease versus continuum.

[158] Which is connected to harmony, internal-external well-being, equilibrium, appropriateness (the aforementioned relation between terms such as the Latin *bonus/bonulus/bellus* and the Greek καλός).

time- and environment- connected,[159] especially in the sense of *Erlebnis*)
ground, to an essential – both personal as well as social – ground. Thus, health
means understanding and (self) knowledge of identity and role in life as opposed to disease, or loss of (part of)[160] identity. Again we are investigating the
connection between these spheres of human action/interaction and the (effec-
tiveness/non-effectiveness on) healing process.

---

[159] Certainly also in a Hegelian, as well as Heideggerian sense, although there are important in-
ferred hypothesis of *absolute* value in this discussion, in particular the focus on human suffering, meaning and healing process.

[160] Especially in psychiatric-psychological terms, as addressed for instance by psychotherapeutic activities such as grieving process and analysis of losses.

Chapter 3
Between Neuroscience and Phenomenology

3.1 Hegel, Merleau-Ponty and Natural Religion: where are we now?

What is the right approach of scientific enquiry within Medical Philosophy? What elements, theories, observable data should be considered the reality, the basis, the necessary evidence in medical practice? According to Hegel, there are degrees of reality within various phenomena. Historically, the concept itself refers to what Plato used to distinguish mere temporal appearances from the eternal *Noumena* of the Ideal Realm. For Hegel, the phenomena partially hide (as appearances) and partially reveal the truth of reality (thus opening up the reality of mind/spirit) in a specific way. Distinguishing between material phenomena and mental phenomena, and focusing on the latter, is the core and scope of this phenomenology, which is indeed a study of appearances, images and illusions filtered by and through the lenses of history and evolution of human awareness and consciousness. This study is an analysis of the dialectical life of the spirit, a process of spiritual advancement (i.e. advancement of the mind) which is built upon thesis, antithesis, and synthesis. The Hegelian perspective is particularly evident in the words by Christopher, Wendt, Marecek and Goodman: "Science –whether in the form of methodological controls or evidence-based practice guidelines– cannot produce "pure" forms of knowledge unaffected by the knowers' place in historical time and geographic space."[161] The question arising from this viewpoint is then how to quantify, and caliber, the perceptual response in the pursuit of this knowledge. Following the examples of Husserl and Heidegger, and in part drifting apart from their analysis, including the dialectic conception, we could investigate the problem with helpful elements provided by the *Phenomenology of Perception* by Maurice Merleau-Ponty. If we are talking about a patient as part of (his) history (time) and material (in the sense of *here-and-now*, geographical, contextual) space, we understand through Merleau-Ponty's work how the body-

---

[161]   Christopher, J.C., Wendt, D.C., Marecek, J., D.C., Goodman, D.M. 2014. *Critical Cultural Awareness. Contributions to a Globalizing Psychology*. In *American Psychologist*. Vol. 69, Num. 7: 645–655 Washington, DC: APA, p. 653

subject is also a body-object. Thus, if we do have a specific ontology of medicine focused on the *here-and-now* of the patient's body, we also need to observe some dualistic elements of this analysis. This perspective contains a partially critical attitude toward the Cartesian dualism as solution of the mind-body problem, and it replaces it with the "primacy of perception", a dialectical, intersubjective concept of consciousness which explains how we as patients, doctors, as well as human beings in general, first perceive the world, and then do philosophy. To be sure, we need to remember the notions of "bodily intentionality" and "motivation" to explain the centralized view of "bodiliness", which ultimately states that we perceive our world through our bodies, in an embodied consciousness perspective, which is existence-based.[162] Is this a form of philosophy of mind? According to Foglia and Wilson:

> "Traditional views in philosophy of mind and cognitive science depict the mind as an information processor, one whose connections with the body and the world are of little theoretical importance. On the contrary, mounting empirical evidence shows that bodily states and modality-specific systems for perception and action underlie information processing, and that embodiment contributes to various aspects and effects of mental phenomena [...]. By challenging mainstream accounts of mind and cognition, embodiment views offer new ways of conceptualizing knowledge and suggest novel perspectives on cognitive variation and mind-body reductionism."[163]

Merleau-Ponty moves between two poles; in fact, the very concept of a body-subject indicates an embodied, corporeal genesis of (human) consciousness, and yet suggests what could be considered its ontological opposite, the world-object. Is this the world of time and history? Is it the embodied world of the Spirit? For Hegel, Spirit defines a conceptual entity encompassing all reality,

---

[162]   This is especially important in our analysis, due to the resulting philosophical implications regarding concepts such as connectedness, loneliness, sense of belonging, sense of purpose, and meaning. A good example of embodied perception/cognition research focusing on the aforementioned elements is found in Wortman, J., Donnellan, M.B., and Lucas, R.E. 2014. *Can Physical Warmth (or Coldness) Predict Trait Loneliness? A Replication of Bargh and Shalev (2012)*. Archives of Scientific Psychology, Washington, DC: APA, American Psychological Association, pp. 13–19.

[163]   Foglia and Wilson 2013. *Embodied Cognition*, Focus Article. Volume 4, Issue 3, abstract from pages 319–325. In this regard, Bunge writes: "I submit that modern biology and medicine are *emergent materialist* rather that either vitalist or reductionist. That is, those disciplines not only regard organisms as systems endowed with physical and chemical properties, but also with typically biological properties. [...] physicalism and chemism were primitive but perhaps unavoidable phases of materialist philosophy, biology, and medicine." Bunge, M. 2013. *Medical Philosophy. Conceptual Issues in Medicine*, Singapore: World Scientific Publishing, pp. 34–35.

thus comprehending a multi-faceted whole, with both universal and specific sides, or "facets". Thus, if thesis represents the dual concept of unconscious and unity, and antithesis is defined by conscious and separation (which is also self-alienation or separation from itself), synthesis is the union of the two, conscious and unity. In the stage of unconsciousness, the Spirit has not yet acquired mind. In the second stage or consciousness, the Spirit acquires mind (a conscious mind, since we have to understand the dual meaning of "Geist") but misinterprets everything it perceives as something separated, divided, other than itself. The third stage of self-consciousness is the realization of the Spirit of the meaning of reality, through an evolution from more childish elements onto more and more mature approaches. This reality includes all human minds, thus including the "divine" or "God", though not identified with the supernatural God of theism. Some viewed this very structure of writing as a "concealed" atheistic dialectic,[164] which is obscure and obscurantist on purpose, especially considering the strong pro-Christian regime of Frederick Wilhelm II.

The conceptual complexity of the term "mind" throws us back to the contemporary research on human soul, especially when comparing physicalist perspectives with theories of immortality. For instance, Warren Brown draws his very belief in what could be viewed as mere materialism, in the sense that there is nothing else beyond the physicality of our selves, including (or substituting the term with it) the mind. Thus, when "we" die, we die completely. This view is especially well described in works such as *Did My Neurons Make Me Do It? Philosophical and Neurobiological Perspectives on Moral Responsibility and Free Will*, as well as the collection of perspectives in *Whatever Happened of the Soul? Scientific and Theological Portraits of Human Nature*. The author extensive work in experimental neuropsychological research on the implications of agenesis of the *corpus callosum*, and in general on its functions and relation with higher cognitive processes in humans, is also the basis for a broader dialectical debate on the lack of immortality of the soul, in the sense that we, as human beings created by God, are monistic in structure, thus every part of our body is the origin and creation of our self. This does not necessarily lead to a reductive causal relation between brain and action, however it is clear that our real "self" has its roots in our bodily features, thus a claim for a separated soul that continues after or physical death does not make sense according

---

[164]   A "platonic dialogue [...] between the great systems of history" in the words of Alexander Kojève. For further reference, see Kojève, Alexander, *Introduction to the Reading of Hegel*, chapter 1.

to Brown. However, the author is ready to explain that this view does not diminish his belief in a creator God, who will recreate us after our physical death "from scratch", although not in the sense of a *tabula rasa*, but as a complete new, reborn, recreated, reformed-remorphed *version* of us.[165] In fact, Brown's perspective presents enough similarities (and, to be fair, possibly as many differences) with the Religious Naturalism of Eric Steinhart,[166] in particular his defense of an elaboration on original Christian (as well as a more personal, "digitally and computationally" translated) perspective on resurrection as opposed to reincarnation:

"According to the classical cosmological and design arguments, God is the creator-designer of our universe. One popular atheistic response to those arguments is simply to assert that if God created our universe, then there is some prior deity who created God. The result is an endless regress of ever greater deities. This regress of deities resembles the regress of engineers in the iterated simulation hypothesis. One problem with this regression is that it has no initial premise—no foundational deity whose necessity transmits existence further down the chain to our universe. Another problem is that earlier deities are more divine than later deities; hence the explanatory burden increases without bound in the regression. The regression of ever greater deities has no explanatory power. Digitalists solve the problems with this endless regress by inverting it: each previous deity is less divine than the next deity. [...] Digitalists argue that intelligent computers have a natural tendency to recursive self-improvement. Every god can design and create a more divine version of itself. And since self-improvement is morally obligatory, every god wants to design and create a more divine version of itself. Hence every god does design and create a more divine version of itself. Every god makes itself more divine in all possible ways. All increases in divinity, for the sake of continuity, are minimal. A minimal increase in divinity is an improvement. Although the initial digital god has little divinity, it has enough to create all possible improved versions of itself. [...] Every god is surpassed by a plurality of successor gods. Hence there is an endlessly ramified tree of ever more divine gods. One of these successor gods supports our universe; but our local god is merely finitely perfect and is surpassed by many more divine gods. The tree of digital gods runs into the transfinite. [...] Every progression of gods is surpassed by a plurality of limit gods. Hence there are infinitely divine digital gods. [...] But there is no maximal digital god—there is no God. The tree of digital gods is an atheistic structure. It does not rise towards any sun; it rises only into greater light. Every digital god supports a universe. Universes are to gods as software to hardware. Thus every universe is a software process running on some god. All digital gods are impersonal machines that ground but do not penetrate their universes [...] A comparison with recent resurrection theories shows that body-uploading is a kind of resurrection. It is the resurrection of your body in a computer-generated universe (which is nested inside our universe). This computer-generated

---

[165]   For further reference, please see bibliography, as well as the interview of Warren Brown with Robert Lawrence Kuhn for the series *Closer to Truth*, available on http://www.closertotruth.com/interviews/1904

[166]   Steinhart, E.C. 2014. *Your Digital Afterlives: Computational Theories of Life after Death (Palgrave Frontiers in Philosophy of Religion)*. New York, NY: Palgrave McMillan.

universe is a habitat for your body and the bodies of other humans. Since our bodies evolved to function in an earthly network of relations, this habitat will be an earthlike environment. Anyone who designs a habitat for persons is ethically obligated to design it for human flourishing. You will actualize more of your positive potentials. But not for very long: the sun will eventually incinerate the earth. Our universe will eventually run down into heat death. The laws of thermodynamics entail that digital replication cannot be everlasting life. Digital replication is a good step towards your digital afterlife. But it isn't enough."[167]

Steinhart's view, albeit partially vague and not offering specific reasons for claims such as "scanning kills you,"[168] literally throws us back into the problem of a connection between mind and body, brain, self, and life as a whole, including our perception of us in/as part of it, our consciousness. What has been described as Hegelian method, consists of actually examining consciousness' experience of both itself and of its objects while focusing (*reine Zusehen* or "pure looking at") on the dynamic evolution creating contradictions. If consciousness' attention is concentrated only to what is actually present in itself and its relation to its objects, it will see that what looks like fixed (in terms of stable forms of existence) will dissolve into a dialectical movement. Hegel describes the first form of consciousness as "sensory" (also intended as childish or infantile), in which we draw general conclusions from a particular (individual) sample/example. The author focuses on this universality of perception in the Preface of the book:

> "Because philosophy has its being essentially in the element of that universality which encloses the particular within it, the end or final result seems, in the case of philosophy more than in that of other sciences, to have absolutely expressed the complete fact itself in its very nature; contrasted with that the mere process of bringing it to light would seem, properly speaking, to have no essential significance."[169]

---

[167] From the description of Steinhart's philosophy as discussed in *Your Digital Afterlives: Computational Theories of Life after Death*, on the author's personal website: http://eric steinhart.com/FLESH/flesh-chabs.html.

[168] Ibid.: "Many digitalists argue that it is technically possible for advanced body-scanners to make exact maps of your body at the molecular level of detail. But to obtain this high precision, those scanners must destroy your body as they scan it—scanning kills you. Fortunately, your death in the scanner produces an exact molecular map of your flesh—it produces your body-file. After scanning, your body-file can be installed on a digital computer to make an exact digital replica of your body. And, since you are your body, this is an exact digital replica of you. This is body-uploading. Body-uploading is body-copying—it is the duplication of the flesh in another medium. Since the mind is a part of the body, body-copying includes mind-copying. Minds are copied; but they are not moved."

[169] Georg Wilhelm Friedrich Hegel, *Phenomenology of Mind*, translation by J. B. Baillie, Blackmask Online Edition, 2001, p. 5.

Through experience, the Spirit's Sensory Consciousness evolves in to Perceptual Consciousness. This type of knowledge allows us to understand, and therefore classify into a comprehensive System of (natural—from an Aristotelian memory) Science, the natural relationships between objects. This passage from a sensory level onto a perceptual one is directly connected to the very presence of humanity in history. As Montgomery observes, "[…] Like history or evolutionary biology, clinical medicine is fated to be a retrospective, narrative investigation and not a Newtonian or Galilean science."[170] Thus, medicine needs to rediscover those (phenomenological) aspects of human nature which lie beyond or (as we will see in the following chapters) at the base of biological evidence and interpretation.

From a perspective of "created world" Hegel writes about the "awakening" of human spirit, since both the philosopher-scientist, i.e. the observer, and the observed (perceived object) are essentially Spirit. In this sense we understand the author's statement: "*Die Phänomenologie des Geistes ist die romantisierte Geschichte des Bewusstseins, das sich mit der Zeit als Geist erkennt.*"[171] How can the spirit transcend this perceptual form of consciousness? Following Kant's theory of Pure Understanding, Hegel introduces the concept of "Understanding Consciousness" as mind's own image of itself, thus seeing itself as a unifying principle, an omnicomprehensive Greater Self in which the separation/diversity/diversification of subjects/objects becomes one, embraced by its very singleness. This is the very step to and further step to science, in logical

---

[170]   Montgomery, K. 2006. *How doctors think: clinical judgment and the practice of medicine*. New York, NY: Oxford University Press, p. 6. "[especially] in the United States, where the idea of medicine as a science is perhaps strongest". (Ibid.). It is interesting to consider the external/*aesthetically* perceived levels of professionalization of the practice of medicine, and investigate the conceptual and perceptual components of the *habitus / habitat / habitudo* of the traditional white coast, which (again, especially in the USA and especially in terms of length) represents a visual coding of achieved professional level. For further reference, see Giardina, S., and Spagnolo, A.G. 2014. *I medici e il camice bianco. Note storico-culturali e implicazioni per la formazione dello studente di medicina*. Medicina e Morale 2014/2, Rome, I: Università Cattolica del Sacro Cuore. Illich is especially critical of the medical institution, especially in the western world, and writes in his *Limits to Medicine; Medical Nemesis: The Expropriation of Health*: "The layman in medicine, for whom this book is written, will himself have to acquire the competence to evaluate the impact of medicine on health care. Among all our contemporary experts, physicians are those trained to the highest level of specialized incompetence for this urgently needed pursuit". Illich, I. 1976. *Limits to Medicine; Medical Nemesis: The Expropriation of Health*. London, UK: Marion Boyars Publishers, p. 6

[171]   "The Phenomenology of Spirit is the romanticized history of consciousness that recognizes itself over time as a ghost", in: Hegel, Georg Wilhelm Friedrich, *Phänomenologie des Geistes*, Suhrkamp Verlag Frankfurt am Main, I. Auflage (edition), 1986 , p. 37.

and theoretical terms. In comparison to the impersonal element of Kant's theory, so perceived by Hegel because of its description of the Self, which has no personality, the author of the Phenomenology of Mind introduces the Self Consciousness. This discussion is actually a combination of four narratives containing hidden dialectics. Hegel focuses on Master and Slave (Lordship and Bondage), Stoicism, Skepticism, and the Unhappy Consciousness.[172] If Kantian theory is guilty of missing the mark of realism, this type of Consciousness is linked to a "real" person, evolved in sub-moments, thus drawing ontological elements from philosophical tradition predating kantian speculation.

More specifically, Self Consciousness evolved within the domain of politics through several stages. The Desiring Self-Consciousness is indicative of the way primitive humans attempted to meet their needs and the needs of their families. This desiring self-consciousness has socio-political implications in the progressive growth of interpersonal, interfamiliar and world wars due to specific practical application of a certain type of self-interest. This stage evolved in the Lordship-Bondage term, as expressed in Mastery Self Consciousness and Servant Self Consciousness. In this regard Hegel writes:

> "Die Doppelsinnigkeit des Unterschieden liegt in dem Wesendes Selbstbewußtseins, unendlich oder unmittelbar das Gegenteil der Bestimmtheit, in der es gesetzt ist, zu sein. Die Auseinanderlegung des Begriffs dieser geistigen Einheit in ihrer Verdopplung stellt uns die Bewegung des Anerkennens dar. Es ist für das Selbstbewußtsein ein anderes Selbstbewußtsein; es ist außer sich gekommen. Dies hat die gedoppelte Bedeutung; erstlich, es hat sich selbst verloren, denn es findet sich als ein anderes Wesen; zweitens, es hat damit das Andere aufgehoben, denn es sieht auch nicht das Andere als Wesen, sondern sich selbst im Anderen."[173]

---

[172] The conceptual parallel between Unhappy Consciousness, Melancholia and Depression is quite evident from this point of view. As related to the identity and structure of (a personalized, individual) Self, it is very interesting to monitor the implications, in terms of quantifiable physical effects on this form of consciousness as it related to psychiatric disorders. In the case of depression, and interesting perspective is offered by the clinical research of Darin Dougherty, a Harvard Medical School associate professor of psychiatry at Massachusetts General Hospital, who was principal investigator of a study of five of the world's first implantations (through surgical insertion of electrodes into the brain's ventral capsule/ventral striatum, ever attempted to control depression. For further reference, see Dougherty, E. 2011. The depths of despair. Medicine tackles melancholia with new tools and understanding. In: Byron, P.B. (Ed.) 2011. *The Science of Emotion*, Boston, MA: Harvard Medicine, p. 26.

[173] "The ambiguity of the difference (the different/the differentiated) lies in the actual (actualized, self-creating and present) self-consciousness, infinite and immediately the opposite of the determinateness in which it is set, to be. The explication of the concept of this spiritual unity in its duplication introduces us to the movement of recognition. It is for the self-consciousness another self-consciousness, it became "Out of itself". This has a

In particular, Mastery Self Consciousness brings the demand and the fear to daily life, as a stimulus for progress. At the same time, this very progress is non-existent for the Ruler, since his job is to fight for and retain his Mastery, without any further development and without thanking or praising anyone, thus isolating himself. Servant Self Consciousness is the creator of progress through his job for the Master, whom he serves by producing new science and technology, though with and through struggle and pain. These torments provide in turn the basis for new philosophical speculation (which is also justification for his role and subordinate position), so that the Servant has in the end all the creative power of inventions and new ideas: *"[...] der Herr aber, der den Knecht zwischen es und sich eingeschoben, schließt sich dadurch nur mit der Unselbständigkeit des Dinges zusammen und genießt es rein; die Seite der Selbständigkeit aber überläßt er dem Knechte, der es bearbeitet."*[174] Out of his condition, the Servant develops his Stoic Self Consciousness, the perfect ideal of work ethics, honesty and virtue. Against this ideal, the children experience the hard truth of reality, which teaches them that good is not always rewarded and wickedness not always punished, and hard work is often merely exploited. Through this process of progressive awareness, the child develops the Skeptic Self Consciousness, through which he approaches reality with cynicism, disbelief, resignation, and mockery of the tender-hearted. This is only a temporary truth, yet undeniable. A further step is represented by the Unhappy Self Consciousness, which determines at first a complete separation from the world, in an ascetic or meditative, monastic way, sometimes through prayer or desperation: "[...] although the unhappy consciousness does not possess this actual presence, it has, at the same time, transcended pure thought, so far as this is the abstract thought of Stoicism, which turns away from particulars altogether, and again the merely restless thought of Skepticism."[175] This exercise can bring some relief, especially in the case of attaining Iron will over subjective, individual, human weakness, which can also lead to joy. It is the case of Free Will, a truth that helps them develop a clearer vision, sometimes by comparison with

---

double meaning: first, it has lost itself, for it finds itself as another being, and secondly, it has thereby eliminated the other, because it does not look at the other(ness) as being but himself in the other(ness)." In: Ibid., pp. 144–145.

[174] "[...] but the Lord, who inserted the servant between that and himself, closes himself only with the lack of independence of the thing altogether and enjoys it completely: [still] he leaves the side of independence to the servant who elaborated it." In: Ibid., p. 151.

[175] Georg Wilhelm Friedrich Hegel, *Phenomenology of Mind*, translation by J. B. Baillie, Blackmask Online Edition, 2001, p. 77.

fellow humans, a vision "clearer than anyone else". Thus, man experiences a progressive awareness of power of the mind and ideas, from which the Idealist Consciousness emerges. This consciousness has a poetic, creative strength, the ability to make all ideas into the real, in contrast with mastery, servitude and the retreat from the world of the ascetic, meditative type of consciousness. However, this all-comprehensive feature specific to the Idealist Consciousness still misses all-inclusiveness, by excluding the non-ideal half of reality. In coming to terms with this problem, Rational Consciousness is born. That is how we (and Hegel as well) understand Schelling's perspective on "the Great Other", the natural element which Idealism has to acknowledge.

To move pass this stage and raise this type of awareness, we need to arrive at the Empirical Consciousness, which not only provides a better tool for our understanding of the issue, but projects the concept of a reason "embodied" in the very object of our analysis, thus denying that reason is in the subject, as reflected onto the world. This type of knowledge is very close to the modern conception of empirical science and its focus on the observed data, monitors through evidence-based methodology, experimentations, statistics, and disciplines such as public health epidemiology, biology etc. Thus, life itself becomes one of these analyzed[176] objects, more specifically an object of various branches of science, from natural to social sciences. At the same time, Hegel argues strongly against the epistemological emphasis of philosophical speculation from Descartes through Kant. The weak point of such positions is the methodology. The author stresses the importance of first establishing the nature and criteria of knowledge prior to actually knowing anything. The reason behind this statement is to be found in the infinite regress that such philosophical method would imply; a foundationalism that Hegel maintains is self-contradictory and impossible. That is exactly why we have to examine actual knowing as it occurs in real (human) knowledge processes. Because Empirical consciousness seeks absolute objectivity, for that very reason the study of the subjective Self could be considered beyond scientific investigation. In regard to the relation between observation and (inner) perception Hegel writes:

"When the unreflective consciousness speaks of observation and experience as being the fountain of truth, the phrase may possibly sound as if the whole business were a matter of tasting, smelling, feeling, hearing, and seeing. It forgets, in its zeal for tasting, smelling, etc.,

---

[176] Although we should certainly be careful in assessing the analytic philosophy-component (as opposite to a continental philosophy-component) of such paradigm, as evidenced in the following discussion.

to say that, in point of fact, it has really and rationally determined for itself already the object thus sensuously apprehended, and this determination of the object is at least as important for it as that apprehension. It will also as readily admit that its whole concern is not
simply a matter of perceiving, and will not allow, e.g. the perception that this penknife lies
beside this snuff-box to pass for an "observation". What is perceived should, at least, have
the significance of a universal, and not of a sensuous particular 'this'."[177]

Is there a way to comprehend a more "holistic" approach to the study of human
knowledge? Hegel writes: "The nerves themselves, no doubt, are again organs
of that consciousness which from the first is immersed in its outward impulses.
Brain and spinal cord, however, may be looked at as the immediate presence of
self-consciousness, a presence self-contained, not an object and also not tran-
sient."[178] Ethical Consciousness overcomes this *empasse* and focuses on the
concept of family begins with the immediate fact of a family, without which a
Self does not exist. A child leaves home and often marries, where male and
female, both antithetic, join in synthetic union, and produce offspring to carry
on the family estate. Where the female is the domain of Divine Law and the
male is the domain of Human Law, the synthesis is a practical ethic which
expands to include the whole community. A family participates in the social
economy, where honesty, thrift and reliability are highly valued virtues. When
the object before consciousness is determined, consciousness possesses reason.
Consciousness, as well as self-consciousness, is in itself properly reason in an
implicit form; but only that consciousness can be said to have reason whose
object has the character of being the category. From this, however, we must
still distinguish the knowledge of what reason is. Let us remember that Hegel
states that "science, in the very fact that it comes to the scene, is itself a phenomenon."[179] That is why Phenomenology deals with (these) phenomena,
which are indeed linked to "the life of the Spirit" according to the 'two movements" or stages of thesis and antithesis. The dialectical movement at the base
of this correlation, which is also correlation between *inner* and *outer* (well
expressed by both Kojève and Verene in their analysis), is the core of this science. The ultimate focus of this science is to show (the path, the method to)
absolute knowledge, which the spirit can attain by getting rid of its own aliena-
tion in the correlation/comparison between object and subject, through self-

---

[177]   Georg Wilhelm Friedrich Hegel, *Phenomenology of Mind*, translation by J. B. Baillie,
        Blackmask Online Edition, 2001, p. 90.
[178]   Ibid., p. 117.
[179]   Ibid., p. 28. See also Trejo, P. , *Summary of Hegel's Philosophy of Mind*, Carnegie Mellon
        University, Pittsburgh, PA, 1993.

realization. This analysis is first, at the beginning of the *Introduction* to the *Phenomenology of Spirit*, a critique of the Kantian *Unterscheidung zwischen den Dingen an sich und den Dingen für uns*. As we saw, this distinction is the core problem blocking the way to this Absolute Knowledge, which is also Knowledge of the Absolute. How can the spirit move beyond this stage? We covered some of the elements, terms and concepts linked to the process, but ultimately, the core of this process is what Hegel defines *Weg der Verzweiflung*, which is conceptually, etymologically and in a practical sense the way of "despair", in which there are two different ways, a pair of opportunities, a separation.[180] That is why this awareness, this consciousness has to take different forms, see their (its) forthcomings and re-morph into a different shape in order to see itself, *als Ende und Anfang*. That is the Absolute Spirit. To continue in our comparison, how can we understand this embodied perspective from the broader view on existence?

3.2 Theoretically grounded, empirically supported: The mind-brain problem

a) An analysis of terms

One of the most important questions in Medical Philosophy is a philosophical question *par excellence*: what is the relationship between our minds and our brains? In particular, we need to investigate the conceptual weight of "brain" and (as well as *versus*) "body" so that we are better prepared to appropriately analyze the dichotomy of the coupled terms mind-body and mind-brain problem. This is fundamental from the embodied cognition perspective, as we previously discussed in regard to science: "The concept of a rational science implies an inherent mind-body split, with the mind providing superior information to that from the body on all counts. A rational science certainly adheres to the old adage, 'I think, therefore I am', and adds to it, 'I measure, therefore I can predict and control'."[181] In this regard, Le Guin writes:

> "People crave objectivity because to be subjective is to be embodied, to be a body, vulnerable, violable [...] . [The language of science] began to develop when printing made written language common rather than rare, 500 years ago or so, and with electronic processing and

---

180   We should note that *Zweifel* is translated as 'doubt' and again represents 'two cases' (*Zwei Fälle*).

181   Schaef, A.W. 1992. *Beyond Therapy, Beyond Science*. New York, NY: HarperCollins, p. 203.

copying it continues to develop and proliferate so powerfully, so dominatingly, that many believe this dialect -the expository and particularly the scientific discourse- is the *highest* form of language, the true language, of which all other uses of words are primitive vestiges.

And it is indeed. Newton's Principia was written in it in Latin, and Descartes wrote Latin and French in it establishing some of its basic vocabulary, and Kant wrote German in it, and Marx, Darwin, Freud, Boas, Foucault, all the great scientists and social thinkers wrote it. It is the language of thought that seeks objectivity.

I do not say it's the language of rational thought. Reason is a faculty far larger than mere objective thought. When either the political or the scientific discourse announces itself as the voice of reason, it is playing God, and should be spanked and stood in the corner. The essential gesture of the father tongue is not reasoning, but distancing – making a gap, a space, between the subject of self and the object or other. Enormous energy is generated by that rending, that forcing of a gap between man and World. So the continuous growth of technology and science fuels itself."[182]

To what extent, can we as human beings relate to one another and to ourselves and be able to understand the connections of the realm of the preconscious,[183] conscious and subconscious, given the impact of our individuality, of our personal experience and perception? Should we apply the same hypothesis to other living being as well? And what about non-living beings? We could follow the scientific approach of linguistics, semantics and etymology and move to more spiritual, mythological, even metaphysical grounds. For instance, we could start by asking ourselves why do Romance languages, plus the English word (itself a Romance borrowing) *Animal* contain the Latin term for "soul"? Is the German translation *Tier* a connection with the corresponding divinity of Germanic paganism? Recent studies have shown a possible connection with the same concept, through a reconstructed Proto-Indo-European *dʰewsóm*, all the way to the Slavic *δγuα*. Interestingly enough, the English term *deer* is related to the same word, and connected to the Old Norse *dýrr*, in turn identifying concepts such as "expensive, costly, valuable and precious". Focusing for a moment on the English language, it is very easy and natural to see the common root in words like "health, wealth, holy and whole". This observation alone could provide some very useful hints in the discovery of deeper meanings and

---

[182]   Le Guin, U. 1989. *Dancing at the Edge of the World*. New York, NY: Grove Press, p. 148, as cited in: Schaef, A.W. 1992. *Beyond Therapy, Beyond Science*. New York, NY: HarperCollins, pp. 205–206.

[183]   See Volk, S. 2011. Fringe-ology: How I tried to Explain Away the Unexplainable—And Couldn't, New York, NY: HarperCollins In particular, *Introduction: What We Talk About When We Talk About the Paranormal* and Chapter 3: *Consciousness Outside the Brain*.

interpretations for the combination visible-invisible, conscious-subconscious and similar. Still, if we want to keep a scientific approach, based on empirical evidence (at least for these first steps in the discussion), we have to be able to apply our findings in a cross-cultural and cross-linguistic viewpoint. Thus, moving towards other language groups, can we see the same connection between a symbolic, omnicomprehensive, absolute, divine, transcendental (and, in some cases, transcendent) realm and the earthly, chthonic, dia-bolic (dichotomous and binary), sensitive/sensible/aesthetically perceived of the realm we live in, by some viewed as the "Veil of Maya"? Throughout history, we can see an alternation between separation and unification of these two opposites, from far eastern philosophies, to some more familiar "Western" approaches, bearing elements of (just to quote some) neoplatonic, manicheic and bogomilistic elements.[184] This relation is definitely visible in Latin, for instance *Doma/Domina/Donna/Donum/Dare* or *Patrimonium/Matrimonium/Munus*, all the way to its deviant form of Medieval Latin and Italian *soldo/soldato/assoldato*. Continuing with Latin, this etymological approach is probably explained at its best by the Italian Giambattista Vico; let us remember his famous quote "Latinis *verum* et *factum* reciprocantur, seu, ut scholarum vulgus loquitur, convertuntur."[185] Now, we could use this exact same sentence to analyse the connection between "Faith" and "Fact", maybe by exploring the Italian *Fatto/Fedele/Fedeltà/Fiducia* or transferring this approach to a different language. To this day, the Italian term for 'Wedding ring' is *Vera*. The connection with the Slavic *Вера* is too evident to be avoided in our analysis. If these assumptions are true, we *should* be able to take the above mentioned paired combination of "health-wealth-holy-whole" and simply summarize/translate it to *богатство*. If we could prove this hypothesis, and successfully apply our statement also beyond the realm of Indo-European studies,[186] we still have to face the chronological impact that history (again, also in Hegelian terms) had

---

184   Malcolm, N. 1996. *Bosnia: a short history*. New York, NY: New York University Press; with special reference, in Chapters 1 through 5, to the work of Ангелов, Д. 1969. *Богомилството в България*, София. and Solovjev, A.V. 1997. *Svedočanstva pravoslavnih izvora o bogumilstvu na Balkanu*, Sarajevo, BiH: Nacionalna i univerzitetska biblioteka Bosne i Hercegovine, Sarajevo and *Bogumilentum und Bogumilengräber in den südslawischen Ländern*, in Gülich, W. 1959 (Ed.) *Völker und Kulturen Südosteuropas*, München. With regard to the manicheic perspective, see also Loos, M. 1974. *Les Derniers Cathares de l'occident et leurs relations avec l'église patarine de Bosnie*, Prague.

185   Vico, G. 1971 (Ed.). Opere (Works), Florence: Sansoni Ed. Vol. I, pp. 63–64.

186   Villar, F. 1996. *Gli Indoeuropei e le origini dell'Europa* (The Indoeuropeans and the origins of Europe), Bologna: Società editrice Il Mulino, 1997—Original Edition: *Los Indoeuropeos y los origenes de Europa. Lenguaje e historia*, Madrid: Gredos, Madrid.

on the evolution of cultures, ethnicities and languages. Change is the challenge. We could benefit from the attentive and detailed analysis of Scholars like Francisco Villar or Vladislav Markovich-Illyich-Svitych, but, in our analysis of the relation between conscious and unconscious we would still have to answer the following question: "is conscience knowledge"? Can we rely on our body-mind connections, our emotions, feelings, sensations, memories to create a valid exegesis, a pure and absolute (also in the theological sense) interpretation of reality?

In regard to the Cartesian approach, Vico already stated that "*coscienza non è conoscenza.*"[187] Is the Latin *cum+scio* similar in meaning and function to the Greek γνῶσις, transferred into *cognosco*? We could use a more empirical, yet alternative (from the historical institutionalized scientific viewpoint) approach. In comparing Newton and Goethe (as well as his impact on personalities like Gustav Klimt, Rudolf Steiner and Elena Petrovna Blavatsky) we should ask ourselves whether there is some sort of reliability in our physical and sensitive perception of the true data. In Goethe's research on light and colour, we should take in consideration the cultural background he was born and educated in. In the German idiomatic sentence "*das scheint gut zu sein*" (roughly translated as "that seems to be good") we are actually depending on our bodily sensation (in terms of analysis through the sense of sight) to formulate a hypothesis. Here, we are focusing on the power of physical appearance to create our model. At this point we should compare the verb *scheinen* with its Germanic brother *to shine*, in English. To what extent does this attitude toward the relationship between body and perception, as well as *propriocezione* (especially regarding the feeling to/from one's body and parts of it to-ward/from one's soul), apply in the Germanic/Anglo-Saxon cultural environment? Could we say the same for the Romance Languages? Italian alchemists used to say "*non è tutto oro quello che luccica*"; an idiomatic expression still in use as a confutation of what we just said, *id est* the proof that "what shines is not necessary the truth". Is this only a product of culture? Are the Germanic *Shine* and the Latin *Scio* related? If we are considering the alchemic process and Gold as

---

[187] Abbagnano, N. and Fornero, G. 1986. *Filosofi e filosofie nella storia* (Philosophers and Philosophies in history), Torino: Paravia, II ed. 1992; for a further analysis on the body-mind related debate, see in particular Vol. I, Chapters 2–6 and Vol. II, part 2; for the analysis on the contemporary logical debate on the relationship conscious-unconscious, please see Vol. 3, Chapter 5. For further reference, see also Vico, G. 1971 (Ed.). *Opere* (Works), Florence: Sansoni Ed. Vol. I, especially the analysis between his position in his *De antiquissima* and the concept of "Human Mind vs/atque Divine Mind."

physical element as well as metaphysical, figurative and metaphorical way to define the reached enlightenment, shall we move onto distant cultures and geographical places? What about the Pre-Indo-European ethnical backgrounds, what about the Arab, Persian, Turkic, and Ural culture? Would the Egyptian Black soil of *al kēme* (alchemy) be a candidate for the Proto-Baltic word **žemē* (for some at the origin of the Ugro-Finnic endonym *Suomi*) and its Slavic cousin Земля? This connection would help us work toward a mutual understanding and increasing tolerance in areas of philosophical, anthropological as well as political challenge, without sacrificing scientific evidence. To remain in that area and focus on the sometimes difficult interaction between Germanic Swedes, Ugro-Finnic Finns and Slavic Russians, let us just think for a moment about the way these people define one another. The term *Finn* is a borrowing from the Anglo-Saxon and Gaelic heritage, a word defining "fairness" "light colored" (as in the Gaelic Fin-na-ghan). So, while in some Scandinavians sayings and jokes people define and differentiate the Finns by associating them with "some sort of archaic land in the east, probably mixed with Russians, Tatars, or Mongols", the Finnish refer to Swedes as "Ruotsi", or "*People of the Русь*". This is obviously just an example of historical mutation of perception of "the other, the diverse, the defined as alternative" and it is fundamental in our anthropological and philosophical analysis. In this context, it is quite interesting to observe the combination and evolution of exonyms and endonyms: for the Greeks and the Romans, the rest of Europeans were people unable to speak their language, every person belonging to this group was simply a βάρβαρος.

The Germanic tribes applied the same concept to Celts and Rheto-romans as well, using the term *Walsche*, which remained almost intact to define Wales and Welch (a Celtic stronghold in the midst of Anglo-Saxon conquers) but also the *Walser* community in Switzerland and France or the term *Wälsch*, defining a member of the Italian speaking minority in the historical Tyrol. From the Slavic perspective,[188] someone who doesn't know how to speak "our" language is, again, нъмьць, "German" by default, with some exceptions in areas under German(ic) or Austrian control, for example Bosnia (especially *Herceg*ovina), where the Germans are representatives of the "Schwäbischer Kreis", the *Šva-*

---

[188]   Since the scope of this writing is not historical etymology, I will skip the analysis of the relation between Slaves and Slaves (Σκλαβηνοι vs Славяни), though I personally consider this term very interesting, especially in the context of psychological and social (self) perception.

bi.[189] Without completely leaving behind this approach, let us concentrate our efforts in understanding if or how our conscience could be part our perception or how our soul could enter our body. Though the modern technology allows us to reach a precision and quality of scientific proof in fields like string theory, quantum physics and antimatter in a wonderful way, unthinkable just few decades ago, to demonstrate the presence of a "soul", whether divine or completely human, remains a very hard task. What we can do is looking at the problem by comparison and confrontation, just like what we did in regard to language, culture and ethnicity. How does the soul relate to our body? Is the soul that makes us (feel) alive? Can we become who we are through a divine spirit? For the Greeks, *ψυχή* was a butterfly traveling through space and time (in the sense of *Aion, Kronos* and *Kairos*), a perfect image of the modern medical term for Psyche, as well as soul. This concept involves motion, movement, rhythm, for example in "breathing", just like in the Latin *Spiritus* and *respirare* (to breath) and *spirare/expirare* (to die). The German equivalent is *atmen*, possibly related to the Hindu *Atma*, the "higher self" in Hindu, Buddhist, and Jain traditions. The same applies to the "great soul" in the Sanskrit *Mahātmā.*[190]

The distinction between Soul and spirit, and its relation to more recent philosophical, as well as psychoanalytic approaches, like in the Freudian *Ich, Es, Super-Ich* or the Junghian Archetypes moves us forward and deeper into an observation of our role and purpose in this world and among other human beings. What is the effect of or conceptualization of the term and our adaptation to a broader system? In looking at the problem of conscious-unconscious, is the *Karma* equivalent and/or comparable to the *Dharma*? Is our personal experience a good reference in jumping from soul to spirit?

The Latin term *Individuum* refers to the concept of "indivisible", similar to the Greek ἄτομος (atom). "Single" (Lat. *Sin-gulus*) refers to the term *sine* (without, as a privative) or *sa/sam* (Greek *σύμ*, as in Symbol), which means unity. The Latin term "Persōna" (Etr. φersu) is linked to the value that a particular element has on the individual. Etymologically speaking, the term is a combination of per + sona, i.e. the mask/face the individual wears, in order to change the sound of his voice and his physical appearance (Greek πρόσωπον).

---

[189]   For a complete list on the historical and anthropological perspectives of medieval Bosnia and pre-Slavic Western Balkans settlements and their relationship with modern linguistic and cultural debate see Živković, P. (Ed.) Topalović, V. 1982. *Bibliografija objavljenih izvora i literature o srednjovjekovnoj Bosni.* Travnik, BiH: Zavičajni Muzej Travnik.

[190]   Certainly it would be interesting to investigate the relationship between the term and the Arab *Muhammad.*

Moreover, borrowing some elements from the field of epidemiology, in order to further analyze the relationship between body and soul, as well as monitoring the effects of this approach on a strictly scientific research, we could focus on the term "personalized" as an *effect modification*, a possible *confounder* in our study of the corresponding cause-effect relation between soul/spirit and their efficacy/entrance/presence in the human body.[191]

b) Suggesting a model

To apply this approach to our analysis, we could view the relation between our body $y(i)$ and our soul $x(i)$ as a straight line, where the beta coefficients play the role of *incognitae*, the scope of our research, plus a standard error or identify possible effect modifications due to the individual/personal impact on the process of the single human being.

$$y_i = \beta_0 + \beta_1 x_i + \varepsilon_i, \quad i = 1, \ldots, n.$$

Would this model really work if all our assumptions were correct or should we take in consideration other elements, *figures* or *shapes* of reality? For years the modern Western world viewed history using a linear model, even though we were challenged in our assumptions both from a philosophical perspective (for instance in Nietzsche, Evola, Eliade, Guénon) as well as through scientific theories such as famous examples like the relativity model or the string theory. Should we therefore apply some sort of curve to our model, bending the line to fit a conceptual empty space or black hole in our framed space? What if we could simplify our model by taking in consideration a huge amount of straight lines, each identifying a single human being, group, culture or ethnicity and "summarize" our dataset into a linear regression model, and then only focus on confidence intervals? We could sum up each individual and use a similar equation:

$$\widehat{\beta_1} = \frac{\sum(x_i - \bar{x})(y_i - \bar{y})}{\sum(x_i - \bar{x})^2} \text{ and } \hat{\beta}_0 = \bar{y} - \widehat{\beta}_1\bar{x}$$

With a variance linked to a standard deviation like this:

---

[191] In this regard, a beautiful analysis of the mind-body connection, also from the perspective of neuroscience and cognitive science is offered by Mario Beauregard, in Beauregard, M., O'Leary, D. 2008. *The Spiritual Brain. A Neuroscientist's Case for the Existence of the Soul.* New York, NY: HarperCollins.

$$\hat{\sigma}_\varepsilon^2 = \frac{SSE}{n-2}.$$

Our model would reflect some sort of perfect line, with a "cloud" of extra data around it.[192] Would that make sense? The weak point of this approach is the lack of certainty and precision, especially (perhaps, because of) the application to human beings. How could we possibly relate to something lying beyond the physical realm? How can we collect data related to the soul?[193] That is indeed a very difficult task, a seemingly impossible one. We could try to examine the unconscious activity with the modern technologies of neuroscience, such as nuclear magnetic resonance imaging (NMRI), or magnetic resonance tomography (MRT), very useful in providing good contrast between the different soft tissues of the body, especially the brain and the heart, for centuries considered the centre of the activity of the soul by philosopher and scientists alike.[194] We could compare the data obtained through these methods with the information from questionnaires assigned to each individual in our cohort study and search for figures and/or pattern schemes. The comparison of physiological activity and emotional, intellectual and individual system of belief represents only a part of the equation, in our case the body-soul and conscious-unconscious problems. To be more accurate we should also include a third term, which is interpretation of the data and a forth, the environment (both physical as well as spiritual) where the experiment/analysis has taken place. Furthermore, there are studies suggesting that *intuition* (albeit embodied in some cases) might play a fundamental role in hypothesis making and calculus, an important perspective for medical science (in particular genetics, homeostatic regulation and neuroscience) and Medical Philosophy in general. If by "Intuition" we understand a form of immediate (some argue, momentary)[195] knowledge, which

---

192   For further reference, see Boncinelli, E. 2011. *La vita della nostra mente* (Our mind's life), Rome: Editori Laterza – In particular, Pt II, Chapters 18–24: *La coscienza: "La madre di tutti i problemi"* (The conscience: the mother of all problems) (18) *Conscio e Inconscio* (Conscious and Unconscious) (21), *Coscienza e razionalità* (Conscience and rationality) (22).

193   Given the premises of its very existence in this context, for the purpose of this analysis.

194   We refrain, for the present moment, from elaborating on the neurological characterization of neural activity, especially as it relates to the production of neurotransmitters in body areas other than the brain, for instance in the digestive system. We will discuss these aspects in the following chapters.

195   An important aspect which we discussed elsewhere (in particular the apparent preeminence, in chronological-procedural terms, of the right hemisphere), with special regard to the theoretical assumptions and hypothesis making related to the post-evaluation of experimental

could be categorized as pre-, para-, ultra-rational (again, some might argue, anti-rational), thus without rational inference, we should also continue our analysis in etymological terms. This means that *intueor* still carries a reference to the action of literally "enter with the sight", if by sight we are willing to contemplate a higher, deeper translate form of perceptual knowledge. This might very well serve as a basis for the adjective "holotropic" in the sense first coined by Stanislav Grof:

> "In these states, consciousness is changed, but is not grossly impaired. All intellectual functions are intact and the person remains fully oriented. The content of holotropic experiences is often spiritual or mystical. This state involves sequences of psychological death and rebirth and a broad spectrum of transpersonal phenomena, including feelings of oneness with other people, nature, and the universe, past life experiences, and visions of archetypal beings and mythological landscapes as described by C.G. Jung (1960)."[196]

In recent studies, these phenomena have been analyzed by many medical scientist, philosophers, and physicists; good examples are found in the research by Beauregard and (separately) Jansen (whom we will discuss in Chapter 5) on Near-death experiences,[197] Stevenson on Reincarnation,[198] and Penrose-Hameroff on Consciousness.[199] In fact, as we will see, the main problem in addressing these issues is first and foremost philosophical in nature. Therefore, a complete discussion on Nonordinary states of consciousness (NOSC) within the field of medicine, especially in the subfields of neurology/neuroscience and anaesthesiology has to begin with philosophy. In fact, there are ways to induce these states artificially, in the laboratory with synthesized forms of chemical elements, or by using psychedelic substances, (isolated or wholly extracted) from plants. Groff continues:

---

psychology and neuroscience, for instance in the case of the corpus callosotomy in Gazzaniga et al. For further reference, please see Bibliography.

[196] Grof, S. 1998. *Rethinking Basic Assumptions about Psychology and Psychiatry: The Role of Spirituality and Nonordinary States of Consciousness*. In: Bassman, L. 1998. *The Whole Mind: The Definitive Guide to Complementary Treatment for Mind, Mood, and Emotion*. Novato, CA: New World Library, p. 43.

[197] Jansen, K.L.R. 1998. *The Ketamine Model of the Near Death Experience: A Central Role for the NMDA Receptor*. Journal Article, The Maudsley Hospital, Denmark Hill, London.

[198] Stevenson, I. 1974 (2nd Ed.) *Twenty Cases Suggestive of Reincarnation*. Charlottesville, VA: University Press of Virginia.

[199] Hameroff, S.R. 2006. *The entwined mysteries of anesthesia and consciousness*. Anesthesiology 105 (2): 400–412. doi: 10.1097/00000542-200608000-00024. PMID 16871075. See also Penrose, R. 1989. *Shadows of the Mind: A Search for the Missing Science of Consciousness*. Oxford, UK: Oxford University Press.

"Holotropic experiences can be triggered by various forms of systematic spiritual practice involving mediation, concentration, breathing, and movement exercises that are used in different systems of yoga, Vipassana, or Zen Buddhism, Tibetan Vajrayana, Taoism, Christian mysticism, Sufism, or Cabala. Ancient cultures have brought on these states of mind through chanting, drumming, breathing, dancing, fasting, enduring extreme pain, and social and sensory isolation, and ingesting psychedelic plants. Such processes were important parts of shamanic practices, healing ceremonies, and rites of passage."[200]

Does this mean that we do not have control over our brain, and that neurological reactions are the origin, in a causal sense, of these altered perceptual states? As we know from scientific research and medical practice, there are many means of altering consciousness through brainwave biofeedback, sensory isolation and, in a psychiatric sense, techniques such as Transcranial Magnetic Stimulation (TMS), Transcranial Direct Current Stimulation (tDCS) as well as the "reset button effect" of Electro-convulsive therapy (ECT). Furthermore, these states can also occur spontaneously and although we are progressively getting better and better in understanding the neurological basis of our experiences with the help of brain imaging (MRI, fMRI, PET scan, EEG, etc.), in the sense that "the brain can no longer hide from researchers behind the fortress of the skull,"[201] we are far from being able to claim that the brain *generates* these mental experiences. In this regard Satel and Lilienfeld warn us against "mindless neuroscience: the oversimplification, interpretive license, and premature application of brain science in the legal, commercial, clinical, and philosophical domains."[202] Certainly, the authors' perspective is not metaphysical, spiritual or transcendental – in fact, their attitude toward these domains of knowledge is at best agnostic and certainly non-theistic (although not necessarily *a*theist-ic) and non-denominational from a religious point of view – however, they take a stand against strictly scientistic/materialistic/reductionist views:

"In 1996, author Tom Wolfe penned a widely cited essay, "Sorry, but Your Soul Just Died." Neuroscience, he wrote, was on "the threshold of a unified theory that will have an impact as powerful as that of Darwinism a hundred years ago." Almost two decades later, the excite-

---

[200]   Grof, S. 1998. *Rethinking Basic Assumptions about Psychology and Psychiatry: The Role of Spirituality and Nonordinary States of Consciousness*. In: Bassman, L. 1998. *The Whole Mind: The Definitive Guide to Complementary Treatment for Mind, Mood, and Emotion*. Novato, CA: New World Library, pp. 43–44.

[201]   Wade, C., Tavris, C., and Garry, M. 2014. *Invitation to Psychology*. 6th Edition. New York, NY: Person, p. 132

[202]   Satel, S., Lilienfeld, S.O. 2013. *Brainwashed. The seductive appeal of Mindless Neuroscience*. New York, NY: Basic Books, p. 149.

ment surrounding neuroscience continues to grow, as well it should. But the promise of a unified theory in the foreseeable future is an illusion. As with sociobiology and the genomic revolution – two valuable conceptual legacies of Darwinism – we should extract the wisdom neuroscience has to offer without asking it to explain all of human nature."[203]

A neuroscience-reductionist view seems the wrong path to follow in order to understand the problems of mind-brain relation and human consciousness. At the same time, are we sure that "the promise of a unified theory in the foreseeable future is an illusion"? Perhaps, a more holistic approach, encompassing evidence-based and theoretical science, philosophical perspectives maybe even including gnosis and theosis,[204] could bring us closer to a deeper, if not absolute truth in understanding who we really are, especially by comparing opposite approaches: "In a rational, mechanistic approach, one gets an idea and then tries to understand it (through experimentation), and in a postmodern approach, one understands something and then tries to get an idea about it."[205] Furthermore, we could argue that we should indeed look for explanations of human nature, at least in terms of moral-ethical values and social norms, in the debate around neuroscience and genomics, and their relationship with human nature. This should not push us back to reductionist perspectives on what makes us human, but open up the perspective on how our inner nature relates to internal-external factors, such as environment and behavior. For instance,

---

[203] Ibid., p. 153.

[204] In this regard, the analysis by Vladimir Lossky in "The Mystical Theology", in particular the relationship between gnosis and theosis, is particularly interesting. For further reference, see Lossky, V. 1944 *Essai sur la theologie mystique de l'Eglise d'Orient* as discussed in: N. O. Lossky. 1951. *History of Russian Philosophy* (Original: *История российской Философии*). London, UK: Allen & Unwin, London / New York, NY: International Universities Press. In this volume, N.O. Lossky writes about V. Lossky: "The genius of Eastern mystical theology lay, he contended, in its apophatic character, which he defined as the understanding that God is radically unknowable in human, thus philosophical, terms. Consequently, God's special revelation in Scripture must be preserved in all of its integrity by means of the distinction between the ineffable divine essence and the inaccessible nature of the Holy Trinity, on the one hand, and the positive revelation of the Trinitarian energies, on the other. "When we speak of the Trinity in itself," said Lossky, "we are confessing, in our poor and always defective human language, the mode of existence of the Father, Son, and Holy Spirit, one sole God who cannot but be Trinity, because He is the living God of Revelation, Who, though unknowable, has made Himself known, through the incarnation of the Son, to all who have received the Holy Spirit, Who proceeds from the Father and is sent into the world in the name of the incarnate Son." The Trinitarian processions in revelation thus produce the energies which human beings experience as grace and by which they are sanctified or "deified." In his Mystical Theology he argued that the theologians of the undivided Church understood that theosis was above knowledge."

[205] Schaef, A.W. 1992. *Beyond Therapy, Beyond Science*. New York, NY: HarperCollins, p. 205.

Francis Collins draws exactly from his work on the Human Genome Project interesting considerations on a) human nature, b) the divine origin of evolution, genetic (sub)structure of creation (including us humans), and c) moral law (as perceived by us humans) and altruism. In discussing the position of Richard Dawkins in this matter, he writes:

> "The major and inescapable flaw of Dawkin's claim that science demands atheism is that it goes beyond the evidence. If God is outside of nature, then science can neither prove nor disprove His existence. Atheism itself must therefore be considered a form of blind faith, in that it adopts a belief system that cannot be defended on the basis of pure reason (not necessarily in Kantian terms –A/N). [...] Science cannot be used to justify discounting the great monotheistic religions of the world, which rest upon centuries of history, moral philosophy, and the powerful evidence provide by human altruism. It is the height of scientific hubris to claim otherwise. If the existence of God is true (not just tradition, but actually true), and if certain scientific conclusions about the natural world are also true (not just in fashion, but objectively true), then they cannot contradict each other. A fully harmonious synthesis must be possible."[206]

We should follow Collins's effort in addressing the imprecise notions of faith throughout history and in very recent times, for instance the one offered by Mark Twain ("Faith is believing what you know ain't so"),[207] Sigmund Freud ("the belief in God is just wishful thinking")[208] and the one by Dawkins ([Faith is] "blind trust, in the absence of evidence, even in the teeth of evidence").[209] We previously addressed the conceptual implication of the term "Faith", and its relationship with a form of "jumping into the unknown" somewhat required, or at least felt, when discussing issues beyond visible science. But this is not, and ought not to be, a "God of the gaps"-type of argument. Furthermore, the emphasis on "powerful evidence" should be discussed even more when "forcing" discoveries (or perceived discoveries) in cutting-edge neuroscientific research onto argumentations for the ontology of (human) ethics, especially if by "research" we simply mean technological advancement, which is (again) not

---

[206]   Collins, F.S. 2006. *The Language of God. A Scientist presents Evidence for Belief.* New York, NY: Free Press Simon & Schuster, pp. 165–169.

[207]   As quoted in Collins, F.S. 2006. *The Language of God. A Scientist presents Evidence for Belief.* New York, NY: Free Press Simon & Schuster, pp. 164.

[208]   As quoted in Collins, F.S. 2006. *The Language of God. A Scientist presents Evidence for Belief.* New York, NY: Free Press Simon & Schuster, pp. 162. In this regard, we should go back once again to the analysis of the term "to wish (oneself)" and its Germanic relative (German) "*(sich) wünschen*" when discussing human mind, especially in consideration of disciplines such as psychiatry, theology, mythology, and anthropology.

[209]   As quoted in Collins, F.S. 2006. *The Language of God. A Scientist presents Evidence for Belief.* New York, NY: Free Press Simon & Schuster, pp. 164.

synonym of knowledge and/or science (and not even scientific progress in some cases):

> "We are unreserved champions of neurotechnological progress. We are certain that brain imaging techniques and other exciting developments in neuroscience will further elucidate the relationship between the brain and the mind. [...] As we've seen, the illuminated brain cannot be trusted to offer an unfiltered view of the mind. Nor is it logical to regard behavior as beyond an individual's control simply because the associated neural mechanisms can be shown to be in the brain."[210]

Interestingly, the authors talk about an "illuminated brain". All the references to a spiritual, as well as historical and social interpretation of the term "illuminated" cannot but makes us more aware of the complexity of the issue. Does this form of "Enlightenment" of empirical, observable, evidence-based, rational (perhaps an oxymoron in this context, especially since we expect rationality to be based, perhaps even located, in our brain) "*nirvana*" constitute "proof of evidence"? Does it tell us more about our behavior, perception, and values? Bunge writes:

> "As for the harmful effect of certain philosophies on medicine [...] a particular effective offender has been the functionalist view of the mind, that usually comes along with the opinion that everything mental is only information processing, hence equally realizable in brains, computers, or even immaterial souls. This philosophical school ignores neuroscience and discourages experiment, while encouraging wild speculation, like that of the self-styled evolutionary psychologists. By the same token, these fantasists have retarded the development of effective psychiatric treatments"[211].

Although Bunge's statement help us frame the problem, putting (material, physical, biological) brains, computers[212] and immaterial souls in the same

---

[210] Satel, S., Lilienfeld, S.O. 2013. *Brainwashed. The seductive appeal of Mindless Neuroscience*. New York, NY: Basic Books, pp. 149–150.

[211] Bunge, M. 2013. *Medical Philosophy. Conceptual Issues in Medicine*, Singapore: World Scientific Publishing, p. 43. However, Bunge appropriately admits that "we exist on several levels" (Ibid., p. 37).

[212] Interestingly, Bunge writes also that "Except for the marginal school of artificial life in Santa Fe, USA, whose members believe that their computer models are alive, no one believes that organisms are machines, if only because machines, unlike living things, are designed" (Ibid., p. 36). We partially agree with this statement; however we don't subscribe the reasoning justification as its basis. The discussion on the "design" of living things, and the world, the universe in general, is quite more complex than a single statement, which in the end, is based solely on personal opinion. In regard to our cosmos, the Argentinean philosopher writes: "[...] some cosmologist speculate about the creation of the universe out of nothing, or even about the coexistence of many mutually disconnected universes, but these unscientific fantasies are seldom taken seriously because they do not connect with any empiri-

category is a quite reductionist and imprecise summary. Confuting the position of Sam Harris "The more we understand ourselves at the level of the brain, the more we will see that there are right and wrong answers to questions of human values,"[213] Satel and Lilienfeld state that neuroscience is very useful in addressing and answering (from the scientific point of view) questions of neural processes in moral decision making, but it does not focus on the ethical aspects of these decisions: "[...] it is not at all evident how such discoverable facts could ever constitute a prescription for how things should be."[214] Note the language here: first of all we talk about "evidence", a term that, once again, brings us back to the basic concepts of Medical Philosophy and of science in general, as well as (human) perception. Secondly, we follow one of the first mandatory requirements for scientific research: facts have to be "discoverable" –the principle of falsifiability follows quite naturally– together with the (understood by some, misunderstood or completely rejected by others, as we have seen) scientific "faith" in the possibility of finding a result.

Given these premises, we could infer that in this process of "illuminating" the brain, we are attempting to shed more light on the very connection between the entire series of concepts mind-brain-body-soul-spirit, in the sense that, from a purely logical point of view, as well from a correct theoretical analysis of our scientific method in this area of medicine, we cannot simply avoid dimensions beyond the physically evident. The mind-body problem, as well as the focus on embodied cognition can be even better understood, if not partially solved, by realizing that Western medicine, in particular psychiatry and psychology is not only ethnocentric (as we previously discussed), but is also "cognicentric" or "pragmacentric".[215] In fact, from a (Western, evidence-based) scientific perspective, psychiatry does not distinguish between delusions, hallucinations, non-rational ideation etc., and mystical experiences, spiritual "calling", and non-ordinary states of consciousness. Although technically in a dif-

---

cal data" (Ibid., p. 132). Again, we should probably refrain from jumping to conclusions based on approximation, with no real and honest cause-effect relation to scientific research (including the theory of the Big Bang). Furthermore, talking about "empirical data" in regard to the universe in general, presents, from a theoretical as well as from an applied science-related perspective, a series of problems that need to be better addressed.

[213]   As quoted in Satel, S., Lilienfeld, S.O. 2013. *Brainwashed. The seductive appeal of Mindless Neuroscience.* New York, NY: Basic Books, p. 150.

[214]   Ibid., p. 152

[215]   Terms used by Stanislav Grof in: Grof, S. 1998. *Rethinking Basic Assumptions about Psychology and Psychiatry: The Role of Spirituality and Nonordinary States of Consciousness.* In: Bassman, L. 1998. *The Whole Mind: The Definitive Guide to Complementary Treatment for Mind, Mood, and Emotion.* Novato, CA: New World Library, p. 45.

ferent context (which we still consider related) we cannot avoid but to remember the famous quote by Vygotsky: "Inner speech is speech for oneself; external speech is speech for others".[216]

According to Grof, this is where our modern "psychospiritual crises" originates: people who *experience* these states, *suffer* these states according to modern medicine; these manifestations (a term that suggests a vast array of metaphysical and theological interpretations), these symptoms don't need to be fully experienced, perceived, embraced. On the contrary, they need to be suppressed or possibly annihilated. Modern medicine and modern science "emphasize experience rather than talk",[217] a process recently questioned by disciplines such as Narrative Medicine. In fact, we should note her that outside time and space of modern, post-industrial, post-Age of Enlightenment, Western culture, the healing process always involved a spiritual, mystical dimension based on Nonordinary states of consciousness.[218] In this sense the healer, the therapist is the one who does indeed "attend and assist in the healing process." This point of view is almost completely ignored in modern medicine, especially in dealing with human mind-body (forgotten or simply reduced in materialistic albeit imprecise cause-effect terms) connection. On one side we have a biologically analyzed evidence-based data (however wrong this version of *Bios* might be), on the other a systematic, symbolic, introspective as well as transpersonal exploration of the human nature, starting from the psyche. However, since this side of the equation is not "truly" observable with the means of

---

[216]   Vygotsky, L.S. 1962. *Thought and Language*. Cambridge, MA: MIT Press., p. 225

[217]   Grof, S. 1998. *Rethinking Basic Assumptions about Psychology and Psychiatry: The Role of Spirituality and Nonordinary States of Consciousness*. In: Bassman, L. 1998. *The Whole Mind: The Definitive Guide to Complementary Treatment for Mind, Mood, and Emotion*. Novato, CA: New World Library, p. 45.

[218]   The opposite of leaving room for this more open, holistic, even spiritual interpretation (and value) is Iatrogenesis, as defined by Illich: "Social iatrogenesis is at work when health care is turned into a standardized item, a staple; when all suffering is "hospitalised" and homes become inhospitable to birth, sickness, and death; when the language in which people could experience their bodies is turned into bureaucratic gobbledygook; or when suffering, mourning, and healing outside the patient role are labelled a form of deviance". Illich, I. 1976. *Limits to Medicine; Medical Nemesis: The Expropriation of Health*. London, UK: Marion Boyars Publishers, p. 41. The author continues: "Iatrogenesis is clinical when pain, sickness, and death result from medical care; it is social when health policies reinforce an industrial organization that generates ill-health; it is cultural and symbolic when medically sponsored behavior and delusions restrict the vital autonomy of people by undermining their competence in growing up, caring for each other, and aging, or when medical intervention cripples personal responses to pain, disability, impairment, anguish, and death." Ibid. pp. 270–271.

evidence-based science, this represents (and presents, shows) a limitation defining our "real", physical (material) nature. Grof writes:

> "According to the Newtonian-Cartesian paradigm of traditional Western science, these restrictions and limitations are absolutely mandatory and definitive, since they result from the material nature of the world and are determined by physiological laws of perception. However, modern consciousness research has clearly demonstrated that in transpersonal experiences these limitations do not apply and can be transcended. This represents a critical challenge not only for psychiatry and psychology, but for the entire philosophy of Western science."[219]

c) Explanation of the goal

The aforementioned considerations, together with analysis of the psychological background in comparison to the science and practice of medicine, help us reach our target, and provide further explanation of the theoretical model we are investigating. The ultimate goal is, once more, the analysis of a possible combination of evidence-based medicine and a patient-centered medicine, in which the human being (both provider *and* patient) brings important knowledge and interpretative elements to the discussion. From this standpoint, our efforts are similar to the ones found in positive psychology, as discussed by Waterman:

> "From a eudaimonist perspective, making life decisions is not an arbitrary undertaking, nor is it a function of being shaped by the contingencies of one's social milieu. Rather, it is each person's process of discovering their latent talents, strengths, and inclinations and bringing these to fruition. This is reflected in two famous classical injunctions: *Know thyself* and *Become what you are*."[220]

We are therefore investigating the possible existence (and related levels, both in qualitative and quantitative sense and means) of correlations between (self) perception and (self) understanding and sense of meaning and purpose [one own's as well as (one own's) life], especially since there are important ontological considerations in every analysis of meaning. For example, the circle of significance according to which every understanding always (still, already, yet)

---

[219]   Ibid., p. 47
[220]   Waterman, A.S. 2013. *The Humanistic Psychology-Positive Psychology Divide. Contrasts in Philosophical Foundations*. In *American Psychologist*. Vol. 68, Num. 3: 123–196 Washington, DC: APA, pp. 127.

projects a meaning.[221] As we previously discussed, both health and illness are connected to a multilayered structure of signifiers and actors on/in human life, and we want to explore the possibility of a multilayered system of different/diverse paths/pathways to reach a condition of internal/external as well as interior/exterior equilibrium, sense of belonging, sense of wholeness, of completeness, of contentedness, of relation, inclination, connection, and similia. Certainly, we also want to understand to what extend we can infer general ideas on absolute, universal (systems of) values versus a specific individual and subjective pattern of action and interaction. Since our research is both qualitative as well as quantitative, we need to be very careful in formulating our questions, and thereby providing solid data to support our claims. As we discussed in the previous chapters, there are still some unknown, perhaps unknowable, parameters of analysis in searching for a definitive answer to questions on human nature. Nevertheless, we believe that we could reach an increased therapeutic success by following a mature (developed, perfected) combination of:

a) A thoughtful theoretico-philosphical analysis of cognitive processes, clinical/medical reasoning, diagnostic/prognosis, scientific method, evidence-based research, therapeutic intervention and patient-provider interaction/communication;

b) A series of multiple philosophical positions and approaches, including ontological, epistemological-theoretical, phenomenological, hermeneutic, and dialectical (not just in a Platonic/Socratic and Hegelian methodology, but also in the –applied– psychological sense of CBT, DBT, and REBT), as well as more metaphysical[222] considerations;

c) A comparative analysis of different scientific perspectives and (statistical, epidemiological, lab-testing) methods: A double-blind, random-

---

[221] It is Gadamer's *circle's positive significance*. See Gadamer. H.-G. 1960. *Wahrheit und Methode. Grundzüge einer philosophischen Hermeneutik*. Tübingen, D: Mohr Siebeck [Unveränd. Nachdr. d. 3. erw. Aufl. Tübingen 1975].

[222] For instance the relationship between different stages, layers of knowledge, including (but not limited to) a general, non-denominational and (on purpose) not better defined form of gnosis, theosis and a non-specific *third way*. This is especially important since we are dealing with existential questions related to the sense of meaning and purpose in life, including the presence/absence of God. Therefore, every parameter of guide/guidance, freedom of will, God as omnipotent and/or/versus good, and the whole spectrum "Thy will be done" to "Thou what thou wilt" should be included in our analysis. Moreover, from Gadamer's standpoint in comparison-contrast with Heidegger, the transcendental ground is not in *Dasein*'s understanding of *Being* but in the ontological difference between singularity-individuality-essence and plurality-identification-objectivity/objectivization, or between *being* and *beings*.

ized clinical trial would be "the perfect choice in a perfect[223] world"; however, because of the very nature of this study and the ultimate goals of our analysis, this "golden standard" is not entirely feasible or, better stated, not enough.[224] To be sure, since our target goes beyond (or further, deeper) what is generally considered "valid" from the perspective of medical science/art/technique-technology[225], we want to make sure to include in our discussion another comparison, namely: 1) Evidence-Based Medicine vs. 2) Evidence-Informed Medicine vs. 3) Patient-Centered Medicine, in particular from the viewpoint of *Erfahrung* v. *Erlebnis*.[226]

Certainly, the discussion on inductive/deductive/abductive observation and reasoning versus introspection[227] and metaphysical method is another focal point of our debate, but we surely do not want to preclude the possibilities of alternate/alternative validity of opposite approaches on the base of different settings and situations. We decided to conduct an empirical research, albeit focused on a specific target more meaningful according to the very nature of the study,[228] to open up a broader view on those issues, realizing that limiting our discussion on one specific method would also impact, in terms of *limitation* the philosophical validity of our results. In fact, we could draw inferences from Gadamer's *sensus communis*, based in taking the infinite variety of circumstances into account.[229] Moreover, the aesthetic, which is perceptive and proprioceptive,[230] consciousness and representation[231] is essential in the analy-

---

[223] Again, "perfect" in the etymological-conceptual sense directly derived from the Lat. *perficiō*.

[224] Also considering the effects of *Wirkungsgeschichte* and (forced, unavoidable) contextualization of method. This is even more important in the consideration of effect/affect of placebo/nocebo mechanisms of action (if such definition makes sense at all).

[225] Including narrative and interpretative parameters.

[226] Thus bringing the ontological shift of hermeneutics as influenced by applied linguistics, mythology, symbolism, and semantics, from consideration around the *Logos – Verbum*, all the way to Lévi-Strauss, through Chomsky, etc.

[227] From the beginnings of the history of psychology, to the debate on the limitations of reflective philosophy.

[228] Namely, our choice of conducting the research in a psychiatric department in a hospital setting.

[229] Gadamer. H.-G. 1960. *Wahrheit und Methode. Grundzüge einer philosophischen Hermeneutik.* Tübingen, D: Mohr Siebeck [Unveränd. Nachdr. d. 3. erw. Aufl. Tübingen 1975].

[230] Also from a generally neurological, neuro-afferent-pathway, and functional mapping of the sensorimotor cortex perspective, especially considering the most cutting-edge research in perceptual transmission and coding in the brain, which involves multiple areas, as well as

sis of value and impact of subjective aspects onto the possible generalization of the data collected and phenomena examined, in particular due to the nature of our survey, which is ultimately patient-centered, since the questions are directly asked, albeit under the premises of anonymous, non-traceable information.

---

areas previously thought as not related to (that) specific function, as in the case of visual representation in blind people on different areas of the cerebral cortex.

[231] As well as temporality, both in the sense presented by Gadamer, as well through the analysis of embodied cognition parameters. Furthermore, a special place in our debate is represented by Dilthey's viewpoint on the conflict between science and life-philosophy in the analysis of historical consciousness. See Dilthey, W. 1883. *Einleitung in die Geisteswissenschaften. Versuch einer Grundlegung für das Studium der Gesellschaft und der Geschichte*. Bd. 1., Leipzig, D: Duncker & Humblot.

Chapter 4
The patient at the center of therapy

4.1 Patient's communication, perception and self-perception

We are approaching the central part of this volume, and we are ready to start discussing the core concept of perception from the perspective of the patient. In fact, the way a patient interacts with himself and the environment, especially the treatment team, is a fundamentally important part of Medical Philosophy. Communication between patient and physician is a core issue, as evidenced for instance by a study conducted by Dominick Frosch.[232] The research found that patients, regardless of their level of education, often feel intimidated when communicating with their physician, especially due to the fear of potential future negative consequences in their care as result of disagreements.[233] Lack of proper communication and misunderstandings contribute to problems that affect the whole spectrum of patients' care, including patients' tendency to "decline elective surgeries and diseases screenings that could lead to risks from false positives and unnecessary interventions."[234] On the other side, Palliative Care and Advance Care Planning represent a fertile ground for investigating the role of physicians in communicating medical information. Recent studies have shown that, on average, there is a 500% of prognostic overestimation in life expectancy as communicated in person to patients by physicians in the United States of America.[235] Recently, the focus of Medical Colleges throughout the United States has been the improvement of communication, as well as diagnostic perception, in particular through an open and honest dialogue between patient and primary care provider: "[...] both people are bringing different perspectives and skills and levels of communication. If you only focus on

---

[232] Dominick Frosch of the Palo Alto Medical Foundation's Research Institute and University of California, Los Angeles, Research conducted in 2012.

[233] Study discussed in Weir, K. 2012. *Improving patient-physician communication.* Monitor on Psychology, Vol. 43, N.10, Washington, DC.: American Psychological Association, p. 38.

[234] Ibid.

[235] Macauley, B. 2014. *Setting the Stage: The ethical imperative for advance care planning.* University of Vermont College of Medicine / Vermont Ethics Network Annual conference 'Advance Care Planning: It's Always Too soon... Until It's Too Late'. Fairlee, VT.

one of the two people, you may be missing an important piece."[236] Better communication skills are therefore required in medical advice. We surely understand the difference, in terms of prognostic response, between these two formulations of the same question: "Doctor x, would you be surprised if patient y will die within a year from now?" and "Doctor x, how much do you think patient y has left to die?" Certainly, we still need to ask ourselves how much of the paternalistic attitude is still present in modern medicine. Traditionally, medicine has not always been prone to be open to disclose information,[237] as we observe in one of the founding fathers of medicine, Hippocrates, who gave this advice to the "perfect physician":

> "Perform your medical duties calmly and adroitly, concealing most things from the patient while you are attending to him. Give necessary orders with cheerfulness and sincerity, turning his attention away from what is being done to him; sometimes reprove sharply and sometimes comfort with solicitude and attention, revealing nothing of the patient's future or present condition, for many patients through this course have taken a turn for the worse."[238]

In this sense, appropriate models of patient-physician relationships always swing between two opposite poles, beneficence and autonomy which, together with non-maleficence and justice constitute the core principles of biomedical ethics. In fact, we should investigate the patient's ability to understand certain given information, making sure that we draw a line between such ability (including voluntariness, the ability of making decisions) and capacity. Certainly, in order to do that we need to make sure we understand the relation between concepts such as autonomy, happiness, and morality, especially from a philosophical perspective. In a theoretical comparison between Aristotle and Kant,[239] morality is not properly the doctrine of how we may make ourselves happy, but how we may make ourselves worthy of happiness. This is where patient self-perception plays the main role, especially when we include a stoic perspective on life's ultimate purpose, a complete happiness achieved through

---

[236]   Kelly Haskard-Zolnierek of Texas State University, as quoted in Weir, K. 2012. *Improving patient-physician communication.* Monitor on Psychology, Vol. 43, N.10, Washington, DC.: American Psychological Association, p. 38.

[237]   A very good read in this regard is "Nazi Medicine and the Nuremberg Trials. From Medical War Crimes to Informed Consent" by Paul Julian Weindling. For further reference, please see Bibliography.

[238]   Jones W, ed. 1923. *Hippocrates With an English Translation.* Hippocrates. Decorum XVI. ed., Vol. 2. London, UK: Heineman.

[239]   Bliss, S. 2014. *Decision-Making Capacity, Autonomy and Voluntariness.* Vermont Ethics Network Annual conference Advance Care Planning: It's Always Too soon...Until It's Too Late. Fairlee, VT.

a life lived according to ethical and rational principles, including self-reflection, self-perception, and inner and outer virtue. To be sure, this self-perception is directly linked to the relationship between patient's ability for autonomy and capacity for autonomy. Within the ability for autonomy we should list the ability of the person (in this case, the patient) to express and/or make her/his own decisions based on personal (individual) chosen (albeit within a specific cultural framework) principles, values, and goals. This is what we call a respective ability, in comparison to a prospective form of ability, which is simply abiding by conclusions and decisions made, therefore a contract (which needs to take into account the process as in a voluntary consent), like the one between patient and primary care provider. Furthermore, this Ability for Autonomy has a qualitative component and represents voluntariness. On the other side, the capacity for autonomy is quantitative in nature, and needs to follow the four basics of informed consent: understand and communicate; appreciation of and for the decision at hand; reason through risk, benefit and alternative; and choice, made free of coercion or undue influence.[240] Thus the perception of patient and provider determines the autonomy and the ability to find ways to improve shared decision making, especially when dealing with important medical issues such as end-of-life discussion. As an example, we quote a study conducted by Wright, which showed that only 37% of US patients with average survival of 4 months reported having had a discussion about end-of-life issues with physician.[241] Another American study showed that 95% of hospitalized oncology patients believe it is important to have discussions about advance directives/end-of-life care, while only 45% of them have these discussions.[242] Furthermore, on average between 80% and 90% of US patients want information about their prognosis.[243] Patient's perception of clinical information, as necessary for autonomous medical and care-related decision making is corroborated by the combination of four distinct and yet

[240] Ibid.
[241] Wright, A.A. 2008. *End-of-Life Care Discussions in Patients With Advanced Cancer*. Journal of Clinical Oncology, JCO.2008.49.6562.
[242] Dow, L.A. 2009. *Paradoxes in Advance Care Planning: The Complex Relationship of Oncology Patients, Their Physicians, and Advance Medical Directives*. JCO January 10, 2010.28 no. 2 299–304. Another study by Mack (Annals of Internal Medicine, 2012) also showed that 87% of patients who died had end-of-life discussion reported or documented.
[243] Block, S. 2014. *Communication in Serious Illness. Serious Care Program*. Harvard Medical School Center for Palliative Care, Dana-Farber Cancer Institute, Brigham and Women's Hospital, Ariadne Labs, Vermont Ethics Network Annual conference Advance Care Planning: It's Always Too soon... Until It's Too Late. Fairlee, VT.

interconnect areas: medical indications, individual preferences, quality of life, and contextual features.[244] According to Jonsen, Siegler, and Winslade,[245] Medical indications focus on: diagnosis, prognosis, medical history, level of problem (acute, chronic, critical, emergent, reversible), goals and options of treatment, probabilities of success, general care and future/alternative plans in case of therapeutic failure. Within Individual preferences we identify problems related to competent decision-making in terms of capacity/incapacity and ability/inability, informed consent, substituted judgment, surrogate and best interests. Quality of life asks questions related to medical and clinical areas, as well as existential and meaning-related perspectives, comparing the status quo to past and future (hypothetical, discussed, planned) clinical and living situation. Finally, Contextual features deals with financial, legal, social, and religious aspects of care. These perspectives are well taken in consideration in the models of physician-patient relationship as offered by Emanuel and Emanuel,[246] as shown in the following figure:

---

[244] For the complete description, please refer to: Jonsen, A., Siegler, M., and Winslade, W. 2002. *Clinical ethics: a practical approach to ethical decisions in clinical medicine*. New York, NY: McGraw-Hill.

[245] Ibid.

[246] Emanuel E.J., and Emanuel, L.L. 1992. *Four Models of the Physician-Patient Relationship*. JAMA. 1992; 267(16): 2221–2226.

	Informative	Interpretative	Deliberative	Paternalistic
Patient values	Defined, fixed, and known to the patient	Inchoate and conflicting, requiring elucidation	Open to development and revision through moral discussion	Objective and shared by the physician and patient
Physician's obligation	Providing relevant factual information and implementing patient's selected intervention	Elucidating and interpreting relevant patient values as well as informing the patient and implementing the patient's selected intervention	Articulating and persuading the patient of the most admirable values as well as informing the patient and implementing the patient's selected intervention	Promoting the patient's well-being independent of the patient's current preferences
Conception of patient's autonomy	Choice of, and control over, medical care	Self-understanding relevant to medical care	Moral self-development relevant to medical care	Assenting to objective values
Conception of physician's role	Competent technical expert	Counselor or advisor	Friend or teacher	Guardian

Table 1.   The model of physician-patient relationship in *Four Models of the Physician-Patient Relationship*, by Emanuel E.J., and Emanuel, L.L. (1992).

Certainly, within "Conception of physician's role" we could include a figure akin to the one of a philosopher.[247] The question regarding self-perception and self analysis is one of the most important topics not only in contemporary philosophical research, but also from the perspectives of the cutting-edge studies in the realm of neuroscience and developmental psychology. Furthermore, from a historical perspective, the cultural and conceptual shift in the view on man and his relationship with the world in the XV and XVI centuries created an instrumental rationalization of society; from means to ends. This approach was indeed present also before the European Renaissance, for instance in the specifics of the Roman law. How can man really understand himself? Does this question even make sense? We have to ask ourselves, where are the foundations of the assumption of a potential premise to knowledge; *id est* the abil-

---

[247]   In particular, when it comes to decision-making related activities, which present a strong theoretical-philosophical component. Mario Bunge suggests we should eliminate decision theory from medicine "just as it has been expelled from all other fields where it has been tried (Bunge, M. 2013. *Medical Philosophy. Conceptual Issues in Medicine*. Singapore: World Scientific Publishing, p. 172 – See also his discussion on Bayesian theorem and application). However, here we are confusing terms. To be sure, decision theory always works at a given point in time, with the amount of (scientific) knowledge at a (the same) given point in time.

ity to know the answer to these questions. Thus, we have to take into consideration the specifics of philosophical research from both analytical and continental perspectives. The main difference between the two currents would be that analytic philosophy is rather based on a logical analysis, scientific and rational that focuses on the details, while continental philosophy would deal with most of the major concepts in their entirety and interpersonal component and would indeed be more skeptical about the ability of cognitive science. In recent decades though, a demarcation between "analytic" and "continental" tradition, its conceptual premises, methodology and reasons is questioned and criticized.[248] "Continental" is, according to some scholars, an increasingly meaningless label: much of what philosophers do on the European Continent these days is "analytic" philosophy or historical scholarship. In this regard, Brian Leiter states that:

> "While a small minority of philosophers in the U.S. still use the label "Continental philosophy" to demarcate whatever someone suitably obscure has done in Paris recently, the label is best-reserved as a characterization for a group of important historical figures largely in Germany and France in the 19th and 20th centuries; in that respect, the label is much like the labels "medieval philosophy" or "early modern." And as with these other historical groupings, there are some overlapping thematic affinities among the figures so designated, but there are also discontinuities and in some cases profound differences (e.g., Husserl has more in common with Frege than with Nietzsche, and Habermas increasingly has more in common with Rawls than Marx)"[249]

In analyzing the potential approach to a deeper and more accurate evaluation of the characteristics and specific values and weights of self –also in relation to a "post-modern instrumental rationality", which has dominated a more traditional (both from the historical, as well as conceptual viewpoint) value rationality[250]—we should still ask ourselves whether the study of man and society could ever achieve the status of scientific knowledge. Furthermore, regardless if we consider the status of "social science" (in the pure epistemological sense) as "desirable by" and "within the scope of" this analysis of self, we still have to deal with what has been defined by Anthony Giddens as a "double hermeneu-

---

[248]   Fornero, Giovanni; Tassinari, Salvatore: *Le filosofie del novecento*, ed. Bruno Mondadori, 2006, p. 1392–1398.

[249]   Leiter Brian, *The Philosophical Gourmet Report*, Blackwell Ed. 2008, introduction.

[250]   Flyvbjerg, Bent, *Aristotle, Foucault and Progressive Phronesis: Outline of an Applied Ethics for Sustainable Development*; in: Winkler, Earl R. & Coombs Jerold R., *Applied Ethics*, Blackwell Publishers, Cambridge 1993, p. 12.

tic".[251] We have to understand the specific features of natural and social sciences, which are –according to Giddens– distinct. In the realm of natural science, the understanding is focused on the structure of the natural world as an object (single hermeneutic). In contrast to natural sciences, the social sciences study people and society, which represent both studying subject and studied object. Based on this point of view, there is a very important distinction between subject and object. The analysis, provided by Nietzsche,[252] of the very separation between man *and* the world as an "incisive diagnosis of humanism's arrogant premise":

> The whole attitude of 'man versus the world', man as world-denying principle, man as the standard of the value of things, as judge of the world, who in the end puts existence itself on his scales and finds it too light – the monstrous impertinence of this attitude has dawned upon us as such, and has disgusted us – we now laugh when we find 'Man and world' placed beside one another, separated by the sublime presumption of the little word 'and'!"[253]

This perspective also applies to man's attempt to separate himself from a "higher self", often channeled into religion or (as noted by Feuerbach as well) scientific rationalism of the Enlightenment, especially when including debates such as the one around man's insight as "penetrating mental vision or discernment; faculty of seeing into inner character or underlying truth, and understanding of relationships and motivational forces."[254] Nietzsche in particular rejects the idea of an objective reality that simply presents itself to us, and states that our perception of this reality is fundamentally shaped by culture, in particular through language.[255] He continues by saying that there aren't any objects which can be considered "uninterpreted". Thus, there is no absolute, universal, self-justifying, neutral reality we can study, analyze or discover. Therefore, we have to keep an adequate account of subjectivity or consciousness within the realm of science. For Nietzsche, the western metaphysical tradition is engaged in a sophisticates but futile attempt to distort reality to the point that the belief in any rational though guided by the principle of causality

---

[251] See Giddens, A. 1984. *The Constitution of Society. Outline of a Theory of Structuration*, Oakland, CA: The University of California Press.

[252] Nietzsche, F. *Gay Science*, pr. 346, quoted in: Allison, D.B. 1997, *The New Nietzsche*, p. xix and in: West, David, *An Introduction to Continental Philosophy*, Cambridge : Polity Press, 1997.

[253] Ibid.

[254] Bliss, S. 2014. *Decision-Making Capacity, Autonomy and Voluntariness*. Vermont Ethics Network Annual conference Advance Care Planning: It's Always Too soon...Until It's Too Late. Fairlee, VT.

[255] See Nehamas, A. 1985. *Nietzsche: Life as Literature*, Cambridge: Harvard University Press.

and able to understand the concept of "Being" is an illusion.[256] In this sense we understand how the German philosopher considered the Christian values as the victory of the mediocre man over an earlier aristocratic mentality. In particular, he focused on the specific "self" within a specific tradition, culture and ethnicity, with a special attention to Europe and its northerner and southerner components, according to him best expressed in the "Germanic" and "Italic" spirit. He defined the "Italic character" as "the finest" for its ability to be able to express wittily and with paradoxes, "the richest" for creativity and variety of urban settings and architectures, and the "most free" from metaphysical and religious constraints.[257] Nietzsche is thus comparing the Italian "self" to the German one, seeing in the latter an obscurantism and a moralism that arose with Luther's attempts to "prevail over Rome" and is still permeating the modern age.[258] In this regard he also believed that Protestant theology was even worse than the Catholic Church, recognizing that the "Mediterranean mentality" of southern European peoples had its roots in Greek philosophy of the Hellenic period, with its openness to aphorisms and paradoxes, as well as an indulgence towards the passions and instincts.[259] The ethnic component of these statements, for some also viewed as ethno*centric*, leads us to the consideration of environmental influences on the concept of self. Certainly, in his analysis of man, Nietzsche is opposed to the historicism of Marx and Engels; the point of existence lies in the moment, the present experience, thus even the sense of self is better understood through the lenses of *hic et nunc*. Furthermore, and in regard to the statements above, the main focus of man's life could be identified in the cultural, intellectual and personal achievement. This is especially the case of exceptional individuals, who might never be surpassed even in a diachronic sense. Furthermore, Nietzsche advocates race mixture as a stimulus for the development of culture. In this sense, the so-called "Master Race" is an internationally mixed race of philosophers and artists who cultivate an "iron self-control."[260]

---

[256]   West, D. 1996 *Friedrich Nietzsche,* in: *An Introduction to Continental Philosophy,* Blackwell Publishers, Cambridge 1, p. 130–132.

[257]   Perniola, M. 2011. *Introduzione a L'Anticristo,* (Introduction to 'the Antichrist') in: Nietzsche. Roma: Edizioni integrali, Newton, p. 7.

[258]   Ibid., p. 13.

[259]   Ibid., p. 15. See also Vitale, Edoardo. 2005. *Il viaggio di Nietzsche nel Suditalia,* Napoli: L'Alfiere.

[260]   West, D. 1996. *Friedrich Nietzsche,* in: *An Introduction to Continental Philosophy,* Cambridge, UK: Blackwell Publishers.

Culture, race, ethnicity, history and external environment: when we refer to the concept of "self", are we talking about the same thing? We should probably understand the differences, not just in etymological terms, but also in the realm of practical application, between concepts such as "individual", "person", and certainly "Being". Are we allowed to apply the same distinction between *Sosein* and *Dasein* in geographical, cultural and linguistic areas which don't belong to the German(ic) tradition? For example, it is very interesting that the German word for smart, intelligent is the adjective *klug*, while the very concept of *Klugheit* is translated as φρόνησις. Thus, the very conceptualization of knowledge is based on an omnicomprehensive view of Aristotle's views on episteme, techne and phronesis.[261] Hegel suggested that we should all taking into consideration the particular feature of culture and language in studying the self, which is better expressed through the *Volksgeist*.[262] In this sense we understand how he and Herder were skeptical of Enlightenment assumptions of a universal human nature. If human self and human being are deeply connected, and if the self is not universal, what can we say about the individual? Is the individual really indivisible or there are several parts of the self (several selves?) which are contributing to the image that one has of self, or that others have of him? According to Sartre, "man is nothing else but that which he makes of himself,"[263] but "the absolute truth is one's immediate sense of one's self,"[264] which in turn is the same as "the sense of others' selves," especially since I cannot obtain any truth about myself, except through the mediation of others.[265] If these assumptions are true, how can we objectivize ourselves and become an observable, a thinkable 'thing'? Beyond the etymological speculation on the closeness between those two terms, we could remember the principles of Thomas von Erfurt, who stated that between thought and thing lies an abyss of difference, better expressed as "heterogeneity", but we also find ho-

---

[261] Flyvbjerg, B. 1993. *Aristotle, Foucault and Progressive Phronesis: Outline of an Applied Ethics for Sustainable Development*; in: Winkler, Earl R. & Coombs Jerold R., *Applied Ethics*, Cambridge, UK: Blackwell Publishers, p. 13.

[262] In this regard, similar considerations apply to the term *Heimat*, expressing a concept which ultimately presents difficulties in translation, especially in English and modern Romance languages.

[263] Sartre, J-P. 1997. *Existentialism and Humanism*, translation and introduction by P. Mairet, Brooklyn, NY: Haskell House Publishers, p. 28.

[264] Ibid., p. 40.

[265] Ibid., p. 46.

mogeneity, or common ground.[266] Does this mean that we can create a bridge between ourselves and the thought, the image, perhaps the *idea* we have of ourselves? According to Thomas von Erfurt, this bridge is called "analogy". Where is the connection, if we could find one, between the analytical method presented and the practice of philosophers of the Continental schools of thought? Certainly, Husserl already made the distinction between the act of intention, of *Noesis* and the content of intention, or *Noema*. We can see how this perspective still reminds of the statements listed above, as well as the phenomenological distinction between *prima intentio* and *second intentio* of Duns Scotus.[267] So is it the same self, who operates this process, or are we talking about something or someone else? According to Heidegger, if we approach a "subject" in order to discover what this subject is, or if we want to comprehend its *Seinsinn*, we must first get into the *Vollzugssinn*, from which alone its Being-Meaning can be derived.[268] Thus, if Heidegger and ontological hermeneutics left an imprint on existentialism, in particular the works by Jean-Paul Sartre, he remains a reference for poststructuralism, deconstruction and postmodernism; as well as a link to the philosophical hermeneutics of Gadamer and Derrida. In particular reference to the historical impact on the analysis and perception of self, Heidegger's view is similar to Hegel's and is also better understood in his perspectives on Enlightenment. A viewpoint shared by Gadamer, who talks about the error of the Enlightenment "prejudice against prejudice" or "the refusal to recognize the significance of our own insertion in a tradition that, at some level, we already understand."[269] Thus we see how the particular, contextual, personal, individual element plays again a major role in our analysis, and the particular filter and perception of reality emphasizes the "effective history" or *Wirkungsgeschichte* that underlies any potential "fusion of horizons" we hope to achieve.[270] So, how can we distinguish between bias and prejudice? According to Gadamer, the concept of prejudice is closely con-

---

[266]   Safranski, R. 1999. *The Outbreak of World War I: Habilitation, War Service and Marriage*, in: *Martin Heidegger. Between Good and Evil*, Harvard University Press, p. 60.

[267]   Ibid., p. 61.

[268]   We could translate *Seinsinn* as "the sense of being", which is indeed also the "meaning" of this being, and in a more extensive and extended way, also the meaning of Being in general, a "Being-meaning". See Safranski, R. 1999. *The Outbreak of World War I: Habilitation, War Service and Marriage*, in: Martin *Heidegger. Between Good and Evil*, Harvard University Press, p. 123.

[269]   Kearney, R.; Rainwater, M. 1996. *Hans-Georg Gadamer* in: *The Continental Philosophy Reader,* New York, NY: Routledge, p. 109.

[270]   Ibid.

nected to the concept of authority,[271] and yet the way our prejudice *works* is finally related to the scope and focus of our analysis. In this sense, and in reaction to the accusation of subjectivism, Gadamer states that "My real concern was and is philosophic: not what we do or what we ought to do, but what happens to us over and above our wanting and doing."[272] The philosopher further expresses this concept:

> "the purpose of [my] investigation is not to offer a general theory of interpretation and a differential account of its methods, but to discover what is common to all modes of understanding and to show that understanding is never subjective behavior toward a given 'object', but towards its effective history – the history of its influence; in other words, understanding belongs to the being of what which is understood."[273]

The concept of effective history is also linked to the analysis of Edmund Husserl, who does appreciate the achievements of theoretical attitude of natural sciences following the tradition of Socrates, Plato and Galileo, but also criticizes the arrogant tendencies of natural scientific reason in the area of moral and cultural value. Thus, philosophy must be free of all presuppositions; a statement better expressed in the assumption and role of modern epistemology: "the content of consciousness represents our only certain knowledge."[274] We could certainly apply this point of view to the subject-object of our analysis, the "self", and understand how all these considerations create a very broad picture of the concept. A view of the very definition of reality and our perception of it can be obtained following the Kantian thought, according to which we can only have knowledge of a phenomenal world as things appear to us. We don't really know if our perception creates just an image of these things – our self included– or we are indeed able to "know" how things are in "themselves". In this sense the very linguistic distinction between semblance and illusion creates a fertile ground for further considerations. The German *Apparenz* is in this sense a mere borrowing from Latin, while *Schein* (as we previously discussed) is the illusion, which is also bringer of light, therefore enlightened vision, knowledge. Thus, even the *Erscheinungen* are testifying not only the presence of our self in this world, but also the value and specific (in-

---

[271] Ibid., p. 115.
[272] Kearney, R. (Ed.) 1998. *Continental Philosophy in the 20th Century*, Routledge History of Philosophy, Volume 8, pp. 295–296.
[273] Ibid., p. 296.
[274] West, D. 1996. *Historicism, Hermeneutics and Phenomenology,* in: *An Introduction to Continental Philosophy*, Cambridge, UK: Blackwell Publishers, p. 89.

dividual, particular) characteristics of our being. Certainly, the concept of value can be quite problematic, especially from the philosophical perspective on (self) perception. According to Talcott Parsons,[275] there are four main (fundamental, structural) variables which build up the map of socially recognized values in modern culture; in particular, the author defines *Action* as formed by values (cultural perspective), norms (social perspective), motivation (as originating in personality), and energy (as produced by the organism). Furthermore, he defines the core concept as the *Unit Act*, involving an actor/agent (in our case patient, physician, or person in general) motivated to action; an end (focus, goal, mission, scope) toward which the previously mentioned action is oriented in order to achieve this goal; a specific situation where this action takes place; and finally norms and values that shape the choice of means to ends. According to Clyde Kluckholm, values possess three dimensions; the affective, the cognitive, and the selective.[276] Generally speaking, human (personal) values incorporate (and/or are generated by) moral and ethical components, qualities, objects and ideas, and can be absolute or relative and serve as a basis for desirable and ethical behavior, action, point of view, worldview and ideology, also from an axiological perspective. From a medical perspective, especially within the framework of end-of-life discussion, value can be expressed as quality over cost. Certainly, there are more complex issues in assessing the results of such equation, especially because both serious and terminal illnesses and care planning are indeed complex processes, involving dimensions of personal, intersubjective, community-related and family-related, cultural, rational, pre-rational, para-rational, and even transcendental and metaphysical value. In fact, a good example comes from human relationships in general, which are "palliative for anxiety, as shown by psychological and medical research, as well as by personal insight."[277] In philosophy, the continental tradition, with its attention to the metaphysical debate around understanding/Verstand and reason/Vernunft helps us contextualize the discussion on the concept of "self" and open the perspectives of methodology and application of

[275]   Marra, R. 2004. *Talcott Parsons. Valori, norme, comportamento deviante*. In: *Materiali per una storia della cultura giuridica*, XXXIV-2, pp. 315–327.

[276]   Hills, M.D. 2002. *Kluckhohn and Strodtbeck's Values OrientationTheory*. Online Readings in Psychology and Culture, 4(4) International Association for Cross-Cultural Psychology.

[277]   Block, S. 2014. *Communication in Serious Illness. Serious Care Program*. Harvard Medical School Center for Palliative Care, Dana-Farber Cancer Institute, Brigham and Women's Hospital, Ariadne Labs, Vermont Ethics Network Annual conference Advance Care Planning: It's Always Too soon… Until It's Too Late. Fairlee, VT.

different philosophical positions. In this regard, the research of Alessandro Pagnini is particularly relevant. In particular, the reflection on the differences between *Verstehen* and *Erklären* within opposite traditions in medicine bring us to the problematic classification (now overcome and useless according to the author) of the Galilean and/versus the Aristotelian (and Platonic) tradition.[278] The contributions of experimental neuroscience, as well as the theoretical debate of modern neurophilosophy are in this sense main contributors to a better understanding of the issue. We have therefore the scientific and moral duty to combine and confront these positions in order to have a deeper and broader understanding of our self and of our ability to perceive it. In this sense we can relate to the skeptical view of Franz Brentano in regard to "introspectionist psychology" intended as exploration of specific and distinctive properties of consciousness, but we also take into consideration his descriptive psychology as a tool to move forward and combine his concept of "intentionality of consciousness". We have to isolate the distortions of context and personal filter, but at the same time evaluate and value their specific weight and influence in order to understand the differences in perception of reality. This is fundamental to a process of personal analysis which becomes both analysis of self and self-analysis; an integrated and integrative approach to understand ourselves and each other within the reach and realm of our abilities; through sharing, debate, confront and intellectual-conceptual mirroring activity of our being in this world.

4.2 The search for meaning

a) Human, All Too Human

Medical Philosophy is indeed focused on the basic questions of Iatrophilosophy. In particular, considering that we are dealing with human beings and their multilayered complexity in terms of spheres of influences and (medical) intervention in the real, perceived and in the here-and-now acting world, we need to contemplate:

> "[...] a profession that incorporates science and scientific methods with the art of being a physician. The art of tending to the sick is as old as humanity itself. Compared with its long and generally distinguished history of caring and comforting, the scientific basis of medicine is remarkably recent. Further the physician is advised to understand the patient as a person.

---

[278] See Pagnini A., (Ed.) 2010. Filosofia della medicina. Roma: Caroce editore.

Three fundamental principles are important to practitioners. They are primacy of patient welfare, patient autonomy and social justice."[279]

According to Jean-Paul Sartre, the existentialist position linked to the relationship between reality and action[280] states that "I cannot obtain any truth whatsoever about myself, except through the mediation of others." At the same time, Kirkmayer notes that, in modern Western medicine "the literature on evidence-based practice is grounded in individualistic notions of the person and the categories used to identify problems, measure outcomes, and organize interventions may not fit specific cultures well."[281]

To what extent can we define ourselves as (human) beings on a base of mutual knowledge, derivative of a previous (*a priori*?) trust and validation of others' judgments and appearance?[282] We could move towards an analysis of the conditions of thought and existence; toward social, cultural and historical perspectives. For instance, Heidegger's position defines the 'I' as rooted in an earth experience (*Dasein* vs *Sosein*).[283] His historical view closely connects interpretation and communication with a specific criticism of the "all-pervasive influence" of scientific reason (and, to some extent, method and methodology) on Western culture.[284] According to Heidegger, *Dasein* is reserved for human existence, therefore for "being" in general. And still, the context of conditions, learning filters and patterns play an important role in the definition of human being and human experience in general. The concept of human being, its meaning and self-perception are in this sense shaped by action; his own as well as collective (in the existentialist view), and created or edited by circumstances an external or internal factors, such as psychic or or-

---

[279]   Goldman, L., and Ausiello, D.. 2004. Cecil Textbook of Medicine, Philadelphia, PA: Saunders, p. 45.

[280]   "There is no reality except in action" in: Sartre, Jean-Paul. 1997 *Existentialism and Humanism*, translation and introduction by P. Mairet, Brooklyn, NY: Haskell House Publishers, p. 48.

[281]   As discussed and quoted in: Christopher, J.C., Wendt, D.C., Marecek, J., D.C., Goodman, D.M. 2014. *Critical Cultural Awareness. Contributions to a Globalizing Psychology*. In *American Psychologist*. Vol. 69, Num. 7: 645–655 Washington, DC: APA, American Psychological Association, p. 652.

[282]   Ibid., p. 40 – Human beings are indeed free to choose, and in doing so they are filtering information and informer on the base of their (free) will; yet human beings cannot base their confidence in human beings they don't know, especially in the case of movements and revolutions.

[283]   Heidegger, M. 2006. *Sein und Zeit*, Tübingen: Max Niemeyer Verlag, p. 64.

[284]   Ibid., p. 46. See also West, D. 1996. *An Introduction to Continental Philosophy*, Oxford, UK: Polity Press, pp. 97–99.

ganic factors or by the action of environment upon the person (for instance in the view of Zola). Certainly, this conclusion leads us back in time to the Kantian conclusion "*Der Mensch kann nur Mensch werden durch Erziehung. Er ist nichts, als was die Erziehung aus ihm macht*" (Man can only become man through Education. He is nothing but what education makes of him).[285] Kant is regarded by some as the founding father of European philosophical anthropology, especially through his lecture on the concept of human ethnicity and race (*Von den verschiedenen Racen der Menschen*, 1772, published in 1775), as well as because of his conception of *pragmatic* anthropology, according to which the human being is studied as a free agent. This viewpoint puts the human being at the center of a balancing process between self-determination and social/cultural influence. This influence is better understood if we take into account the historical component of the learning process. The most current research in the field of developmental psychology seems to confirm the relation between human (and, in a broader sense, animal) sensation and the perception of surroundings, whether we are focusing on the pure physical or a social environment. Herder follows Heidegger (and, from this perspective, also Hegel) in linking what we said above to considerations around language and reason. In this sense, man can relate to the world through language (which makes him what he is) and channel his sensation into an objectivization of the world around him, leading to self-reflection. This aspect is perhaps forgotten in the discussion around modern medical education, according to Philip Overby:

> "Many writers have argued that art and literature should have a place in the medical curriculum on the grounds that art helps doctors understand experiences, illness and human values and that art itself can fulfill a therapeutic role. At its best humanistic education will help doctors at the bedside by forcing them to grapple with the kinds of existential question that their patients can avoid."[286]

This very reflection on (the) self and (its) (one own's) existence allows man to create himself freely: "*Der Mensch ist der erste Freigelassene der Schöpfung, er steht aufrecht. Die Waage des Guten und des Bösen, des Falschen und Wahren hängt an ihm; er kann forschen, er soll wählen.*" (Man is the first release-*d* / liberated being of creation, he stands upright. The balance between good and bad, between false and true depends on him; he can (re)search, he *should* choose). Considering the variety of methodological approaches to this

---

[285]   Kant, I. *Über Pädagogik (On Pedagogy)*, first published by Friedrich Nicolovius in Königsberg, p. 23.

[286]   Overby, P. 2005. *The Moral Education of Doctors*. The New Atlantis; 10: 17–26.

act of creation, the statement could be shared by researchers belonging to either continental or analytical philosophy, with various degrees of possible application.

A criticism to the application of anthropology in a philosophical debate (or the pure comparison between anthropology and philosophy) comes from Hegel, who still follows the above presented process of self-reflection through objectivization of the world, but thinks of history as the preferred channel to understand human beings. In this sense his position makes us go back to Sartre, who doesn't share a historical perspective, but a more pure existential view of the relationship between (self) knowledge, essence and existence. According to the French philosopher, man is not an object, and therefore he cannot be "objectivized".[287] Existentialism criticizes materialism also through the concept of a human kingdom as a pattern of values in distinction from the material world. If, according to Sartre there is no such thing as human nature, but there is a *condition*, and this condition is universal also in the epistemological sense, we need to explore, and possibly redefine or challenge existentialist positions. In this sense, philosophical anthropology is the attempt to unify disparate ways of understanding behavior of humans as both creatures of their social environments and creators of their own values, with the added value of opening up discussion on the very foundation of moral law. In this regard, Francis Collins writes that:

> "A religious person will see [the principles of bioethics – Respect for autonomy, Justice, Beneficence, and Nonmaleficence] as principles clearly laid out in sacred texts of the Judaeo-Christian, Islamic, Buddhist, and other religious traditions. In fact, some of the most eloquent and powerful statements of these principles are to be found in such sacred texts. But one need not be a theist to agree to these principles. Even a person untrained in musical theory can be transported by a Mozart concerto. The Moral Law speaks to all of us, whether or not we agree on its origins. Basic principles of ethics can be derived from the Moral Law, and are universal. But conflicts can arise in a situation where not all of the principles can be satisfied at the same time, and different observers attach different weights to the principles that must be somehow balanced".[288]

We will analyze in the following chapters the relationship between moral law and the belief in God; for now it is important to notice that even the very position of Sartre toward God is somewhat problematic, depending on (among

---

[287]   Sartre, J-P. 1997. *Existentialism and Humanism*, translation and introduction by P. Mairet, Brooklyn, NY: Haskell House Publishers, p. 42.

[288]   Collins, F. 2006. *The Language of God: A Scientist Presents Evidence for Belief*. New York, NY: Free Press Simon & Schuster, pp. 243–244.

other things and for instance) our decision to accept some accounts of the alleged conversion of the French philosopher in the last moments of his life, and the following criticism to such claims, from De Beauvoir an others. In this context, I am reporting only one comment on the issue, and refer to the bibliography for further readings. Stephen Wang writes:

> "There is an urban myth that Sartre had a death-bed conversion, called for the priest, and died in the bosom of the Catholic Church. It's not true. But it is true that in the last few years of his life he re-evaluated some of his core existentialist convictions, and in particular became more open to the idea of God and the significance of religion. He was undoubtedly influenced – some would say coerced – by Benny Lévy, a young Egyptian Maoist who was rediscovering his own Jewish inheritance at the time he was working as Sartre's secretary and interlocutor. Their conversations were published just weeks before Sartre's death".[289]

Sense of meaning and purpose in life are strictly related to what we define "positive affect" and "full affect" in psychiatric assessments.[290] In particular, there is a correlation (we will examine the possible relation of cause and effect) between the terms. Certainly, positive mood in general refers to feelings of different levels of happiness, from being cheerful, pleased, satisfied, and even content. According to Vaillant, happiness is:

> "A conscious state of mind, rooted in the neocortex, the region of the brain responsible for thinking, planning, and decision-making. Joy is all about our connection with others. It's a subconscious, almost visceral feeling that appears to stem from the brain's limbic system, which is believed to control emotions, including pleasure. Unlike happiness, joy involves little cognitive awareness [...] but it's more enduring."[291]

As we discussed in the previous chapters, the use of the verb "stem" in a causal-mechanistic way is imprecise and represents a subjective (philosophical, but

---

[289]   Wang, S. 2010. *Sartre's death-bed conversion?* In: Bridges and Tangents. Looking across the landscape of contemporary culture, available at https://bridgesandtangents.wordpres s.com/2010/07/31/sartres-death-bed-conversion/.

[290]   On these themes, Magdalena R. Naylor, a professor and physician at the University of Vermont Medical Center, wrote with her husband Thomas H. Naylor (Professor Emeritus of economics at Duke University and a founder of the secessionist Second Vermont Republic) and pastor William H. Willimon "The Search for Meaning". Dr. Naylor brought interesting elements to the discussion, especially from the perspective of her native Poland and the relationship between the Soviet Socialist system and the Catholic Church. For further reference, see Naylor, T.H, Willimon, W.H., and Naylor, M.R. 1994. *The Search for Meaning*. Nashville, TN: Abingdon Press.

[291]   Cerretani, J. 2011. *The contagion of Happiness. Harvard researchers are discovering how we can all get happy*. In: Byron, P.B. (Ed.) 2011. The Science of Emotion, Boston, MA: Harvard Medicine, p. 12.

also personal) position, not proven by any scientific research so far, although, to be fair, the author adds the verb "appears". It would be interesting, from the perspective of evidence-based Science to discuss the parameter of this (visible, tangible, monitorable and quantifiable) appearance. Moreover, there is a difference between mood and affect (starting from the traditional perspectives of Hippocrates of course), but generally speaking studies have suggested that meaning in life, or more accurately, the belief in and/or perception of the existence of such meaning, is consistently positively correlated with positive affect.[292] To be sure, there are plenty of studies that indicate a very strong correlation between happiness and good health, both within communities as well as in single subjects.[293] Also, good mental health slowed the deterioration of physical health.[294] Furthermore, as Heintzelman and King note, induced positive mood leads to higher meaning in life, and even mild experiences that enhance positive affect such as listening to certain music or reading certain literature can promote a sense of meaning in life.[295] Finally, the authors argue that the cause-effect interaction between happiness and life's meaning works both ways.[296] This type of research obviously involves self-reports and it requires a specific definition of "meaning", which generally includes at least three common themes:

---

[292] Heintzelman, S.J. and King L.A. 2014. *Life is pretty meaningful*. Vol. 69 N.6, p. 562.
[293] Cerretani, J. 2011. *The contagion of Happiness. Harvard researchers are discovering how we can all get happy*. In: Byron, P.B. (Ed.) 2011. The Science of Emotion, Boston, MA: Harvard Medicine, p. 13.
[294] Ibid. The study focused on male subjects, and yielded positive results even after adjusting for genetics, obesity, and tobacco and alcohol use. Furthermore, and very interestingly, the authors speculate that "good feelings continue to move from person to person", thus presenting a model very similar to the one used for airborne droplets, such as flu.
[295] Heintzelman, S.J. and King L.A. 2014. *Life is pretty meaningful*. Vol. 69 N.6, p. 562.
[296] Ibid. The authors discuss three important aspects/potential answers to the questions on meaning, or lack of, in life. In particular, they list social exclusion, positive mood, and environmental pattern and coherence as main elements. The latter is explained through this analysis: "[...] our research has shown that meaning in life reports are sensitive to the presence of reliable pattern or coherence in environmental stimuli. Drawing on the cognitive component of meaning in life noted above, we hypothesized that meaning in life would be higher after an experience with stimuli characterized by pattern or coherence than after experiences lacking such pattern or coherence. Put simply, we predicted that when stimuli make sense, life should be more meaningful [...]" To be sure, the authors also indicate the difference between the perception of life's meaning and the ultimate existence of meaning in life (regardless or disconnected from the person-al perspective and belief).

a) A meaningful life is one that has a sense of purpose (motivational/existential theme)
b) A meaningful life is one that matters or possesses significance (motivational/existential theme)
c) A meaningful life makes sense to the person living it, it is comprehensible, and it is characterized by regularity, predictability, or reliable connections (cognitive theme).[297]

Heintzelman and King discuss meaning in life also from the perspective of its social absence, in terms of "existential vacuum":

> "The notion that the meaningful life is relatively rare is also reflected in the science of psychological well-being. Meaning in life is typically considered emblematic of eudaimonic well-being. Eudaimonia has been described variously as happiness that emerges as a function of the satisfaction of orgasmic needs (Ryan & Deci, 2001), self-realization (Waterman, 1993), or actualizing one's potentials (Ryff, 2012; Ryff & Singer, 2008). In a sense, eudaimonia is conceived of as something greater that plain old happiness (Kashdan, Biswas-Diener, & King, 2008). As part of Eudaimonia, then, the meaningful life would seem to be a true (and potentially rare) human accomplishment. Certainly compared to say, the happy life, the meaningful life has been characterized as relatively scarce (Seligman, 2002, 2011). Research has shown that most people rate their levels of happiness or satisfaction as above the midpoint on self-report rating scales (Diner & Diener, 1996). Thus, from the eudaimonic perspective, we might expect meaning in life to be at least less common than happiness, so we might tally a vote for relatively low levels of meaning of life."[298]

---

[297] Baumeister et al. as cited in: Heintzelman, S.J. and King L.A. 2014. *Life is pretty meaningful*. Vol. 69 N.6, pp. 561–562. In the same article, on p. 562, the authors quote Steger's definition of meaning as "the web of connections, understandings, and interpretations that help us comprehend our experience and formulate plans directing our energies to the achievement of our desired future. Meaning provides us with the sense that our lives matter, that they make sense, and that they are more than the sum of our seconds, days, and years." Certainly, we are more than the sum of (our) parts.

[298] Diener, E., and Diener, C. 1996. *Most people are happy*. In: Psychological Science, 7, 181–185; Kashdan, T.B., Biswas-Diener, R., and King, L.A. 2008. *Reconsidering happiness: the costs of distinguishing between hedonics and Eudaimonia*. Journal of Positive psychology, 3, 219–233; Ryan, R.M., and Deci, E.L. 2001. *On happiness and human potentials: a review of research on hedonic and eudaimonic well-being*. Annual Review of psychology, 52, 141–166; Ryff, C.D. 2012. Existential well-being and health. In: P.T.P. Wong (Ed.). *The human quest for meaning: theories, research, and applications* (2nd ed., pp. 233–247). New York, NY: Routledge/Taylor & Francis Group; Ryff, C.D., and Singer, B.H. 2008. *Know thyself and become what you are: A eudaimonic approach to psychological well-being*. Journal of Happiness studies, 9, 13–39; Seligman, M.E.P. 2002. *Authentic happiness*. New York, NY: Free Press; Seligman, M.E.P. 2011. *Flourish: A visionary new understanding of happiness and well-being*. New York, NY: Free Press; Waterman, A.S. 1993. *Two conceptions of happiness: Contrasts of personal expressiveness (Eudaimonia) and hedonic enjoyment*. Journal

Another analysis comes from Charles Leslie Stevenson, who examines the cognitive use of language, and therefore the viewpoint of a human self-knowledge through communication with other human beings in a specific context. The first pattern analysis focuses on the two parts of ethical statements, the speaker's declaration (more specifically the declaration of the speaker's attitude) and an imperative to follow it in a specular way; to mimic, copy, mirror it. If we are asking about the way human beings shape their meaning and significance, whether to or through self-reflection or external (environmental) factors, we have to keep in mind that Stevenson's translation of an ethical sentence remains a non-cognitive one.[299] Still, this analysis reconnects to the specific requirements of existentialist position in terms of personal responsibility and action. Since imperatives cannot be proven, they can be supported, and the purpose of this process is to make the listener understand the consequences of the action they are being commanded to do. Whether we are allowed to take these considerations and move onto a more general (absolute) principle, depends on the second pattern analysis. In this process, the relation between figure *a* and figure *b*, between speaker and listener (who is also judge in this case) changes according to the rules and requirements of this principle.

From a pure anthropological perspective, especially the *intersubjectivity* perspective of anthropology of interpersonal relationships,[300] we could further focus on the impact and value of the external factors on the speaker as well as on the whole process. Would a different listener (or group of listeners) change the system of values (and, most important, evaluation) of the speaker? This question certainly raises an entire new and broad list of considerations, in particular the meaning and weight of diachronic perspectives. Furthermore, we have to analyze the possibility of practical application of theories and methods next to and beyond the realm of philosophical speculation. For instance, Brinton used evolutionary theory in his analysis of Native American languages, in order to prove the inferiority of their culture on the base of pervasive vocalic inconsistency.[301] Franz Boas criticized this position and in doing so, he was

---

of Personality and Social psychology, 64, 678–691. In: Heintzelman, S.J. and King L.A. 2014. *Life is pretty meaningful*. Vol. 69 N. 6, pp. 561–574.

[299] See Stevenson, C.L. 1944. *Ethics and Language*, New Haven, CT: Yale University Press, 1944; in particular pp. 21–28.

[300] See for example Jackson, M. 2005. *Existential Anthropology—Events, Exigencies, and Effects (Methodology and History in Anthropology)*, California: Berghahn Books.

[301] See the response to the paper published by Brinton, D.G. (University of Pennsylvania, 1888), in Boas, F. 1889. *On Alternating Sounds*.

able to give an important contribution not only to anthropology, but to the foundation of linguistics as a science, especially in the United States.[302] The ethnographer's bias, the emotional factors as well as the ontological assumptions (analyzed by Jackson as well) were at the center of Boas' research. In this sense, we can say that the German-American anthropologist made a shift from pure anthropological linguistics to the analysis of perception, entering therefore in the realm of cognitive and developmental psychology. This is obviously crucial in our analysis of self-perception and presence of human beings in the world. In particular, descriptive linguistics focuses on the way we relate to these external factors and make them our own. More specifically, how are we to note (and know) the sounds we perceive onto a schematic and structured system, which we can use to express ourselves, and relate to other human beings? In this sense, we are viewing the previously expressed evolutionary theories (as well as empiric and analytical methodologies) through the lens of cultural relativism. It is in German Enlightenment that the epistemological claims that led to the development of cultural relativism have their origins. The Kantian perspective tells us that all our experiences are filtered through the human mind and its perception of universal structures according to concepts of time and space given *a priori*. Therefore we as human beings are not capable of direct and unmediated knowledge. Herder took this perspective and stated that those very experiences could be mediated also by particular, national and cultural structures. All these considerations created the fertile milieu where modern anthropology and ethnography build their research. All the steps are important to a wider and deeper perspective on human (self) perception, from the perspective of philosophical anthropology. Already Wilhelm von Humboldt tried to bridge the gap between Kant and Herder's ideas, and William Graham Summer summarized the impact of one's culture (and limitation—those external factors due to the environment also analyzed in existentialist positions) on one's perception with the principle of Western ethnocentrism.[303] The exploration of human nature and human condition, leading to the definition of philosophical anthropology as a specific field of philosophy though the work of Scheler, Plessner and Gehlen, is exactly what lies at the base (and to some ex-

---

[302]   In his native Germany, and in the rest of continental Europe, the situation was different, mostly because of the historical and academic element of scientific research and literary tradition. The best example is probably the contribution of the analysis and laws of *Lautverschiebung* by von Schlegel, Rask and Grimm.

[303]   See for example Summer, W.G. 1963. *Social Darwinism: Selected Essays* , ed. Stow Persons—Englewood Cliff, NJ: Prentice-Hall.

tent, as basis) of our analysis. Since we saw how human are both the product of their social, cultural, ethnic, geographic, external environment as well as creators of their own perception and values, we could analyze our equation from two separate and yet mutually influenced perspectives. The first view postulates that man objectivizes the world around him and within himself. The second, also explored in Jackson's notion of "control", states that human beings anthropomorphize inanimate objects around them in order to enter into an interpersonal relationship with them. This process has diverse possible interpretations. Human beings could be potentially trying to erase, or at least reduce the distance between himself and the objects, as well as between himself and what he perceives as "self", between two or more parts of self. Or, in Jackson's view, he could use this process to feel as if he had control over situations or inanimate objects; and this view could lead us into more specific areas of linguistics and philosophy of neuroscience. We could for instance ask ourselves how do we, as human beings part of a certain culture, ethnic background or even tradition, define and understand the difference between objects, especially in the organic and biologic realm, for instance when we relate to animals, plants and non-anthropic and environmental elements such as lakes, rivers or mountains, in assigning names and definitions. The act of separation is already a movement toward ourselves (se-*parare*), is it therefore possible to isolate all these terms and concepts from our interpretation of them? We could go back to the beginning of this analysis and argue that true knowledge of man's meaning and presence in the (this) world is only possible through a combination of perspectives. It is therefore necessary to relate to actions and outcomes to understand oneself, and human being-s (also understood as "other-s from me") and their presence, values, evaluations play a major role in defining who I am as an in-dividual. Thus, we could apply structures and methods of analysis of communication and language, dividing our perspectives in two halves (not necessarily from a chronological perspective, certainly not form a perspective of value and weight) following the model of grammar and syntactic analysis, or integrating more perspectives at the same time, in a concentric scheme, in which meaning is at the center, and language, community of practice, and culture are the outer layers.[304]

---

[304]   This is the case of the model developed by Loftus, in which the conceptualization of language happens through the investigation of embedded concepts such as Ritual, Rhetoric, Hermeneutics, Narrative, Metaphor, Categories, Utterances, and Heuristics. See Loftus, S.F. 2006. *Language in clinical reasoning: using and learning the language of collective clinical*

b) Experimental Philosophy

Bringing together all these perspectives into one cohesive discussion on Medical Philosophy is certainly a complex task, and among the most problematic issues in monitoring the effectiveness of such effort, there are purely methodological considerations to analyze. As we previously discussed, the ultimate purpose of this study is to open up the discussion and generate new questions, inferring information from the data examined as well as the reasoning process, in particular the patient-provider relationship, the scientific approach and existential considerations at the base of patient perception in diagnostics and therapy. First of all the decision to include in a philosophical analysis an empirical study could create some misunderstandings, perhaps even a general sense of disappointment or skeptical disbelief in what should be considered "true philosophy" in comparison with scientific areas of field research.[305] However, beside the necessary consideration on analytic vs. continental philosophy (which we previously discussed), an honest debate on Medical Philosophy needs, in our opinion, a thorough examination of possible new methodological combinations and a realistic and practical awareness of the whole historical paradigm and the most cutting-edge research in both empirical science and philosophy. In fact, the very field of experimental philosophy originates in the scientific debate around natural philosophy in the early 2000, focused in particular on areas of medical research, especially psychology and psychiatry. Certainly, there is strong evidence for a special influence by analytic philosophers in these efforts, but the very core of the philosophical debate goes be-

---

decision making. Sydney, AUS: Faculty of Health Sciences, School of Physiotherapy, University of Sydney, p. 237.

[305] Anthony Appiah writes: "It's part of a recent movement known as "experimental philosophy," which has rudely challenged the way professional philosophers like to think of themselves. Not only are philosophers unaccustomed to gathering data; many have also come to define themselves by their disinclination to do so. The professional bailiwick we've staked out is the empyrean of pure thought. Colleagues in biology have P.C.R. machines to run and microscope slides to dye; political scientists have demographic trends to crunch; psychologists have their rats and mazes. We philosophers wave them on with kindly looks. We know the experimental sciences are terribly important, but the role we prefer is that of the Catholic priest presiding at a wedding, confident that his support for the practice carries all the more weight for being entirely theoretical. Philosophers don't observe; we don't experiment; we don't measure; and we don't count. We reflect. We love nothing more than our "thought experiments," but the key word there is thought. As the president of one of philosophy's more illustrious professional associations, the Aristotelian Society, said a few years ago, "If anything can be pursued in an armchair, philosophy can." See, Appiah, A.K. 2007. The New Philosophy. New York, NY: The New York Times, direct link: http://www.nytimes.com/20 07/12/09/magazine/09wwln-idealab-t.html?_r=2&

yond (and, in some cases, against) a purely analytic perspective. In fact, at the center of experimental philosophy is simply the use of empirical data. Some have argued that the very use of an empiric approach goes against a "pure" philosophical methodology, relying mainly on thought experiments or aprioristic justification.[306] Although the traditional divide between analytic and continental philosophy seems to support this claim, we could argue that perspectives from dialectic (Hegelian for sure, but not only), as well as postmodern literature do not necessarily discard the use of empirical data. To be sure, the data we are talking about is gathered through surveys and questionnaires, thus on philosophical questions originating in, and directed at, (the very essence of) man, since the core of our analysis is patient's perception. Furthermore, the very origin of the empirical method in philosophy as a combination of "classical" philosophy with the perceived experimental rigor of (social) sciences is linked to psychological research. And we all know how a very big part of classical and modern psychology is still based on cognitive perspective on critical thinking, especially in the form of the so-called Socratic method, definitely a "true" philosophical form of inquiry. In trying to defend one side (at the far end) of the research spectrum against the other, we risk to miss an important opportunity to understand the "patient at the center of therapy", with his complexity, his mystery, and multilayered phenomenology of possible interpretation.[307] For instance, completely discrediting a contemplative approach in philosophy and an observative (evidence-based) approach in experimental science would be a terrible mistake. To be sure, we need to keep in mind that there are other elements we need to add to these perspectives, in order to obtain a more "realistic" picture, an image of our patient (and, in a translated sense, of human beings, as well as of ourselves). As we previously discussed, examining what we can perceive with our basic sense represents an important first step in our analysis, a very good support to our study, as long as we don't allow ourselves to be trapped in a positivistic, reductionist, nihilo-ultra-materialistic approach which ignores the importance of a strong theoretical debate, to satisfy ego-

---

[306]   For further reference, see for instance Fulford, K.W.M. 1991. The potential of medicine as a resource for philosophy. *Theoretical Medicine*. Dordrecht, NL: Kluwer Academic Publishers, 12: 81–85.

[307]   This is true for the whole spectrum of medical intervention, not just in psychology and/or psychiatry: "We may speculate that different problems require different medical paradigms and that no single theoretical model is sufficient for so complex an activity as clinical medicine." Elstein, A. S., Schulman, L. S., & Sprafraka, S. A. 1978. *Medical problem solving: An analysis of clinical reasoning*. Cambridge, MA: Harvard University Press, p. 228.

ist(ic) and self-righteous, self-justifying needs, instead of the ultimate goal of (Medical) Philosophy, a more accurate and comprehensive account of truths in our understanding of man.[308] Among the areas of research in experimental philosophy we find the debate on consciousness (including the mind-brain/body problem), cultural and ethnic-religious diversity, determinism and moral responsibility (including the discussion on neuroscience), epistemology, intentional action, and predicting philosophical disagreement (including personality traits).

---

[308] This especially true in biased, often inaccurate and imprecise accounts of what philosophers *actually* do; according to Jon Lackman "Philosophers have ignored the real world because it's messy, full of happenstance details and meaningless coincidences; philosophy, they argue, has achieved its successes by focusing on deducing universal truths from basic principles. X-phi, on the other hand, argues that philosophers need to ask people what and how they think. Traditional philosophy relies on certain intuitions, presented as "common sense," that are presumed to be shared by everyone." See Lackman, J. 2006. *The X-Philes. Philosophy meets the real world*. Slate Magazine. Furthermore, the discussion at the beginning of this volume, brings us back here in this contextual analysis of the role of philosophy in (*id est* within) medicine. James Marcum offers a very attentive and comprehensive analysis, which is worth reporting, at least in part: "[...] Edmund Pellegrino took issue with Shaffer, claiming that Shaffer in an effort to deny a relationship or interface between philosophy and medicine has "philosophized about medicine" (1975, p. 231). Pellegrino also made a distinction between a philosophy in medicine and a philosophy of medicine. The first relationship between philosophy and medicine, philosophy in medicine, is unproblematic and involves using philosophical methods to address philosophical problems such as causality in medical knowledge and practice. The second relationship, philosophy of medicine, Pellegrino admitted is problematic because of the nature of medicine. However, according to Pellegrino medicine is, contra Shaffer, more than simply the sum of the sciences that constitute it. Philosophy of medicine involves defining the nature of medicine per se or in terms of its essence. A few years later, Pellegrino (1976) added a third relationship between the two disciplines, philosophy and medicine, in a lead article to the first issue of a new journal entitled The Journal of Medicine and Philosophy. This relationship involves problems that overlap between the two disciplines. "Philosophy in medicine," according to Pellegrino and Thomasma, "refers to the application of the traditional tools of philosophy—critical reflection, dialectical reasoning, uncovering of value and purpose, or asking first-order questions—to some medically defined problem" (1981a, p. 29). Pellegrino and Thomasma admitted that philosophy of medicine is the most problematic of the three relationships and needs careful explication. In philosophy of medicine, genuine philosophical issues concerning medical knowledge and practice are examined. [...] According to Pellegrino and Thomasma, this relationship is defined as "a systematic set of ways for articulating, clarifying, and addressing the philosophical issues in medicine" (1981a, p. 28). The philosopher's role vis-à-vis medicine is to apply a critical and dialectical methodology to address philosophical issues in medicine, especially the clinical encounter. The aim of the philosophy of medicine is to account for "the whole domain of the clinical moment" (Pellegrino and Thomasma, 1981a, p. 28) (Marcum, J.A. 2008. An introductory philosophy of medicine: humanizing modern medicine. New York: Springer, pp. 1–2.

There is certainly an extensive literature on human perception of an ultimate understanding, structure, (pre)destination (in an etymological sense),
purpose and meaning. The aim of this study is to combine the empirical results
and theoretical approaches produced in scientific and philosophical analysis
and readdress them in a more specifically oriented medical setting, to provide a
more *stable* and efficient support to diagnostic and therapy. Special attention is
paid to those realms of medical and scientific analysis which are still difficult
in terms of clinical understanding, *thus* psychology and psychiatry. An interesting anecdote (which is however related a fairly common patient's viewpoint
in my clinical work every day) is represented by the following account by a
friend and colleague from Harvard Medical School, whose identity I will re-
spectfully keep private, and who recently shared with me that: "If I had mental
problems and depression, I would certainly look for a philosopher to help me. I
think they are much better trained in existential questions than the average
physician in this country, including psychiatrists." To be sure, there is an underlying irony in this statement, especially since the doctor who expressed this
point of view does indeed work in a medical/academic setting. At the same
time, this form of anecdotal knowledge could at least help raise questions and
curiosity around what lies "beyond" the effectiveness of therapeutic intervention. As we previously discussed, and we will further analyze in the chapter on
alternative medicine, there are still many unanswered questions in addressing
the effect of placebo and patient-physician relationships. Many of these questions are closely connected to patient's (and provider's) perception, opinion and
belief on the ultimate purpose, goal and task of (his/her) life.[309]

---

[309]   In the aforementioned article by Heintzelman and King, the authors discussed these important factors from a very interesting comparative and epidemiological perspective, which
is definitely worth citing (with the inclusion of statistical data) in this context: "[...] These
descriptive data strongly support two conclusions: first, that life is meaningful [from the in-
terviewed person's perspective, as we have seen above, A/N], and second, that the level of
meaning in life experienced is pretty high. Two surveys using dichotomous response options
show that most people find their lives to be meaningful. First, in its 2002 wave of data
collection, the Health and Retirement Study, an ongoing longitudinal study of Americans
over age 50 [...], included, for some participants (n 1,062), two items regarding the
meaningfulness of their lives during the past 12 months. In response to the question "Did
you feel that your life has meaning?" 95% answered "yes." For the item "Did you feel that
there's not enough purpose in your life?" 84% said "no." Second, Oishi and Diener (2013)
[See Bibliography for further reference, A/N] recently reported on data collected from 132
nations (N 137,678) in 2007 by Gallup Global Polls. This assessment included the item "Do
you feel your life has an important purpose or meaning?" Averaging across the 132 nations,
the percentage responding in the affirmative was 91%. Life was considered to be meaningful
by 90% or more of those surveyed in nations as diverse as Cuba, Kosovo, Malawi, Sierra

In clinical research, two of the most interesting surveys addressing these aspects in the form of established measuring systems, are the *Purpose in Life Test* or *PIL* by Crumbaugh and Maholick and the *Meaning in Life Questionnaire* or *MLQ* by Steger et al.[310] From a philosophical and scientific perspective, it is important to address the questions of conceptual definition of meaning (which we briefly discussed in the previous paragraph), as well as the validity, in terms of general applicability/generalization, of the statistical data, especially within descriptive statistic and the analysis of means (for premeas-

---

Leone, Sri Lanka, and the United States. Even among the nations defining the lowest levels of endorsement (e.g., Hong Kong, Slovenia, Japan, and France), the percentage of individuals doing so was over 60% (Oishi & Diener, 2013). [...] In the 2007 Baylor Religion Survey (Baylor University, 2007), conducted by Gallup, respondents (N 1,648) rated the single item "My life has a real purpose" on a scale from 1 (strongly disagree) to 5 (strongly agree). Just 1.1% strongly disagreed, 9.1% disagreed, and 6.1 % were undecided. The remaining respondents (over 83%) agreed (54.9%) or strongly agreed (28.7%) that their lives had "a real purpose" (Stroope, Draper, & Whitehead, 2013). Although the mean for the rating is not provided in the original article, the extrapolated mean based on these percentages is 4.01 (above 3, the scale midpoint). In the Americans' Changing Lives survey (House, 1986, 2008), respondents (N 1,660) rated two items relevant to meaning in life on a scale from 1 (strongly agree) to 4 (strongly disagree). The items included "I have a sense of direction and purpose in life" and "In the final analysis, I'm not sure that my life adds up to much." With reverse coding so that higher scores indicate higher meaning in life, the means were 3.50 (SD 0.76) and 3.44 (SD 0.86) for the two items, respectively [...].The distributions of the ratings show that these means are not driven by a few extreme cases. For the "purpose" item, 90.4% somewhat agreed (27%) or strongly agreed (63%); for the "final analysis" item, 84.4% somewhat disagreed (20.2%) or strongly disagreed (64.2%) (House, 2008). Two representative U.S. surveys included the 3-item Purpose subscale of the Psychological Well-Being Scales (Ryff, 1989). Unlike the other scales included in this analysis, none of these items explicitly mention meaning or purpose in life. A sample item is "Some people wander aimlessly through life, but I am not one of them." Items are rated on a 1 to 6 scale. The means for both samples suggest that life is pretty purposeful. In one sample (N 1,108) the mean sum ($\alpha = .33$) of the items was 14.4 (SD 3.2; Ryff & Keyes, 1995). Converting this value to the average rating over the three items, the mean is 4.8 (above the scale midpoint, d 1.22) [...] in 2008, the Centers for Disease Control administered three items from the Meaning in Life Questionnaire's Presence of Meaning subscale (Steger, Frazier, Oishi, & Kaler, 2006) to a large national sample (N 5,399; Kobau, Sniezek, Zack, Lucas, & Burns, 2010). The items included "My life has a clear sense of purpose," "I have a good sense of what makes my life meaningful," and "I have discovered a satisfying life purpose." See Heintzelman, S.J. and King L.A. 2014. *Life is pretty meaningful*. Vol. 69 N.6, pp. 564–555.

[310]   See bibliographic references: Crumbaugh, J. C., & Maholick, L. T. 1964. *An experimental study in existentialism: The psychometric approach to Frankl's concept of noogenic neurosis*. In: Journal of Clinical Psychology, 20, 200–207; Steger, M. F., Frazier, P., Oishi, S., & Kaler, M. 2006. *The Meaning in Life Questionnaire: Assessing the presence of and search for meaning in life*. In: Journal of Counseling Psychology, 53, 80–93 ; Frankl, V. E. 1984. *Man's search for meaning* (3rd ed.). New York, NY: Washington Square Press. (Original work published 1946).

ured or as outcome measures) in correlational studies of meaning in life, as discussed by Heintzelman and King. In the authors' analysis of mean PIL and MLQ scores, it important to note that "[...] two potential concerns with the PIL are the extremity of some items and the conflation of purpose in life with positive affect, enjoyment, vitality, or zest [...]. These means, then, might be inflated by momentary positive mood or general positive emotionality."[311] Any claim of scientific objectivity, in the sense of EBS-Western science, is in this context, very imprecise, perhaps even oxymoronic in conceptual validity; but if we want to open up the epistemological discussion on the application of the term "science" within the framework of philosophical understanding of life's meaning, then it becomes apparent how not only the data collected are indeed affected by *fluctuations* in the person's (patient's) response, but that these fluctuations are the very ground of investigation we need to focus on. In fact, these variations in output might represent a differentiation, (perhaps even a *differànce* as in Derrida), in internal (inner) and external (environmental, contextual, historical as in Hegel) factors. Among these factors we might include a general sense of biased weight, both in negative or positive terms (especially in diagnostics, both from the patient's as well as the physician's viewpoint), even a form of "wishful thinking" that might produce (or even be produced, from a psychological, and/or evolutionary/biological perspective) an *adaptive* mechanism,[312] which we have to understand in diagnostics and therapeutic intervention. Furthermore, this mechanism might be founded on the very nature of our existence as human beings, in the sense of a continuous striving (this time also in the French existentialist viewpoint) for meaning, because the (at more brief or extended times) lack of (perception, awareness) of meaning might be a stimulus underlying the very experience of life on this earth, the same way we perceive/feel sensations/cravings of thirst and hunger, which need to be continuously satisfied as part of our (physical-biological) life. At the same time, we need to keep in mind the correlational aspects of this relation between biology and meaning, and not jump to the (reductionist) conclusion that the biological aspect causes the existential one, and that we need to address the question of whether the origin of our perception of meaning, and of meaning itself, mat-

---

[311]   Heintzelman, S.J. and King L.A. 2014. *Life is pretty meaningful.* Vol. 69 N.6, p. 567.

[312]   Which, regardless of its connection with reality, could promote a better outcome, both in medical/health-related as well as generally existential (including ethical and moral) perspectives, as the authors note: "We leave it to others to consider whether, given the association between meaning in life and many positive outcomes, it would be a good idea to divest individuals of this particular illusion." See Ibid., p. 568.

ters in this context; and if it does matter, to what extent it influences/contributes to the outcomes in our analysis (and in life's unfolding and structure in general).

c) Mirror, Mirror on the Wall

The aforementioned considerations bring us straight to a very important part of Medical Philosophy, and of medicine in general, the relationship between internal and external environment, in the form of interactions between gene, meme, and environment. Staring from the definition by Richard Dawkins, as inspired by the work by Cavalli-Sforza (in particular the Dual inheritance theory or DIT),[313] Cloak and Cullen, the "meme" follows the evolutionary (also cultural) structure according to which the core of significance in explaining human behavior lies in the self-replicating unit of transmission.[314] A harsh criticism not necessarily of the conceptual basis of the meme itself, but of the use by Dawkins in terms of causal and structural aspect to justify and explain human behavior, comes from within the scientific community, and it is mainly focused on the claim of scientific validity (versus philosophical and conceptual hypothesis) of what has been defined as "pseudoscientific dogma"[315] that forces (the absence of) an organic/biochemical/biological substructure (similar to the DNA code) to be the basis of such an explanation. Certainly, the connections between genes and environment are fundamental in trying to examine behaviors related to neurogenetic basis, especially in psychiatry and psychology. In fact, the combination of research by psychological scientists and psychiatric geneticists has shown that both genetic and environmental factors (including education and support) contribute to psychiatric disorders. We could argue

---

[313]   Original "*ipotesi dell'ereditarietà duale*". A further detailed explanation can be found in Cavalli-Sforza, L. L. and M. Feldman. 1981. *Cultural Transmission and Evolution: A Quantitative Approach*. Princeton, New Jersey: Princeton University Press.

[314]   Dawkins, R. 1989. *The Selfish Gene* (2 ed.), Oxford, UK: Oxford University Press, pp. 191–193: "[...] We need a name for the new replicator, a noun that conveys the idea of a unit of cultural transmission, or a unit of imitation. 'Mimeme' comes from a suitable Greek root, but I want a monosyllable that sounds a bit like 'gene'. I hope my classicist friends will forgive me if I abbreviate mimeme to meme. If it is any consolation, it could alternatively be thought of as being related to 'memory', or to the French word même. It should be pronounced to rhyme with 'cream'." According to the Merriam-Webster Dictionary, the word was first used in 1977, and expresses "an idea, behavior, style, or usage that spreads from person to person within a culture."

[315]   See Benitez Bribiesca, L. 2001. *Memetics: A dangerous idea*, Interciencia: Revista de Ciencia y Technologia de América. Venezuela: Asociación Interciencia, 26 (1): 29–31.

that genes represent the general *given*[316] background, and environment helps turn these genes "on" and "off". Studies have also shown that a single gene or genetic variant connected to any specific mental disorder has yet to be found, and that most likely, each psychiatric disorder is influenced by thousands of genetic variants.[317] Furthermore, these variants are often found outside the human protein coding genes. The mechanism of genetic influence on mental health and general behavior is still very unclear, and might be direct or indirect (especially in the product of those variables, in the case of epistasis), as well as interactive. Plus, most of psychiatric research on phenotype has been focused, on adult subjects, even in the case of childhood-onset cases, following a binary (yes/no presence/absence) diagnostic analysis, which ultimately is (retrospective confirmation) biased/based on the DSM, the Diagnostic and Statistical Manual of Mental Disorder. This has a fundamental philosophical impact on the very validity of psychotropic medications, which are assumed to target specific neurotransmitter systems, believed to be connected to a specific mental health disorder. In fact, the mores specific the (definition of) mental disorder, the more valuable, in terms of economic market perspective, is a specific

---

[316]   In this sense, we could extend the term in a theological examination of (divine, God-personal) behavior, according to the definition of *The Given* by Brightman: "[God's] consciousness is an eternally active will, which eternally finds and controls The Given within every moment of his eternal experience. The Given consists of the eternal, uncreated laws of reason and also equally eternal and uncreated processes of nonrational consciousness which exhibit all the ultimate qualities of sense objects (qualia) disorderly impulses and desires, such experiences as pain and suffering, the forms of space and time, and whatever God is the source of surd evil. The common characteristics of all that is "given" [...] is, first, that it is eternal within the experience of God and hence had no other origin than God's eternal being; and, secondly, that is not a product of will or created activity. For The Given to be in consciousness at all means that it must be process; but unwilled, nonvoluntary consciousness is distinguishable from voluntary consciousness, both in God and man. [...] God, finding The Given as an inevitable ingredient, seeks to impose ever new combinations of given rational form on the given nonrational content. Thus The Given is, on the one hand, God's instrument for the expression of his aesthetic and moral purposes, and, on the other, an obstacle to their complete and perfect expression. [...] the will of God, partially thwarted by obstacles in the chaotic Given, finds new avenues of advance, and forever moves on in the cosmic creation of new values." See Brightman, E.S. 1940. *A philosophy of Religion*. New York, NY: Prentice-Hall, pp. 336–338, cit. in Bertocci, P.A. A theistic explanation of evil. In: Ferré, F., Kockelmans, J.J., Smith, J.E. 1982. *The Challenge of Religion. Contemporary Readings in Philosophy of Religion*. New York, NY: The Seabury Press, pp. 340–341.

[317]   More specifically, the estimated heritability (population variance in liability to the disorder that is due to genetic variation) for schizophrenia, bipolar disorder, and autism is likely in excess of 70%, whereas heritability for depression and anxiety disorders is estimated to be 30%–40%. See Sullivan, P. F., Daly, M. J., & O'Donovan, M. 2012. *Genetic architectures of psychiatric disorders: The emerging picture and its implications*. Nature Reviews Genetics, 13(8), 537–551.

medication that targets that very psychiatric issue.[318] Finally, the medical/scientific understanding of risk loci for mental health disorders is quite problematic from the perspective of gene-gene and gene-environment interaction. In fact, analysis following Genome-Wide Association Studies (GWAS) need to take into account important factors such as immediate data (results/outcomes), interpretation of such data, polygenicity, cross-disorder effects/pleiotropy, rare variants, missing and phantom heritability, and epigenetics.[319] Given these premises, what lies beyond the surfaces of gene-

---

[318]   For a thorough analysis of these aspects, see Bibliography, in particular: Whitaker, R. 2010. *Anatomy of an Epidemic: Magic Bullets, Psychiatric Drugs, and the Astonishing Rise of Mental Illness in America*, New York, NY: Crown, and Breggin, P.R. 1991. *Toxic Psychiatry: Why Therapy, Empathy, and Love Must Replace the Drugs, Electroshock, and Biochemical Theories of the "new Psychiatry"*, New York, NY: St. Martin's Press. Partially against this view, Mario Bunge writes "Half a century ago, when psychotropic drugs replaced psychoanalytic myths, the psychiatric profession gained in pills and in grateful patients" (Bunge, M. 2013. *Medical Philosophy. Conceptual Issues in Medicine*. Singapore: World Scientific Publishing, p. 88). However, the Argentinean author is ready to add "Scientific psychiatry is still so backward, that it even lacks a good categorization of mental diseases; the standard one is symptomatic, [...] there are no reliable biomarkers of mental disorders; only behavioral and subjective symptoms." (Ibid.).

[319]   "Beyond methods that identify specific risk variants, approaches that examine collective contributions of hundreds or thousands of single nucleotide polymorphisms (SNPs) at once, such as polygenic risk score profiling (Purcell et al., 2009) and SNP heritability estimates (Yang, Lee, Goddard, & Visscher, 2011), are now yielding additional clues about the genetic architecture of psychiatric disorders. Consistent with decades of results from family studies, it has now been confirmed with molecular data that psychiatric disorders are highly polygenic (Sullivan et al., 2012). These new approaches are also yielding novel insights. For example, it has been demonstrated that the combined effects of common genetic variants are responsible for a substantial portion of liability to schizophrenia (Ripke et al., 2013), ruling out the possibility that only rare variants contribute to schizophrenia. This represents a fundamental discovery in the emerging picture of the genetic architecture of psychiatric disorders. [...] due to the very small effect of any individual locus on population-level risk for a disorder, sample sizes in the tens of thousands are often necessary to detect risk loci. [...] New polygenic modeling techniques have made it possible to estimate the number of common loci contributing to a given disorder, which, for schizophrenia, has been estimated at 8,300 common variants (Ripke et al., 2013; Stahl et al., 2012). Thus, it is clear that—for schizophrenia at least—there are many thousands of risk loci and that dramatic increases in sample sizes led to the detection of a large number of specific risk loci. Third, molecular data now provide more evidence for pleiotropy, the phenomenon in which individual genetic variants yield more than one phenotypic effect (Cross Disorder Group of the Psychiatric Genomics Consortium, 2013a, 2013b; Purcell et al., 2009; Solovieff, Cotsapas, Lee, Purcell, & Smoller, 2013). These findings are relevant to psychiatric disorder nosology, and recent reports have largely confirmed findings from twin studies (Cross-Disorder Group of the Psychiatric Genomics Consortium, 2013a). The strongest overlap in genetic influences identified to date (using molecular methods) is between schizophrenia and bipolar disorder, but the state of genome-wide research varies widely across disorders, so a complete understanding of pleiotropy awaits studies that combine large samples of individuals across multiple

environment interactions? Since our focus is on Medical Philosophy, and on

---

psychiatric disorders. [...] A rare variant refers to a variant whose minor allele is present in a very small proportion of the population (typically less than 1%, though definitions vary). [...] Additionally, using exome sequence data and trio designs, a role for de novo point mutations has also been established for autism (Neale et al., 2012; O'Roak et al., 2011; Sanders et al., 2012). [...] Missing heritability refers to the gap between how much phenotypic variance has been explained by specific genetic variants and how much has been explained by heritability estimates from twin or other *suitable* studies [Author's cursive—See Bibliography: Breggin, N/A]. For schizophrenia and many other complex phenotypes, the gap is substantial. For example, in the seminal article on this topic, Manolio et al. (2009) noted that only 5% of the variance in height had been explained by the approximately 40 known loci for height, compared with a population estimate of 80% heritability for height. The gap of 75% was referred to as missing heritability, and extensive discussion of possible explanations for it and potential avenues for solution have been offered (e.g., Manolio et al., 2009; Parker & Palmer, 2011). Sources of missing heritability undoubtedly include undetected common and rare variants but may also include structural variants not well captured by existing arrays, nonadditive genetic effects (dominance and epistasis), and gene–environment interactions (Manolio et al., 2009). Regarding GxE [Gene-Environment product/interaction, N/A] effects, it's worth noting that the nature of the environmental variable involved in a GxE determines whether the effect of a particular G₁ E contributes to the additive genetic (h2, narrow-sense heritability) or nonshared environmental variance component in twin models (Purcell, 2002), so it is unclear whether—on balance—GxEs may have inflated or reduced heritability estimates from twin studies. Further, the effect of G₁ Es on heritability estimates may vary across traits. For an argument that heritability estimates may be inflated due to interactions, thereby leading to "phantom heritability,". See Zuk, Hechter, Sunyaev, and Lander (2012), and for a relevant counterpoint, which predates Zuk et al., see Hill, Goddard, and Visscher (2008). [...] Epigenetics refers to heritable changes in gene expression or cellular phenotype that are caused by factors other than sequence changes in DNA.4 Common mechanisms of epigenetic effects are methylation and histone modifications. Unfortunately, epigenetics seems particularly susceptible to gross misunderstandings vis-à-vis genetic effects on psychiatric phenotypes. One problem is that epigenetics is in its infancy and may prove even more complex than the study of genetic sequence itself. Thus, efforts to explain psychiatric phenotypic variation via a small number of epigenetic variables (e.g., two variables out of millions possible) will likely encounter the same pitfalls evident in candidate gene and candidate G₁ E research. Another challenge is that epigenetic marks vary across and within tissues. Thus, peripheral (e.g., blood) measures of epigenetic variation may not reflect brain epigenetic states." Cit. from Duncan, L.E., Pollastri, A.R., Smoller, J.W. 2014. *Mind the Gap. Why Many Geneticists and Psychological Scientists Have Discrepant Views About Gene–Environment Interaction (GxE) Research*. In *American Psychologist*. Vol. 69, Num. 3: 218–324 Washington, DC: APA, American Psychological Association, pp. 259–260. Epigenetics represent evidently an immense help in understanding mental health disorders. It is important to remember, and we agree with Bunge in this regard, that "[...] the only important and robust finding of medical genetics, until recently the wunderkind of medicine, is that the one disease-one gene principle is just one more failure of genetic reductionism." (Bunge, M. 2013. *Medical Philosophy. Conceptual Issues in Medicine*. Singapore: World Scientific Publishing, p. 173). Perhaps, the terms "only important and robust" are not completely correct. Plus, we suggest here we extend the same judgement to the one disease-one cause of many modern Western medical researchers and practitioners, to open up the perspective to the interconnectedness of everything living, including the human organism.

patient self-perception, it is evident that understanding the scientific basis of human behavior is a fundamental requirement. The realization of the importance of environment, especially in human behavioral action-reaction goes beyond the poetic and aesthetic discussion, although those aspects are strongly connected to our analysis; it is a thoroughly scientific discovery that allows us to shed light to the poetic (this time, in term of creative, morphing/forming) aspects of sympathy/empathy in our philosophical analysis. We are talking about the Discovery of Mirror Neurons by Italian neurophysiologits in the early 1990s, one (perhaps the most) fundamental discovery in modern neuroscience in regard to the understanding of human nature, perception, and behavior.[320] The vast challenges that science has encountered in defining the origin of human behavior, were certainly worthy of effort, especially since discoveries such as mirror neurons and neurogenesis opened new perspectives on the gene-environment interactions, including our (human) ability to influence and be influenced by life experience. In fact, we could argue that the wonderful aspects of the research on interaction between genes and internal-external environment is one of the most important parts of Medical Philosophy, since they

---

[320] We are obviously talking about Giacomo Rizzolatti, Giuseppe Di Pellegrino, Luciano Fadiga, Leonardo Fogassi, and Vittorio Gallese at the University of Parma, Italy, between 1980 and 1990. By placing electrodes in the ventral premotor cortex of the macaque monkey, the scientist were studying neurons specialized for the control of hand and mouth actions. The researchers allowed the monkey to reach for pieces of food and recorded from a single neuron in the monkey's brain. Therefore, they were able to measure the neuron's specific response to specific movements. The Italian scientists found that some of the neurons they recorded from would respond when the monkey saw a person pick up a piece of food as well as when the monkey picked up the food. Interestingly, the discovery was initially sent to *Nature* but was rejected for its "lack of general interest". A few years later, the same group published another empirical paper, discussing the role of the mirror-neuron system in action recognition, and proposing that the human Broca's region was the homologue region of the monkey ventral premotor cortex. While these papers reported the presence of mirror neurons responding to hand actions, a subsequent study by Ferrari Pier Francesco and colleagues described the presence of mirror neurons responding to mouth actions and facial gestures. Further experiments confirmed that about 10% of neurons in the monkey inferior frontal and inferior parietal cortex have "mirror" properties and give similar responses to performed hand actions and observed actions. In 2002 Christian Keysers and colleagues reported that, in both humans and monkeys, the mirror system also responds to the sound of actions. See Rizzolatti, G., and Craighero, L. 2004. *The mirror-neuron system*. Annual Review of Neuroscience 27: 169–192; Rizzolatti G., and Sinigaglia C. 2006. *So quel che fai. Il cervello che agisce e i neuroni specchio*. Milan, I: Raffaello Cortina Editore; Rizzolatti G., Sinigaglia C. 2010. *The functional role of the parieto-frontal mirror circuit: interpretations and misinterpretations*. Nature reviews neuroscience, 11(4) 264–274; Keysers, Christian2010. *Mirror Neurons*. Current Biology 19 (21): R971–973. doi: 10.1016; Fogassi et al. 2005. *Parietal Lobe: From Action Organization to Intention Understanding*, In: Science, Washington, D.C: American Association for the Advancement of Science.

are closely related to our direct understanding of what it means to be human in the healing process, in particular through the realization that our interaction, *id est* perception of the world within and around us has a straightforward effect on how we feel, physically, mentally, emotionally, and spiritually. To be sure, at the center of therapy there is communication, perception and self-perception. Ultimately, there is a relationship between patient and provider, as we previously discussed. Our investigation must therefore take into account the implications of these aspects in the analysis of both the best possible methodological strategies in therapy, as well as the best predictors for positive outcomes in the healing process. A special place in this debate is represented by the analysis of quality and quantity of provider's care, as well as the patient' role, also in terms of direct *effector*, in (his) health. This brings us to one of the central elements in defending the hypothesis discussed in this study, namely the scientific outcomes resulting from reopened discussion on the very nature and structure of medicine: again, the combination of evidence-based medicine and a patient-centered medicine, both supported by a strong theoretical (philosophical-scientific) basis, is key in producing positive outcomes in clinical-therapeutic settings, in particular diagnosis, prognosis, and treatment. This central element is represented by the complex, and to some extent mysterious, mechanisms underlying doctor-patient interaction. In the next chapter, we will be directing our attention to these mechanisms and to those therapies which complement, or integrate, the evidence-based biomedical science upon which Western Medicine is based.

Chapter 5
Complementary, Alternative, Traditional Medicine

5.1 I shall please, I will please

"Data showed that, with the exception of intense psychotherapy, people were spending far more time each year with alternative practitioners than they were with other health care providers."[321]

According to many defenders of the scientific and therapeutic superiority of modern conventional Western biomedicine, the positive results of alternative therapies are entirely due to the placebo effect. Generally speaking, the term (and its opposite *nocebo*) indicates a simulated and/or clinically ineffective treatment (procedure, substance, including pharmacological interventions) for a specific disease in the absence of patient's awareness-knowledge of the presence of the treatment itself.[322] Thus, the placebo/nocebo's respectively positive or negative effect, when proven (observed) existent, happens without a recognized, in terms of evidence-based science, activity. Therefore, a causal mechanism connected to the beneficial or detrimental outcomes of the therapeutic intervention is not observed. Alternative forms of medicine include those therapies, for which such a mechanism is not found and proven, and which are therefore justified, in terms of therapeutic effectiveness, by virtue of this placebo effect. Aside from the social and ethical considerations related to the use of *placebos* in medical settings, we need to understand the role of this effect in our discourse on patient-provider relationship as basis for positive outcomes in

---

[321] Quote by Dr. Carl Marci, a Harvard Medical School assistant professor of psychiatry at Massachusetts General Hospital, as cited by Cameron, D. 2011. *The Look of Love. Love's many splendors begin with empathy and attachment.* In: Byron, P.B. (Ed.) 2011. *The Science of Emotion*, Boston, MA: Harvard Medicine, pp. 28–30. Dr Marci studied the placebo effect in medicine, focusing in particular on alternative therapies such as acupuncture, homeopathy, and Reiki.

[322] More precisely, the term derives from the Latin *placēbō*, "I shall/will please" from *placeō*, "I please", in particular from the medieval funeral functions in which people used to pray (following Psalm 116,9 in the Latin Vulgata Clementina) "*placebo Domino in regione vivorum*", or "I will please the Lord in the land of the living (ones)".

therapeutic interventions. The fields of medical neuroscience and health psychology, in particular the biopsychosocial approach, have provided a great number of research studies showing the great importance of a more comprehensive analysis of these interactions, especially on neurological level and with a special medical importance in the field of psychoneuroimmunology. For instance, we know that empathy, not just in term of patient-provider relationship, but in a more general and universal (social) sense, triggers two important neurochemicals, dopamine and serotonin, associated with the emotion center of the brain, which is in turn connected to the brain's reward center. This is even more evident in the medical-scientific analysis of neurological development in children: "Human babies have the most postnatal neuronal growth of any species. Without empathy, there is no attachment, and attachment is essential for survival."[323] These aspects contribute to the understanding of similar models of human interaction, for instance the mother-infant connection. Research has suggested that mothers directly impact their babies' cortisol levels by their reaction to internal and external stressors (and related hormonal levels), thus causing different responses in the modulatory ability of their children.[324] The most important lesson here is that our physical health depends on our sense of connectedness with others, or, in other terms, our perception of (our)selves *in relation to* others, including health providers.[325] In the following chapters we will see how this "sense" of connectedness, especially from the perspective of the dopaminergic reward center, can be triggered/stimulated by pharmacological intervention, although this does not completely explain the aforementioned

---

[323]   Dr. Carl Marci, as cited by Cameron, D. 2011. *The Look of Love. Love's many splendors begin with empathy and attachment*. In: Byron, P.B. (Ed.) 2011. *The Science of Emotion*, Boston, MA: Harvard Medicine, p. 30.

[324]   See in particular the research by Dr. Karlen Lyons-Ruth, in: Cameron, D. 2011. *The Look of Love. Love's many splendors begin with empathy and attachment*. In: Byron, P.B. (Ed.) 2011. *The Science of Emotion*, Boston, MA: Harvard Medicine, p. 30.

[325]   "When you're disconnected, your immune system goes to hell. [...] If we know that loneliness affects our immune response, it's not surprising that it would happen at the level of DNA expression", according to Richard Schwartz. Jacqueline Olds further explains "[...] we now know that social connectedness and the feeling of being loved also activate [...] [the] reward center. If you lack the relationships needed to stimulate that part o your brain, you'll likely find it in a drug." Both researchers are discussed in: Cameron, D. 2011. *The Look of Love. Love's many splendors begin with empathy and attachment*. In: Byron, P.B. (Ed.) 2011. *The Science of Emotion*, Boston, MA: Harvard Medicine, p. 31. Furthermore, we could argue that the correlation between the empathetic understanding on the other's emotions, feelings, and ultimately, (physical, mental, spiritual, etc.) suffering has a lot of internal value as a founding element in the series of conceptual elements imagination-ideation-fantasy/phantom(izing)-ghost-*Geist*.

complexity of these interactions, and certainly not the more subtle, and yet very present and apparent, effects of the so-called "placebo response mechanism", a true conceptual oxymoron which Medical Philosophy attempts to reframe and rephrase on a theoretical level, by further analyzing the scientific data available.[326] To be sure, we need to realize that the very use of a term such as "placebo" is a logico-conceptual fallacy, a not-so-hidden scientis*tic* escape from a not-yet-understood (under the lenses of modern Western medical science) underlying healing mechanism, philosophically related to the famous *Vis medicatrix naturae* of Naturopathic Medicine.[327] This healing power is understood and used as methodological basis for therapeutic interventions in alternative therapies such as art and music therapy.[328] Furthermore, the concept of a

---

[326] For further reference and current scientific data see Miller, A. 2014. *Friends wanted. New research by psychologists uncovers the health risks of loneliness and the benefits of strong social connections.* Monitor on Psychology, Vol 45, No. 1 Washington, DC: American Psychological Association, pp. 54–58.

[327] The phrase is itself a Latin rendering of the Greek *Νόσων φύσεις ἰητροί* or "Nature is the physician(s) of diseases", as wrongly attributed to Hippocrates, rightfully credited for the *Primum non nocere*. For further reference, see Bibliography, in particular: Hiroshi, H. 1998. *On Vis medicatrix naturae and Hippocratic Idea of Physis.* In: Memoirs of School of Health Sciences, Faculty of Medicine, Kanazawa University 22: 45–54. For current research, see for instance Donia M.S., Cimermančič P., Schulze C.J., et al. 2014. *A systematic analysis of biosynthetic gene clusters in the human microbiome reveals a common family of antibiotics.* Cell.; 158(6): 1402–1414.

[328] One of the most recent examples of research in the analysis of the effects of music training in children neurological development is the study by Hudziak and Albaugh, as described by Dr. David C. Rettew, MD, a child psychiatrist at the UVM Medical Center and director of the Child & Adolescent Psychiatry Residency Program: "The subjects for the study were 232 typically developing children without psychiatric illness between the ages of 6 and 18, all of whom received structural MRI scans at up to three different time points. With these serial MRI scans the examiners were able to see how the thickness of the brain cortex changed with age. Prior studies have indicated that the cortex generally thins across adolescence as the brain undergoes a normal "pruning" process that may be related to more efficient brain functioning. A delay in this cortical thinning process, particularly in regions such as the prefrontal and orbitofrontal cortex, which are thought to be important for "executive control" functions such as inhibiting impulses and regulating attention, has recently been shown among those with clinical attention problems and ADHD. The amount of musical training a child had was also measured to see if this variable interacted with age in its association to cortical thickness. The average time playing an instrument was about two years. The main result of the study was that years of musical training were indeed related to age-related cortical thinning. Specifically, more musical training was associated with accelerated thinning, not only in the expected motor cortices but also in some of the very same regions implicated in those with more pronounced attention problems. "What was surprising was to see regions that play key roles in emotional regulation also modified by the amount of musical training one did." The authors concluded that musical training was associated with more rapid cortical maturation across many brain areas, and they hypothesized that musical training may have beneficial effects on brain development for children whether or not they suffered from

healing power pushes us to considerations touching upon the metaphysical sphere, especially from a dualistic versus monistic perspective:

"At first sight, the placebo effect supports the dualist belief in the power of the immaterial mind over the material body. Actually, it does just the opposite. Indeed, recent studies with fMRI [...] have shown that a placebo object activates the same brain regions that are stimulated with opiates, among them the endorphins synthesized by the brain itself. That is, the placebo response is a brain process."[329]

---

attention or executive function difficulties. [...] Dr. Hudziak, who has done research on the genetic influence of various traits and abilities, notes that our culture seems to have it backwards in promoting certain activities only for children who seem born to excel at them. He questions why "only the great athletes compete, only the great musicians play, and only the great singers sing," especially as children age. He and his team have worked to improve local access to musical training through research studies and mentorship programs. The need is still high, however, and is now underscored by the increasing data linking wellness activities to measurable changes in brain development." See: Rettew, D.C. 2014. *A Prescription for Music: Study Finds Musical Training Linked to Enhanced Brain Maturation in Children*. University of Vermont Medical Center Blog, December 17th, 2014. The study discussed: Hudziak JJ, Albaugh MD, et al. *Cortical thickness maturation and duration of music training: Health-promoting activities shape brain development*. JAACAP. 2014; 11: 1153–1161. In terms of therapeutic application of medicine, and interesting article by Amy Novotney appeared on the November 2013 edition of Monitor on Psychology. The author writes: "While music has long been recognized as an effective form of therapy to provide an outlet for emotions, the notion of using song, sound frequencies and rhythm to treat physical ailments is a relatively new domain, says psychologist Daniel J. Levitin, PhD, who studies the neuroscience of music at McGill University in Montreal. A wealth of new studies is touting the benefits of music on mental and physical health. For example, in a meta-analysis of 400 studies, Levitin and his postgraduate research fellow, Mona Lisa Chanda, PhD, found that music improves the body's immune system function and reduces stress. Listening to music was also found to be more effective than prescription drugs in reducing anxiety before surgery (Trends in Cognitive Sciences, April, 2013). "We've found compelling evidence that musical interventions can play a health-care role in settings ranging from operating rooms to family clinics," says Levitin, author of the book "This is Your Brain on Music" (Plume/Penguin, 2007). The analysis also points to just how music influences health. The researchers found that listening to and playing music increase the body's production of the antibody immunoglobulin A and natural killer cells — the cells that attack invading viruses and boost the immune system's effectiveness. Music also reduces levels of the stress hormone cortisol. "This is one reason why music is associated with relaxation," Levitin says". The article also examines interesting aspects of the healing power of vibration, opening new scientific and philosophical perspectives on traditional practices such as chanting, especially in relation to the use of mantras and the connection with chakras. For reference, see Novotney, A. 2013. *Music as medicine. Researchers are exploring how music therapy can improve health outcomes among a variety of patient populations, including premature infants and people with depression and Parkinson's disease*. Monitor on Psychology, Vol. 44, N.10, Washington, DC: American Psychological Association, pp. 46–49.

[329]   Bunge, M. 2013. *Medical Philosophy. Conceptual Issues in Medicine. Singapore*: World Scientific Publishing, p. 162.

Unfortunately, this claim is a classical example of *post (iste) hoc, ergo propter hoc*, and it does not provide any scientific evidence for accepting the causal relation, or even the connection, between the physiological (neurological) level and the visible (evidence/d) of the placebo.[330] In fact, Bunge partially contradicts himself few paragraphs below: "The belief associated with the placebo effect does not arise spontaneously; it only occurs in a brain manipulated by the persons who offer the placebo object."[331] Again, we should first work on the conceptual value of belief in this specific case, and then, make sure that we understand the physical and/or multilayered effector of *mani*pulation, since it is a *person* administering it. Plus, the non-spontaneity of the effect should also push us to further investigations beyond this perspective. This logical fallacy is observable also in accounts such as the following, by Carlson:

> "[Philosophers'] lack of success made it clear that mere speculation is futile. If we could answer the mind-body question simply by thinking about it, philosophers would have done so long ago. [...] We believe that once we understand how the body works – and, in particular, how the nervous systems works – the mind-body problem will have been solved. What we call "mind" is a *consequence* of the functioning of the body and its interactions with the environment. The mind-body problem thus exists only as an abstraction. Because a belief in free will implies that the mind is not constrained by physiology, it is a form of dualism. This belief is unacceptable in the laboratory; physiological research is limited to those things that can be measured by physical means – matter and energy."[332]

We certainly won't argue against the fact that evidence-based research has to focus on observable data; that is the very nature of this type of research. However, if our goal is to understand human beings and *what it mens to be human*, which is part of the focus of this study, we have to realize that this methodology, as precise, accurate and adapt as it may be, it is not enough. In fact, what Carlson writes about philosophers, could be rightfully said about physical scientists as well: The book by Carlson was first published in 1977, and continuously improved until the 5th edition in 1994. Over ten years later evidence-based science alone still did not answer the body problem. Or, more precisely, physical science presented one possible hypothesis, among many others. In

---

[330]   For further reference, please see Jensen K.B., Kaptchuk T.J., Kirsch I., et al. 2012. *Nonconscious activation of placebo and nocebo pain responses*. Proceedings of the National Academy of Sciences. September 10, 2012.

[331]   Bunge, M. 2013. *Medical Philosophy. Conceptual Issues in Medicine. Singapore*: World Scientific Publishing, p. 163.

[332]   Carlson, N.R. 1994 (5th Ed.). *Physiology of Behavior*. Needham Heights, MA: Allyn and Bacon / Paramount Publishing, p. 4, (our Italics). We leave the discussion on whether matter and energy are purely (and entirely) physical *things* to the continuation of this volume.

fact, that is what philosophy does, too, as it has been doing for centuries. Carlson is ready to (re)frame his statement with a certain aura of tolerance, few paragraphs after: "[...] For all practical purposes physiological psychology will never take all the mystery out of an individual's behavior,"[333] thus admitting the possibility of more than one layer of interpretation, perhaps something still not quite understood in between monism and dualism. The main problem and fallacy of this argument can be summarized in the following sentence "Because our techniques are physical, our explanations must also be physical."[334] Again, this is *mettere il carro davanti ai buoi*. We are confusing technology (or technological progress, not methodology) and knowledge/understanding, and in doing that we are using (an inappropriate, imprecise, wrong form of) philosophy, not evidence-based science. These are not-verified assumptions, similar to the one that wants the placebo effect to happen (exclusively) in the brain, due to mechanisms such as cognitive control, conditioning or production and secretion of neurotransmitters, completely ignoring the non-verified causal effect of such mechanisms from brain to *effects* which *affect* the whole person, and the fact that, however this statement might sound accurate, we are still in the realm of philosophical-theoretical speculation, and further proof is necessary. In short, it is still a matter of opinion whether the whole mechanism is a proof of a (-n intelligent, purposeful, meaningful, divine,) design, evolution (which, let's not forget does not necessarily imply "blind" and "random"), or pure chance. Still, we have a lot of work to do, and our work has to be necessarily philosophical, especially since we need to ask the right questions *in the hope* (with all the possible implications that this term may and might contain) to find the right[335] answers. As we previously discussed, the modern conception of medical science, and as medicine in general, is strictly linked to the

---

[333]   Ibid., p. 5. To be sure, Carlson states that "We assume that, in principle, human behavior can be explains down to the last detail by completely understanding its physiology" (Ibid.), and we agree. In the sense that this is *an assumption*, and *in principle*.

[334]   Ibid.

[335]   In fact, the problem is much deeper than the oversimplification used here for explanatory clarity. Bunge writes: "[...] since mutations are random, molecular biology, bacteriology, and virology use probability theory to study them. But the effects of mutated pathogens on cells are causal, not random; whereas some of them will be ineffective, others will provoke the immune system to produce the adequate antibodies, and still others will attack the body unopposed. In sum, randomness on one level of organization will induce causation in the next. This alteration of chance and cause happen in several fields, and it suggests that, although the two categories are interrelated, neither is reducible to the other." Bunge, M. 1951. *What is chance?* Science and Society 15: 209–231, cited in: Bunge, M. 2013. *Medical Philosophy. Conceptual Issues in Medicine*. Singapore: World Scientific Publishing, p. 167.

combination between accurate, precise, non-biased, individual (with generalistic clinical applicability) observation, a strong theoretical approach (which allows for intelligent hypothesizing) and experimentation. In regard to psychological science, a very common view in the Western Medical environment is that autochthonous, aboriginal, tribal, folk, traditional (in the sense of non-school medicine), philosophical and religious perspectives and advice, these have to be first contextualized through a "Westernizing" evidence-based filter, for instance by literally translating them into empirical or theoretical concepts from psychology and medicine.[336] According to Christopher, Wendt, Marecek and Goodman "This unexpected requirement reflects the scientific ideal of sharply separating psychology from philosophy and religion."[337] Although there are positive elements in this sectorialization of knowledge, a division in part derived from the Cartesian and post-Cartesian view of separation between mind/spirit/soul and body/brain, a total separation has negative effects on both disciplines. The first and most apparent is the lowering effect, in terms of scientific value and ethical guidance, of philosophy. The second is the negation of the vast positive improvement of psychological science when the latter uses the methods of evidence-based hard science to add support to its theoretical basis. In the same volume, Albert Katz writes as example:

> "Psychology at Western [Ontario University] separated from philosophy and became an independent administrative unit in 1948, because of, as the story goes, antipathy toward psychology by the then-president of the university, who thought that psychology would wither on the vine by being isolated from philosophy."[338]

Similar problems are also encountered when comparing different psychological schools, approaches and methodologies. According to Christopher, Wendt, Marecek and Goodman:

---

[336]   A filter, as we repeatedly observed, which is itself not immune to those considerations, especially in those typical western evidence-based medical institutions such as hospitals and medical colleges: "[…] The hospital, the modern cathedral, lords it over this hieratic environment of health devotees." Illich, I. 1976. *Limits to Medicine; Medical Nemesis: The Expropriation of Health*. London, UK: Marion Boyars Publishers, p. 79.

[337]   Christopher, J.C., Wendt, D.C., Marecek, J., D.C., Goodman, D.M. 2014. *Critical Cultural Awareness. Contributions to a Globalizing Psychology*. In *American Psychologist*. Vol. 69, Num. 7: 645–655 Washington, DC: APA, American Psychological Association, p. 647.

[338]   Katz, A. 2014. *Obituaries: Mary J. Wright (1915–2014)*, In *American Psychologist*. Vol. 69, Num. 7: 645–655 Washington, DC: APA, American Psychological Association, p. 703.

"[...] beyond learning about other psychologies, psychologists need to be open to learning from them – that is, to reassessing or even revising their own ways of thinking. The psychologies of Buddhism and Yoga, for instance, blur the sharp distinction that Western thought has drawn between religion and philosophy, on the one hands, and psychology, on the other. Moreover, other cultures may yield practices that have useful applications in clinical psychology and behavioral medicine in the United States. Meditation and mindfulness-based practices are ready examples. Learning from other cultures involves being open to practices that may not involve professionalized services, credentialed clinicians, or medicalized or "health"- oriented frameworks."[339]

In fact, we could argue that certain views on multidisciplinary approach versus sectorialization of disciplines are more derived from the cultural milieu of the society that produces them, than a genuine effort to advance scientific research. This is especially true in Western, especially American, politics guiding rules and regulations of academia, medicine, applied science and public policy. One of the most inaccurate cultural and political stereotypes in the United States wants to equate far-right wing, conservative and republican politics with the love of history, tradition and philosophy and left-wing, liberal, progressive and "godless" politics with a generalized lack of "true" values especially in terms of morality, and socio-cultural awareness (in terms of patriotism). This hypersectorialized division between two poles does not serve any of the disciplines in the scientific, cultural, social, religious and philosophical (if we still want to maintain division of subjects) study, application and research, and certainly does not contribute to the search for truth (and its application in practical and ethical terms), which should be the ultimate goals of any of the above mentioned disciplines. Needless to say, the too often present cultural imperialism and self-righteousness of Western science had been proven to discredit knowledge which does not fit in the accepted paradigm of the time. Certainly, one of the best definitions of Post-Galilean Science has to do with science's ability to reconsider its statements in the light of more updated data. However, there are some areas in which not only contemporary science still fails to provide successful and definite explanation, but which also provide some knowledge that has been so far (through the lens of human history) be quite successful and generally "working" in therapeutic sense. This is the area of the healing process, where oftentimes meanings are "so commonplace that

---

[339]   Reference to the work by Csordas, 1997; Echo-Hawk et al., 2011; Gone & Calf Looking, 2011; Kalkar, 1982; in: Christopher, J.C., Wendt, D.C., Marecek, J., D.C., Goodman, D.M. 2014. *Critical Cultural Awareness. Contributions to a Globalizing Psychology.* In *American Psychologist.* Vol. 69, Num. 7: 645–655 Washington, DC: APA, American Psychological Association, p. 652.

they are invisible."[340] To be sure, we should not rely on a "Science of the Gaps" based on a reinterpretation of the previously mentioned definition of "God of the Gaps", thus simply on the sense of awe and mystery of a not yet explained phenomena. This is exactly what science is not, and what should not be(come). In Medical Philosophy, and generally speaking in any philosophy which cares about the methods, purpose and theoretical and epistemological basis of (modern) science, we should avoid certain labeling attitudes which contribute to the misunderstanding and discreditation of traditional perspectives. Bunge's attitude toward this type of medicine is unequivocal: "For example, the Amazonian Indians, who are among the most backward, use several plants to which they attribute healing or magic properties."[341] This attitude is obviously not applied only to traditional healing methods, but even more to all those disciplines, such as Complementary and Alternative Medicine (CAM) which respect and partially use some of the therapeutic methods derived from traditional medicine. Bunge rejects every medical perspective not based on strong empirical, observable data and strong theoretical basis. However, by strongly and rightfully opposing the hyper medication of modern Western (again, especially US-American) society he is willing to accept therapies well grounded in psychological science and theory, such as Cognitive-Behavior Therapy. Certainly, the core problem here is to find a specific mechanism underlying the disease, and not relying on the two extremes of scientific enquiry, pure positivism and gullible attitude toward pseudo-science.

It is also very interesting to note that oftentimes scientific medicine is not perceived as "meaningful" from the perspective of defendants of complementary and alternative medicine, because of its perceived lack of deep spiritual components. This perspective is further corroborated by some proponents of a more 'scientistic' form of medicine, which, far from addressing purely scientific questions, takes on the conceptual purity of medicine as a science in which there is no room for "fantasizing" or "marveling". In this sense both sides are victims of their own sectorialized (in some cases even sectarianized) view, a view that purposely takes away awe and appreciation for the miracle (in the etymological sense) for what is observed and observable within the limits of modern science. We then wonder why the relationship between sci-

---

[340]   Christopher, J.C., Wendt, D.C., Marecek, J., D.C., Goodman, D.M. 2014. *Critical Cultural Awareness. Contributions to a Globalizing Psychology*. In *American Psychologist*. Vol. 69, Num. 7: 645–655 Washington, DC: APA, American Psychological Association, p. 648.

[341]   Bunge, M. 2013. *Medical Philosophy. Conceptual Issues in Medicine*, Singapore: World Scientific Publishing, p. 1.

ence in general and specific branches of medicine focused on mental issues is so problematic, from the perspective of evidence-based analysis. Schaef asks a similar question:

"Why, then, is psychology so wedded to empirical science? The reasons must be political and economic. The intensity of emotion with which psychologists defend the old paradigm strongly suggests that we are not dealing with open-minded science here.

Historically, we have always seen that when an old cultural paradigm is dying and on the verge of collapse, there is a tendency to become more rigid in the old paradigm, to set up progressively stricter controls, and to try to kill off new ideas and dissenters through the use of the regulatory and legal arms of the culture. We are seeing this in the United States today (and in many other parts of the Western world). As the old paradigm is being challenged professionally, politically, and economically, the arm of regulation and control gets stronger and stronger.

Contrary to popular belief, the push to maintain the old scientific paradigm and the Western worldview is very emotional and is based on economics and politics. If the existing worldview falters, we will not be able economically and politically to exploit Third World countries, indigenous people, the animal kingdom, or nature. The existing worldview has permitted and supported rape on every level, and, unfortunately, psychology and the helping professions have contributed to that rape."[342]

---

[342]   Schaef, A.W. 1992. *Beyond Therapy, Beyond Science*. New York, NY: HarperCollins, p. 226. The relation between *psychotherapy* and (social) science is even more complicated. As Tracey, Wampold, Lichtenberg, and Goodyear, have examined, "Essentially, psychotherapy is a process about which the therapist receives little explicit and valid feedback about what actions are productive of a therapeutic outcome. Notwithstanding the above difficulty, there is extensive evidence that psychotherapy is effective. As well, there are documented differences among the outcomes achieved by therapists—some therapists consistently achieve better outcomes than others. Thus, although it appears that there exists such a thing as expertise, little is known about what differentiates the more effective therapists from others; certainly it does not appear to be the type of therapy delivered or the experience of the therapist (Beutler et al., 2004). What has emerged is that more effective therapists appear to be able to form working alliances across a range of clients (Baldwin, Wampold, & Imel, 2007) and have a greater level of facilitative skills (Anderson, Ogles, Patterson, Lambert, & Vermeersch, 2009). [...] Clearly, more research about the process and outcome of psychotherapy is needed (see Kazdin, 2008), including what characterizes expert therapists with better outcomes, because it is clear that better outcomes do not emerge as a function of experience. It is crucial that therapists obtain quality information about both client and therapist outcomes if they are to establish expertise. However, as we have argued, outcome information alone, even if of high quality, does not ensure that expertise will develop. Cognitive heuristics, especially hindsight bias, can minimize the impact of outcome information on future practice. To benefit from quality information, therapists are encouraged to adopt a prospective testing of hypotheses, where the outcome information serves as the criterion." See Tracey, J.G., Wampold, B.E., Lichtenberg, J.W., Goodyear, R.K. 2014. *Expertise in Psycho-*

5.2 Integrating, complementing, completing

a) A logical examination: Central Medicine

Certainly, there are important components of modern science that need to be reanalyzed from the aforementioned perspectives if we want to incorporate all these elements in our effort to overcome the dichotomies between East and West, mainstream and alternative, etc. and create a truly ***Central Medicine.*** Central, in the sense that the patient is at the center of our therapeutic strategies[343], and Central, with respect to the extreme (extremist) opposite sides of what is accepted in terms of Hierarchy of Evidence, (hyper)medication, and healthcare policies. Luckily, more and more research within the accepted fields of evidence-based medicine, and science in general, is yielding very convincing results to support an alternative perspective, to the point that perhaps we will not have to use the term "alternative" in the first place or *in the place of* a perceived opposite side of the scientific spectrum of medicine. Medical Philsopohy helps again to identify the problem and frame the discussion around which the validity of the claims by CAM can be understood, examined, and ultimately supported or rejected. One of the first issues is represented by the very elusive nature of some therapies, take as example homeopathy. To be sure, our analysis needs to challenge preconcepts and prejudices from within alternative therapies, especially when they are faith and/or belief based. At the same time, we also need to remember our previous discussion on metaphysical and theological grounds toward human ability of achieving understanding. In detail, we must reconsider our very concept of *existence*:

> "Heidegger is using the word 'exist' in a technical manner; non-Daseinish things (things like snowflakes and speedboats) do not 'exist', but that does not mean that there are no such things. Instead, it means they have a different mode of being. Something only 'exists' in Heidegger's sense when its way of being is one particular interpretation of how it should be the thing it is."[344]

The last part of this statement is the real core of our analysis. Where should we draw the line between what is considered "existing" and "non-existing" in our search for mechanisms and theoretical ground to support diverse approaches to

---

therapy. *An Elusive Goal?* In: *American Psychologist.* Vol. 69, Num. 3: 217–315. Washington, DC: APA, American Psychological Association, pp. 225–226.

[343]   This is a fundamental aspects, as we should never forget that technology should serve the patient, and not the other way round, as it is sometimes the case with Electronic Health/Medical Records (EHR or EMR).

[344]   Wrathall, M. 2006. *How to Read Heidegger*, W. W. Norton, p. 13.

medicine? Many simply argue that the line is drawn by what is proved through the lenses of scientific experimentation. This is the "real" (connected to the *Res*) evidence, upon which medicine is based. No scientific evidence[345] means no scientific proof, thus, no medicine. Some argue instead, that an empirical approach should be used, even beyond the limits of what is tested in field research or laboratory. From this standpoint, "if it works, it is medicine; if it doesn't, it is not."[346] However, this implies that there is no room, nor need for concepts such as alternative, complementary, integrative, traditional, holistic, etc. Let us see why. First, there is no alternative to therapeutic effectiveness, because (again) if it works is already medicine, the alternative being therapeutic failure. Second, if medicine works and produces (a complete, even if not definite) healing, there is no need to complement it, since the goal has already been achieved. Third, to integrate something means that this something is lacking some parts, and as we just said, if medicine is able to provide healing, all the sufficient and necessary parts are already in place. Fourth, since the very nature of science, in the modern, Galilean, evidence-based, Western (etc.) view of the term, means to continuously and actively looking for hypothesis and related proof, tradition alone should constitute an epistemological oxymoron. History (aside from the related statistical/epidemiological standpoint of monitored, longitudinal studies) has absolutely no value from this perspective. Fifth, what we said about complementing and integrating applies to a holistic approach as well: medicine is already whole, no room for anything else. If this is all true, why more and more people still believe in this form of medicine? Is it all there is, *just* a form of belief?

> "Studies show most patients don't tend to bring up their CAM [Complementary and Alternative Medicine] usage at medical appointments – a problem since some alternative therapies could interfere with conventional medicines. [Dr. Evelyn Y. Ho] and her team conducted a workshop to help patients build four skills: preparing a list of questions before the appointment; being proactive by initiating the CAM conversation; disclosing all CAM use; and

---

[345]   We should most definitely investigate the extent to which the concept of evidence is connected with visibility and perception, in science in general, but especially under the lenses of medical practice: "[...] explaining, in contrast to describing, involves conjecturing or exhibiting mechanisms, most of which are imperceptible, e.g., because they are too small or too big." Bunge, M. 2013. *Medical Philosophy. Conceptual Issues in Medicine*. Singapore: World Scientific Publishing, p. 32.

[346]   Obviously, we should also note that there are problematic issues arising I discussing whether it is necessary and sufficient for a therapy or pharmacological intervention to work in the lab, and in the lab only, from the perspective of tested, replicable, evidence-based research onto its application to the treatment of a patient.

asking relevant questions. After the workshop, more than half of patient mentioned their CAM use within the next two physician visits – a positive sign, Ho says."[347]

Those five points we just covered need to be further expanded and reinterpreted under the lenses of Medical Philosophy. Medicine should be able to address all these issues, in order to provide an even better (as well as *both* even, *and* better)[348] level of care. It should employ conceptual and experimental methods, dual control and double-blind study, randomization, and analysis of placebo/nocebo effects (including true placebo vs. deficient placebo, and non-specific effects), and a strong theoretical analysis to identify (possibly hidden) mechanisms.[349] In the case of CAM, the requirements of above mentioned standard are in some cases, hard to match. On the level of clinical trials, the main problem is the quantifiability of data; on the level of theoretical analysis, the big issue is the verifiability of hypothesis and theories. These problems are directly rooted in the very nature of some CAM therapies, due to the aforementioned problematic categorization of the existence of mechanisms and effects, which are hard to control for external/internal affecting/effecting factors. Certainly, some terminology used in CAM is totally foreign, or simply perceived as naïve, esoteric, imprecise, or completely out-of-context by evidence-based science.

However, the same could be said about conventional medicine, whose terms often make practitioners look, permit the term, "somewhat hard to understand" in comparison to the general, lay public (although this does not usually happen in areas in which Greek and Romance languages are spoken, since the medical terminology used therein simply, rightfully, and appropriately matches anatomy, symptoms, diagnosis, and prognosis)[350]. But what is alterna-

---

[347] Study discussed in Weir, K. 2012. *Improving patient-physician communication.* Monitor on Psychology, Vol. 43, N.10, Washington, DC.: American Psychological Association, pp. 38–40.

[348] We should never forget the social and ethical implication of an even perspective on the subjects of our studies, research and therapies. The focus is not on a *leveling universalization*, a generalization which does not respect the individuality and subjectivity of each person, but on a more fair treatment of every patient.

[349] It is the case of quantum theory applied to science, in particular medical research and therapy. Bunge disagrees, by stating that medicine focuses (starts) only at the macromolecular level, instead of what happens through chemistry and molecular analysis in pharmacology and biology. However, medicine treats the (whole) individual, and we should certainly refrain from jumping to (very imprecise) conclusion in defining this individual only at a macromolecular level.

[350] Regarding the linguistic aspects, "Foucault [...] claimed that the crucial difference between modern and traditional medicine is linguistic, whereas our [writes Bunge] account has fo-

tive medicine? The term comprises a wide range of theoretical and philosophical standpoints, diagnostic assessments, and therapeutic interventions, which are nowadays considered outside the theory and practice of mainstream medicine. However, the very concept of an alternative form of medicine does not apply to conventional forms of medicine from a purely historical perspective, since before the birth of modern evidence-based western medicine a distinction between the two approaches did not make sense. Furthermore, it is evident that other definitions such as "school medicine", mostly used to EBM are also historically correlated, in the sense that they originate from the same cultural background (with obvious ethno-geographical differences) out of which modern complementary and alternative methods were born. In fact, the problem in defining the differences between EBM and alternative medicine is mainly connected with the issue of accreditation and legal aspects. To be sure, practitioners of EBM follow a relatively standardized path, both in terms of education, research, and testing/verifying gained knowledge. Practitioners of alternative therapies instead were, until very recently and by the very nature of the term, outside this standardization. In fact, we could argue that by "alternative" we refer to an approach used *in place / instead of* conventional medicine, while by "integrative" and "complementary" we intend an approach used *in combination with* conventional medicine. Certainly, as we previously discussed, there are also important differences between integrating and complementing.[351] The

---

cused on biological discoveries." (Bunge, M. 2013. *Medical Philosophy. Conceptual Issues in Medicine*, Singapore: World Scientific Publishing, p. 37). This viewpoint starts in the description of Foucault's (again, in the interpretation of Bunge) take on method: "Foucault claimed that modern medicine is empiricist to the point of rejecting theory and philosophy, whereas we have emphasized the role of hypothesis in biomedical research and practice, as well as the strong impact of philosophy on the discipline sicne antiquity." (Ibid.).

[351]   A very interesting note in regard to the debate between integrative and alternative approaches is the decision of the US National center for Complementary and Alternative Medicine (NCCAM) to change its name to the National Center for Complementary and Integrative Health (NCCIH). The change did effectively take place during the writing of this study, and was presented on December 17, 2014: "Why did Congress change NCCAM's name? As part of an omnibus budget measure signed by President Obama in December 2014, Congress has changed the name of NCCAM to the National Center for Complementary and Integrative Health, or NCCIH. The change was made to more accurately reflect the Center's research commitment to studying promising health approaches that are already in use by the American public. Since the Center's inception, complementary approaches have grown in use to the point that Americans no longer consider them an alternative to medical care. For example, more than half of Americans report using a dietary supplement, and Americans spend nearly four billion dollars annually on spinal manipulation therapy. The name change is in keeping with the Center's existing Congressional mandate and is aligned with the strategic plan currently guiding the Center's research priorities and public education activities. Why

historical perspective is even more important when we attempt to define the borders between EBM and CAM. Among the vast criticism of the first to the latter is the non-verifiability of claims, following the rigorous procedures of laboratory and hypothesis testing: Alternative medicine is definitely more empirically and traditionally oriented. To be sure, this statement obviously carries all the complex series of philosophical implications related to the term "Tradition". However, scientific medicine is by definition always changing based on new discoveries and more recent and valid knowledge. Therefore, many practices that *traditionally* were used in CAM are now used within conventional medicine. From a theoretical standpoint, this might sound an oxymoron, but again the historical perspective within Medical Philosophy helps us better frame the problem. In fact, the aforementioned alternative practices (certainly not all of them, but a number which is constantly increasing) that are now part of mainstream medicine were always part of the medical practice, before the split between (let us use these terms for now) folk, traditional medicine and evidence-based medicine. Modern medicine separated itself from the non-verifiable claims of traditional medicine, thus inventing its own tradition, a tradition strongly based on a different type of evidence, based not only on ob-

---

does the new name include "Integrative Health" instead of "Alternative Medicine"? Large population-based surveys have found that the use of "alternative medicine"—unproven practices used in place of conventional medicine—is actually rare. By contrast, integrative health care, which can be defined as combining complementary approaches into conventional treatment plans, has grown within care settings across the nation, including hospitals, hospices, and military health facilities. The goal of an integrative approach is to enhance overall health, prevent disease, and to alleviate debilitating symptoms such as pain and stress and anxiety management that often affects patients coping with complex and chronic disease, among others. However, the scientific foundation for many complementary approaches is still being built". From the NCCIH Website https://nccih.nih.gov/. A further explanation describes the input of Dr. Collins, whose philosophical standpoint and scientific research we already discussed, and will encounter again in the following chapters: "Since its establishment 16 years ago, the center has funded thousands of important research projects. Without this work, the American public would lack vital information on the safety and effectiveness of many practices and products that are widely used and readily available," said NIH Director Francis S. Collins, M.D., Ph.D. "This change by Congress reflects the importance of studying the approaches to health and wellness that the public is using, often without the benefit of rigorous scientific study". "The intent of an integrative approach is to enhance overall health status, prevent disease, and alleviate debilitating symptoms such as pain and chemotherapy-induced nausea, among others. However, the scientific foundation for many complementary approaches is still being built," said Josephine P. Briggs, M.D., Director of NCCIH. "The mission of NCCIH will remain unchanged. We will continue to focus on the study of the usefulness and safety of complementary and integrative interventions, and provide the public with research-based information to guide health care decision making."(Ibid.).

servation, but on testing and statistics. This new paradigm brought an immense amount of new knowledge, technical skills and technologic advancement. In short, EBM brought progress to the art and science of treating illnesses. We have to keep in mind that EBM did not completely reject the practices of folk medicine: it simply discarded what could not be proven through evidence-based testing, and in this sense we should all be grateful for the vast achievements, both in philosophical-theoretical forms, as well as in clinical application, of modern science and modern medicine. With a constantly improving medical science, it is now time to further investigate complementary and alternative forms of medicine using the same rigorous methods of EBM. However, some forms of CAM are impossible to be verified using the aforementioned methods by their very nature, which brings us to the core of the theoretical debate of Medical Philosophy: if we want to verify the claims of CAM can we, should we, must we, apply the same rigorous methods of EBM?

b) Efficacy, Efficiency, Effectiveness

Generally speaking, in modernity the differences between philosophy and science, beside obvious etymological origins, have more to do with perceptions, emotions and feelings attached to the weight of these terms in society, than with a solid theoretical structure. This is absolutely not to say that the two terms are equivalent, certainly not from a philosophical and scientific perspective. Still, since both terms have a form of knowledge as the center, scope and target of their respective investigations, why is there a need to separate them? An analysis in terms of logic, semiotics, epistemology, and linguistics is definitely beyond the scope of this study, and yet, nearly every time we hear about science in the news we all tend to attach to this term a methodological *rigor*. We do not have to be prominent academics in the field of historical linguistics to understand the implications of such concept: (in plain alphabetic order) cold-ness, harshness (and harsh inflexibility in judgment, opinion, temper), inflexibility (and quality of being or inert), numb and numbness, rigor, rigidity, rigidness, severity, stiffness, strictness, stress, torpor, tremor. Interestingly enough, for a term associated with the precision of scientific investigation, this concept is often associated with the quality of being unyielding, and yet scientific evidence means yielding valid results. Furthermore, the Proto-Indo-European root *reyǵ- is translated with to reach, to stretch (out), qualities generally not associated with precise values (to stretch a result in science often means to have some form of bias, or cheating on the results). Now, all the aforementioned considerations might mean nothing to someone interest in

Medical Philosophy and in philosophy of medicine in general. They might even be considered far beyond what the scope of this research *should* be. Medical Philosophy deals with the understanding, in a theoretical and applied, therapeutic discourse, of what it means to be human. And there are not many things in our reality as complex, constantly morphing and less *rigorous* (in the above listed semantic series) then human beings.

Let us be clear; among the main focuses of science we find predictability of results and methodologically accurate forecast. We certainly do not advocate the use of imprecise or too flexible methods in clinical trials targeted at understanding the effect of, let's say, a new medication. We want to be *as rigorous as possible* in our investigation. However, when this very medication will be prescribed and administered to a human being there are many complex issues added in our quest for (in this case) therapeutic efficacy, starting from the previously discussed placebo effect. This is especially true when we are not dealing with modern, western, evidence-based, laboratory-tested, man-made, medicines and medical interventions, but with complementary and alternative medicine, which by its own nature defies some of these categories. Certainly we cannot put all the therapeutic methods usually listed under CAM in the same category, in the same group based on their efficacy, efficiency, and effectiveness.

Notably, *Efficacy* is the capacity to produce an effect. However, the term has different specific meanings in different fields. For instance, in medicine the term is closely related to the therapeutic *effect* of intervention, including physical therapy, a specific (or set of) drug(s), a medical device and/or technology, a surgical procedure, especially in clinical trials or laboratory research (contrary to *Effectiveness*, which is connected to the same meaning, but in applied clinical/medical practice, thus the capability of producing a desired impression, outcome or result.). The same applies for an intervention in the field of public health and/or translational science. From a philosophical perspective, we should also note that an *effective* theory or model focuses on explaining certain (observed) effects without the claim that the theory correctly models the underlying (unobserved) processes, and therefore very similar to a *phenomenological* theory or model. Finally, we define *Efficiency* as the amount of time, effort, or cost is well-used in order to achieve a specific result or outcome, and is thus different from Efficacy in the sense that the latter focuses on the aforementioned goals, not in the process of (in) achieving them. To be sure, "what is effective is not necessarily efficacious, and what is efficacious is not necessarily efficient."[352]

These definitions are the very center of the scientific/philosophical debate on Complementary and Alternative medicine. If we had to summarize the incredible amounts of resources, studies, general opinion, investigations, historical accounts, anecdotes, clinical trials, etc. in one single sentence, the supporters of CAM will say "*it works.*" Obviously, the critics would express themselves in a similar manner, although by morphing the sentence into the negative "it doesn't". We could argue that a great amount of efforts in proving or disproving the scientific validity if CAM still remains stuck in this type of argument. More specifically, many claims *pro* or *contra* this type of medicine originate from a personal belief, opinion, and even bias. Our goal and duty is to use the aforementioned definitions of efficacy, efficiency, and effectiveness to investigate the validity of CAM and understand to what extent a form of scientific rigor *can* be expected and *should* be applied. In order to follow this goal, we should at *least list* the most common and/or known forms and/or definitions within the vast realm of Complementary and Alternative/integrative medicine/health and related therapies and/or practices, with some indications on their proven efficacy, efficiency, and effectiveness as reference to the most current research findings (when available[353]) in the endnotes (here in alphabetical order):[354]

---

[352]   AA.VV. 2011. *Longman English Dictionary Online.* Harlow, UK: Longman, Pearson. Term: "Effective—Definition from Longman English Dictionary Online".

[353]   The reader should be advised that the hereby provided research results come from studies produced mostly in Europe and the USA. Although this might be considered a cultural and ethnocentric bias, we want to address the issue by indicating that the choice is related to the availability (also in terms of access through paper version and/or internet archives) of reliable (*id est* scientifically valid) material, published or translated in English (in few cases this was not possible and the author provided references in original language). Furthermore, the quoted research materials serve as an indication of the current CAM research, and by no means is intended to provide an omnicomprehensive and complete account of all the studies produced so far. The criticism of alternative methods is vastly directed at the lack of scientific evidence, in the sense that until very recently, only few integrative approaches have been submitted to evidence-based scientific evaluation (as in controlled trials), or if they had some were also found "guilty" of providing confirmation bias or imprecise results (a very famous case is the series of studies and articles on homeopathy published on *the Lancet* from 1995 on). Furthermore, the difficulties in producing valid research is due to a series of problems related to subjects' size (even smaller than 10, according to Kunstler, R., Greenblatt, F., & Moreno, N. 2004. *Aromatherapy and hand massage: Therapeutic recreation interventions for pain management.* Therapeutic Recreation Journal, 38, 133–147), and/or selection bias, error, imprecision and non-randomness (Rho, K., Han, S., Kim, K., & Lee, M.

- Acupuncture[355]
- Anthroposophic medicine[356]
- Aromatherapy[357]

S. 2006. *Effects of aromatherapy massage on anxiety and self-esteem in Korean elderly women: A pilot study.* International Journal of Neuroscience, 116, 1447–1455).

[354] Please note that many of these therapies can be comprised within bigger groups or smaller subfields in medicine, as well as associated with several forms of psychotherapy, such as cognitive-behavior(al) therapy (CBT), dialectic-behavior(al) therapy (DBT), acceptance and commitment therapy (ACT), and so on.

[355] Among the most important discoveries of resent research, we should note the effectiveness of "real" acupuncture interventions versus "sham" acupuncture (namely, needles randomly inserted). For further reference, see Vickers AJ, & Linde K 2014. *Acupuncture for chronic pain.* JAMA: the journal of the American Medical Association, 311 (9), 955–956 PMID; Endres HG, Zenz M, Schaub C, Molsberger A, Haake M, Streitberger K, Skipka G, Maier C, 2005. *German Acupuncture Trials (GERAC) address problems of methodology associated with acupuncture studies.* Schmerz. Jun; 19(3): 201–204, 206, 208–210; Leung L 2012. *Neurophysiological basis of acupuncture-induced analgesia–an updated review.* Journal of acupuncture and meridian studies, 5 (6), 261–270; Vickers AJ, Cronin AM, Maschino AC, Lewith G, MacPherson H, Foster NE, Sherman KJ, Witt CM, Linde K, & Acupuncture Trialists' Collaboration 2012. *Acupuncture for chronic pain: individual patient data meta-analysis.* Archives of internal medicine, 172 (19), 1444–1453 Crespin D.J., Griffin K.H., Johnson J.R., Miller C., Finch M.D., Rivard R.L., Anseth S., Dusek J.A. 2015. *Acupuncture Provides Short-Term Pain Relief for Patients in a Total Joint Replacement Program.* Pain Med. Jan 13. doi: 10.1111/pme.12685.Hollifield, M., Sinclair-Lian, N., Warner, T.D., and Hammerschlag, R. 2007. *Acupuncture for Posttraumatic Stress Disorder: A Randomized Controlled Pilot Trial.* The Journal of Nervous and Mental Disease; Kong J., Kaptchuk T.J., Polich G., et al. 2009. *Expectancy and treatment interactions: a dissociation between acupuncture analgesia and expectancy evoked placebo analgesia.* NeuroImage; 45(3): 940–949. Please also note that "Psychologists, even if certified, should not serve as a client's acupuncturist as well as his or her psychotherapist since acupuncture often involves the client removing articles of clothing, a clear boundary violation. Also, in some states, it is illegal for psychologists to provide any forms of treatment that involve piercing of the skin. Yet administering some of these treatments to current psychotherapy clients constitutes an inappropriate multiple relationship (APA Standard 3.05) and a boundary violation" (See Barnett, J.E., and Shale, A.J. 2013. *Alternative techniques. Today's psychologists are increasingly integrating complementary and alternative medicine techniques into their work with clients. Here's an overview of the most popular treatments, the research on their efficacy and the ethical concerns they raise.* Monitor on Psychology. Washington, DC: American Psychological Association, Vol 44, No. 4, p.48). See also the ethical discussion on the factors affecting resilience and vulnerability ("DOVE" or: desire to help, a powerful opportunities, values, and education) in: Tjeltveit, A.C., and Gottlieb, M.C. 2012. *Avoiding ethical missteps. By drawing on the science of prevention, psychologists can develop skills, relationships and personal qualities to bolster ethical resilience and minimize risks related to unethical behavior.* Monitor on Psychology, Vol 43, No. 4. Washington, DC: American Psychological Association, Vol 44, No. 4, pp. 68–74.

[356] Ernst, E 2004. *Anthroposophical medicine: A systematic review of randomised clinical trials.* Wien, A: Wiener klinische Wochenschrift 116 (4): 128–30; Kienle, S.G., Kiene H. und Albonico H.-U. 2006. *Anthroposophische Medizin in der klinischen Forschung. Wirksamkeit, Nutzen, Wirtschaftlichkeit, Sicherheit.* Stuttgart, D: Schattauer.

- Art Therapy[358]
- Ayurvedic medicine[359]
- Biofeedback[360]
- Bioenergetics / Bioenergetic therapy / Vegetotherapy[361]
- Chiropractic[362]
- Christian Faith Healing[363] / Religious & Spiritual healing[364] / Shamanism
- Dance Movement Therapy (DMT)[365]

---

[357]   Kiecolt-Glaser JK, Graham JE, Malarkey WB, et al. 2008. *Olfactory influences on mood and autonomic, endocrine, and immune function. Psychoneuroendocrinology*; 33(3): 328–339.

[358]   Also Art Assisted Therapy, Applied Art Therapy, Clinical/Medical Art Therapy; see Slayton, S.C., D'Archer, J., and Kaplan, F. 2010. *Outcome Studies on the Efficacy of Art Therapy: A Review of Findings*. Art Therapy: Journal of the American Art Therapy Association, 27(3) pp. 108–11.

[359]   Napolitano J.G., Lankin D.C., Graf T.N., et al. 2013. *HiFSA fingerprinting applied to isomers with near-identical NMR spectra: the silybin/isosilybin case. Journal of Organic Chemistry*; 78(7): 2827–2839. Please note that not everything sold as part of alternative medicine is completely safe, as evidence by this research: Saper R.B., Phillips R.S., Sehgal A., et al. 2008. *Lead, mercury, and arsenic in U.S. and Indian-manufactured Ayurvedic medicines sold via the Internet*. Journal of the American Medical Association; 300(8): 915–923.

[360]   Used, with positive results, in the treatment of ADHD, depression, headaches, and pain, among other symptoms, as reported in Fuchs, T., Birbaumer, N., Lutzenberger, W., Gruzelier, J., & Kaiser, J. 2003. *Neurofeedback treatment for attention-deficit/hyperactivity disorder in children: A comparison with methylphenidate*. Applied Psychophysiology and Biofeedback, 28, 1–12; Nestoriuc, Y., Martin, A., Rief, W., & Andrasik, F. 2008. *Biofeedback treatment for headache disorders: A comprehensive efficacy review*. Applied Psychophysiology and Biofeedback, 33, 125–140; and others.

[361]   Lowen, A. 1975. *Bioenergetics*. New York, NY: Coward, McCarin & Geoghen; Reich, W. 1927. *Die Funktion des Orgasmus*. Revidierte Fassung 1982: Genitalität in der Theorie und Therapie der Neurose/Frühe Schriften II, Köln, D: Kiepenheuer & Witsch.

[362]   Haas M., Spegman A., Peterson D., et al. 2010. *Dose response and efficacy of spinal manipulation for chronic cervicogenic headache: a pilot randomized controlled trial*. Spine Journal; 10(2): 117–128.

[363]   There are several branches and sub-branches of Christian Faith Healing, and of Religious healing in general, some of which are definitely more in tune with theories and practices of American Christian Science in general. However, there are areas of investigations which move on the grey area between meditation, self-analysis and reflection, introspection, evaluation, prayer, revision etc. Among the most famous examples in the Christian Catholic tradition, the *Examen* and the Spiritual Exercises by Ignatius of Loyola.

[364]   Vis, J., & Boynton, H. 2008. *Spirituality and transcendent meaning making: Possibilities for enhancing posttraumatic growth*. Journal of Religion & Spirituality in Social Work, 27, 69–86; Cook, C. 2004. *Addiction and spirituality*. Addiction, 99, 539–551. doi: 10.1111/j. For Christian Centering Prayer, see Volk, S. 2011. *Fringe-ology: How I tried to Explain Away the Unexplainable—And Couldn't*, New York, NY: HarperCollins, pp.195–196.

[365]   Earhart, G.M. 2009. *Dance as therapy for individuals with Parkinson disease*. European journal of physical and rehabilitation medicine 45 (2): 231–8.

- Deep breathing exercises[366]
- Energy medicine[367]
- Ethno medicine[368] / Folk medicine[369] / Traditional medicine[370]
- Guided imagery[371]
- Herbal medicine and phytotherapy[372] / Spagyrics
- Hypnosis[373] / Hypnotherapy
- Homeopathy[374]
- Homotoxicology[375]
- Magnetic healing / Mesmerism[376] – animal magnetism

---

[366] Dickinson H., Campbell F., Beyer F., et al. 2008. *Relaxation therapies for the management of primary hypertension in adults: a Cochrane review*. Journal of Human Hypertension; 22(12): 809–820.

[367] Abbot, N.C.; Harkness, E.F.; Stevinson, C.; Marshall, F.P.; Conn, D.A.; Ernst, E. 2001. *Spiritual healing as a therapy for chronic pain: a randomized, clinical trial*. Pain 91 (1–2): 79–89.

[368] Including ethnopharmacology, ethnobotany, ethnopsychiatry, and ethnopsychoanalysis.

[369] For example, the *Phytognomonica* of Giambattista della Porta, the doctrine of signatures, the research of Paracelsus and Jakob Böhme, and forms of humoral and astrological medicine.

[370] Including the scientific analysis of medical anthropology and ethnology.

[371] Utay, J.; Miller, M. 2006. *Guided imagery as an effective therapeutic technique: a brief review of its history and efficacy research*. Journal of Instructional Psychology, 3/06.

[372] Cefalù W.T., Floyd Z.E., Stephens J.M., et al. 2014. *Botanicals and translational medicine: a paradigm shift in research approach. Nutrition.* NIH PubMed. 2014; 30(7–8S):S1–S68.

[373] Effective in the treatment of fatigue and generalized pain, as well as side effect of cancer treatments, such as nausea and vomiting. See Jensen, M. P., Ehde, D. M., Gertz, K. J., Stoelb, B. L., Dillworth, T. M., Hirsh, A. T., Kraft, G. H. 2011. *Effects of self-hypnosis training and cognitive restructuring on daily pain intensity and catastrophizing in individuals with multiple sclerosis and chronic pain*. International Journal of Clinical and Experimental Hypnosis, 59, 45–63.; Lang, E.V., Berbaum, K.S., Faintuch, S. et al. 2006. *Adjunctive self-hypnotic relaxation for outpatient medical procedures: A prospective randomized trial with women undergoing large core breast biopsy*.; and Castel, A., Salvat, M., Sala, J., & Rull, M. (2009). *Cognitive-behavioural group treatment with hypnosis: A randomized pilot trial in fibromyalgia*. Contemporary Hypnosis, 26, 48–59. For cancer and surgery effects therapeutic intervention, see Montgomery G.H., Bovbjerg D.H., Schnur J.B., David D., Goldfarb A., et al. 2007. A Randomized Clinical Trial of a Brief Hypnosis Intervention to Control Side Effects in Breast Surgery Patients. J National Cancer Institute; 99: 1304–1312.

[374] Goldacre, B. 2007. *Benefits and risks of homoeopathy*. The Lancet, Amsterdam, NL: Elsevier Volume 370, No. 9600, p1672–1673. An interesting debate on a very recent study on the effectiveness of a homeopathic treatment can be found on *Science-Based Medicine* (see Bibliography) with the title "The Worst Homeopathy Study. Ever", available at: https://www.sciencebasedmedicine.org/the-worst-homeopathy-study-ever/. The original article has been published on: http://www.ncbi.nlm.nih.gov/pmc/articles/PMC4527103/ Retrieved September 20th, 2015.

[375] Namely, the theory and method developed by Hans-Heinrich Reckeweg.

[376] Kihlstrom J.F. 2002. *Mesmer, the Franklin Commission, and hypnosis: a counterfactual essay*. The International Journal of Clinical and Experimental Hypnosis 50 (4): 407–19.

174   Medical Philosophy

- Massage Therapy[377]
- Meditation[378]
- Mindfulness[379]
- Mind-Body medicine[380]
- Music Therapy[381]
- Narrative Medicine[382]
- Naturopathy[383] / Heilkunde[384] (including the *Neue Deutsche Heilkunde*)
  – Heilpraktiker / Naturarzt

[377]   Cherkin D.C., Sherman K.J., Kahn J., et al. 2011. *A comparison of the effects of 2 types of massage and usual care on chronic low-back pain: a randomized, controlled trial.* Annals of Internal Medicine; 155(1): 1–9.

[378]   See: Slagter, H.A., Lutz, A., Greischar, L.L., Francis, A.D., Nieuwenhuis, D., Davis, J.M., and Davidson, R.J. 2007. *Mental training affects distribution of limited brain resources.* PLOS Biology; Lutz A., Brefczynski-Lewis J., Johnstone T., et al. 2008. *Regulation of the neural circuitry of emotion by compassion meditation: effects of meditative expertise.* PLoS ONE. 2008; 3(3):e1897. For Transcendental Meditation see Nidich S.I., Rainforth M.V., Haaga D.A.F., et al. 2009. *A randomized controlled trial on effects of the Transcendental Meditation program on blood pressure, psychological distress, and coping in young adults.* American Journal of Hypertension. 2009; 22(12): 1326–1331.

[379]   For current research, please refer to: Kaliman P., Álvarez-López M.J., Cosín-Tomás M., et al. 2014. *Rapid changes in histone deacetylases and inflammatory gene expression in expert meditators.* Psychoneuroendocrinology; 40: 96–107 Britton W.B., Lepp N.E., Niles H.F., et al. 2014. *A randomized controlled pilot trial of classroom-based mindfulness meditation compared to an active control condition in sixth-grade children.* Journal of School Psychology. 2014; 52(3): 263–278; Jedel S., Hoffman A., Merriman P., et al. 2014. *A randomized controlled trial of mindfulness-based stress reduction to prevent flare-up in patients with inactive ulcerative colitis.* Digestion. NIH PubMed; 89: 142–155; Desbordes G., Negi L.T., Pace T.W.W., et al. 2012. *Effects of mindful-attention and compassion meditation training on amygdala response to emotional stimuli in an ordinary, non-meditative state.* Frontiers in Human Neuroscience; Hölzel B.K., Carmody J., Vangel M., et al. 2011. *Mindfulness practice leads to increases in regional brain gray matter density.* Psychiatry Research: Neuroimaging; 191(1): 36–43.

[380]   Cotton S., Roberts Y.H., Tsevat J., et al. 2010. *Mind-body complementary alternative medicine use and quality of life in adolescents with inflammatory bowel disease.* Inflammatory Bowel Disease; 16(3): 501–506.

[381]   Brown, L., and Jellison, J. 2011. *Auditory Perception of Emotion in Sung and Instrumental Music in Children with Autism Spectrum Disorders.* AMTA Published Journals Posters Research Catalog. Silver Spring, MD: American Music Therapy Association.

[382]   Although not strictly a form of CAM, Narrative Medicine n is often associated with an integrative approach as a support to conventional medicine. Further reference: Greenhalgh T., and Hurwitz B. 1999. *Narrative based medicine: Why study narrative?* BMJ, 318: 48–50. For research reference, see Conboy L.A., Macklin E., Kelley J., et al. 2010. *Which patients improve: characteristics increasing sensitivity to a supportive patient-practitioner relationship.* Social Science & Medicine; 70(3): 479–484.

[383]   Herman P.M., Szczurko O., Cooley K., et al. 2008. *Cost-effectiveness of naturopathic care for chronic low back pain.* Alternative Therapies in Health and Medicine; 14(2): 32–39.

[384]   As well as *Pflanzen-* (and *Kräuter-*) *heilkunde*.

- Osteopathy[385] / manipulative medicine[386] / Feldenkrais method and Alexander technique[387]
- Pranotherapy, Therapeutic and Healing Touch[388]
- Progressive relaxation[389]
- Qi gong[390]
- Reiki[391]
- T'ai Chi Ch'uan[392]
- Traditional Chinese Medicine (TCM)[393]
- Traditional Tibetan Medicine (TTM)[394]
- Wilderness Therapy[395]
- Yoga[396]

---

[385] Licciardone J.C., Buchanan S., Hensel K.L., et al. 2010. *Osteopathic manipulative treatment of back pain and related symptoms during pregnancy: a randomized controlled trial*. American Journal of Obstetrics and Gynecology. 2010; 202(1): 43.e1–43.e8.

[386] Bialosky J.E., George S.Z., Horn M.E., at al. 2014. *Spinal manipulative therapy-specific changes in pain sensitivity in individuals with low back pain* (NCT01168999). The Journal of Pain; 15(2): 136–148.

[387] Gelb, M. 2004 *Körperdynamik. Eine Einführung in die Alexandertechnik*. Frankfurt, D: Runde Ecken Verlag

[388] Nguyen H.T., Grzywacz J.G., Lang W., et al. 2010. *Effects of complementary therapy on health in a national U.S. sample of older adults*. Journal of Alternative and Complementary Medicine; 16(7): 701–706.

[389] Hofmann, E. 2003. *Progressive Muskelentspannung, ein Trainingsprogramm*. 2. Aufl. Göttingen, D: Hogrefe

[390] Lee M.S., Oh B., Ernst E. 2011. *Qigong for healthcare: an overview of systematic reviews*. JRSM Short Rep 2(2): 7.

[391] McKenzie, E., et al. 1998. *Healing Reiki*. Hamlyn Health & Well Being: Hamlyn; Lee, M.S.; Pittler, M.H., Ernst, E. 2008. *Effects of Reiki in clinical practice: a systematic review of randomized clinical trials*. International Journal of Clinical Practice 62 (6): 947–54.

[392] Yeh G.Y., McCarthy E.P., Wayne P.M., et al.. 2011. *Tai chi exercise in patients with chronic heart failure: a randomized controlled trial*.. Archives of Internal Medicine; 171(8): 750–757; Wang C., Schmid C.H., Rones R., et al. 2010. *A randomized trial of tai chi for fibromyalgia*. New England Journal of Medicine; 363(8): 743–754..

[393] Ritenbaugh C., Hammerschlag R., Dworkin S.F., et al. 2012. *Comparative effectiveness of traditional Chinese medicine and psychosocial care in the treatment of temporomandibular disorders-associated chronic facial pain*. Journal of Pain; 13(11): 1075–1089.

[394] Witt C.M., Berling N.E.J., Rinpoche N.T., Cuomo M.; Willich S.N. 2009. *Evaluation of medicinal plants as part of Tibetan medicine prospective observational study in Sikkim and Nepal*. Journal of Alternative & Complementary Medicine, 2009-01-0115:1, 59(7).

[395] DeAngelis, T. 2013. *Therapy gone wild. More psychologist are using the wilderness as a backdrop and therapeutic too in their work*. Monitor in Psychology, Vol. 44, No. 8. Washington, DC: American Psychological Association, pp. 48–52.

[396] Kiecolt-Glaser J.K., Christian L., Preston H., et al. 2010. *Stress, inflammation, and yoga practice*. Psychosomatic Medicine; 72(2): 113–121.

Based on the above list, it is easy to understand that within the realm of complementary and alternative medicine many different approaches and techniques are found, and that there are many differences between them, in terms of their historical origin, therapeutic applicability and effectiveness, and dedicated research studies. In general however, CAM is vastly used in those geographical areas in which conventional medicine is practiced. In fact, some researchers even claim that there are actually more visits, or more repeated visits to the same provider in CAM versus EBM medicine.[397]

c) Culture and Identity

The modern neuroscientific research has provided new and interesting perspectives on how human beings perceive themselves and the world. Whether we can validate the equation *brain* = *mind* remains an open question, passionately defended by some and equally discarded by others. Thus, the new approaches used in the field also provided the therapeutic assessment and treatment in psychiatric settings, with new clinical practices. In order to understand this approach and add a more philosophical perspective to investigate the validity and applicability of such claims, we could start from the very concept of conscience. At the same time, we should take into consideration how this conscience works in everyday life, thus opening up the analysis of the environment on the conscience and of the conscience of the environment. What is this relation, and how does man and man-made institutions in society and culture perceive these elements? According to Amy Gutmann, "by recognizing that conscience can be either secular or religious, democratic governments avoid discriminating either in favor or against religious citizens."[398] Where is the role

---

[397]   "Eisenberg et al. (1998) determined that people visited CAM practitioners 243 million more times than they visited primary-care physicians in the preceding year. According to 2007 data from NCCAM, 38.3 percent of adults and 11.8 percent of children reported having used a form of CAM in the preceding year (Barnes et al., 2008). This corresponds with nearly $34 billion being spent each year on CAM products and services (Briggs, 2007). Although this amount accounts for only 1.5 percent of the total amount spent on health care, it is nearly 11.2 percent of out-of-pocket health-care costs (Briggs, 2007)." (Barnett, J.E., and Shale, A.J. 2013. *Alternative techniques. Today's psychologists are increasingly integrating complementary and alternative medicine techniques into their work with clients. Here's an overview of the most popular treatments, the research on their efficacy and the ethical concerns they raise*. Monitor on Psychology. Washington, DC: American Psychological Association, Vol 44, No. 4,). For a critical perspective of the statement above, see Gorski, T.N. 2002. *The Eisenberg Data: Flawed and Deceptive*. Quackwatch, article posted on March 16, available on http://www.quackwatch.org/11nd/eisenberg.html.

[398]   Gutmann, A. 2003. *Identity in Democracy*, Princeton University Press, Princeton, New Jersey, p. 26.

of the individual in this analysis and related application of the individual's own identity and conscience? Is the individual really free to choose or to be chosen by this category or are there other elements and influences we should control for, the same way we would do in a clinical trial? This is absolutely important when we want to address issues of bias, prejudice, labeling and stigma, often associated with mental health issues. The question of belonging to a group is therefore at the center of our investigation of patient's perception, toward himself/herself and toward the environment. The latter can be medical, especially in the case of a locked unit of a psychiatric ward, but also familiar, social, cultural, religious, etc. Questioning the relationship between patient and environment, patient and group is discussing the very basis of our democratic society, thus opening up the conversation on those public policy and sociological issues which are analyzed in translational science, as we will see in Chapter 7. From an ethical perspective, Gutmann states that there are three principles we should focus on, in order: 1) civic equality, or the obligation of democracies to treat all individuals as equal agents in democratic policies and support the conditions that are necessary for their equal treatment as citizens. 2) equal freedom, the obligation of democratic government to respect the liberty of all individuals to live their own lives as they see fit consistent with the equal liberty of others; and finally 3) basic opportunity, the capacity of individuals to live a decent life with a fair chance to choose among their preferred ways of life.[399] The author continues by stating that:

> "Without any identities, defenders of group identity say individuals are atomistic, not autonomous. Psychological experiments demonstrate that something as basic as self-image changes when individuals identify with others. And a difference in self-image can be based on a seemingly irrelevant identification with others."[400]

This intellectual imprint seems to be very different from other psychoanalytical speculations, in which 'genetic predestination' seems to play a bigger role. For instance, we could quote Hans Jürgen Eysenck, who stated that "All the evidence to date suggests the [...] overwhelming importance of genetic factors in producing the great variety of intellectual differences which we observe in our culture, and much of the difference observed between certain racial groups."[401] This psychological statement, which is arguably more of a philo-

---

[399] Ibid., pp. 26–27.
[400] Ibid., p. 2.
[401] Eysenck, H. J., *Race, Intelligence and Education*, Temple Smith Ed., London, 1971, p. 130.

sophical position, if not a 'mere' personal opinion, leads us to the consideration of the major issues related to ascriptive groups. As the definition itself states, there is no choice for members of ascriptive groups of being identified with that specific group. This is very important also in relation to the cultural, religious and social implication of the perception and self-perception of the individual, especially when the very definition of the above mentioned characteristics don't match the actual status (again, cultural, social, even economic and professional, or just geographical) of the individual. In this context Illich writes:

> "More and more people subconsciously know that they are sick and tired of their jobs and of their leisure passivities, but they want to hear the lie that physical illness relieves them of social and political responsibilities. They want their doctor to act as lawyer and priest. As a lawyer, the doctor exempts the patient from his normal duties and enables him to cash in on the insurance fund he was forced to build. As a priest, he becomes the patient's accomplice in creating the myth that he is an innocent victim of biological mechanisms rather than a lazy, greedy, or envious deserter of a social struggle for control over the tools of production."[402]

The sense of self in relation to others, especially when these others are associated with specific professional roles in society, contributes to the person's identity in a clinical setting. More specifically, there is an important shift between self-perception as a *general individual* versus a *generalized patient*. The apparent oxymoron of general individual is definitely a core concept in our analysis of the relation between evidence-based medicine, patient-centered medicine and evidence-informed medicine; and helps us distinguish between shifted identity positions when a person is part (by personal choice or not) of a group.[403] This is better explained by taking a closer look to the current research on refugee resettlement programs and immigration policies all over the world.[404] To be sure, we should investigate how much this 'born-in', which is also a 'born-with' identity shapes not only the self-perception of the individual but also his self-perception in relation to others, in relation to the perception of

---

[402]   Illich, I. 1976. *Limits to Medicine; Medical Nemesis: The Expropriation of Health*. London, UK: Marion Boyars Publishers, p. 123.

[403]   In this regard, the author also discusses "[...] the proposal that doctors not be licensed by an in-group does not mean that their services shall not be evaluated, but rather that this evaluation can be done more effectively by informed clients than by their own peers [...]". Illich, I. 1976. *Limits to Medicine; Medical Nemesis: The Expropriation of Health*. London, UK: Marion Boyars Publishers, p. 255.

[404]   A topic unfortunately always current and modern, let us think for instance at the Syrian refugee crisis in Europe and elsewhere.

others and finally in relation to other' self-perception(-s). What are the practical and social implications of these considerations? Gutmann argues that the very 'absence of freedom' defines this type of identification, and raises criticism.[405] More specifically, the author writes that "to say that racial, gender, ethnic and national identities are social constructions, as David Laitin recognizes, is not to say that they are any easier to change than our genetic inheritance or physiognomy."[406] Can we thus define the problem in terms of physical perception? What about the theories of ethnic or racial superiority? In another essay,[407] Gutmann adds that "if a liberal democracy need not, or should not respect [such] "supremacist cultures, even if those cultures are highly valued by many among the disadvantaged, what precisely are the moral limits on the legitimate demand for political recognition of particular cultures?"[408] To what extent can we talk here about 'supremacist *cultures*'? If culture is indeed a necessary condition for human freedom, as analyzed by Bent Flyvbjerg in his essay on phronesis and by comparison with Aristotelian position,[409] we should focus on the distance, in terms of relation, between the individual and his (own?) culture. If this *relationship* is very close, the individual can even develop pride[410] toward his 'given' culture, in terms of ascriptive identity. Now, we should be careful in putting ascriptive identity and close culture in the same basket. First of all, if we identify this closeness in cultural terms, with something that is 'pre-given', 'pre-formative'. Thus, we are relying on the assumption of the truthfulness of the equation 'genotype x environment', in a conception quite similar to specifically neo-Darwinist positions, such as the one offered by Richard Dawkins.[411] Furthermore, identification by Ascription often

---

[405] Gutmann, A. ed., 1994. *Multiculturalism*, Princeton University Press, Princeton, New Jersey, p. 118. In particular, the author uses examples of cultural-national origin, as well as purely physical, from aesthetic perception (color of skin, dimensions, etc.) to more specifically medical conditions (ex. To be born deaf or blind).

[406] Ibid., p. 120

[407] Gutmann, A. 1994. *Introduction*, in: Gutmann, Amy, ed., *Multiculturalism*, Princeton University Press, Princeton, New Jersey.

[408] Ibid., p. 5.

[409] Flyvbjerg, B. 1993. *Aristotle, Foucault and Progressive Phronesis: Outline of an Applied Ethics for Sustainable Development*; in: Winkler, Earl R. & Coombs Jerold R., *Applied Ethics*, Cambridge: Blackwell Publishers, p. 18–19.

[410] As observed by Gutmann in Gutmann, A. 2003. *Identity in Democracy*, Princeton University Press, Princeton, New Jersey, p. 136: "pride in ascriptive identity if you have to overcome social obstacles."

[411] Though we should mention here the value and concept of human beings as media in this process, as well as further specify the role of the *meme* from this intercultural—ethical perspective.

informs interest, which can be cultural, social and/or personal.[412] Therefore, we see here a combination of internal and external physical factors on one side, and internal and external cultural factors on the other. The conscience of the individual, and the related form of identification work in a context of space and time, although "*Sed fugit interea fugit irreparabile tempus.*"[413]

The physical, cultural, social environment plays a key role in shaping the individual and it is in turn shaped by the individual himself, by his own individuality. The concept of space here is therefore physical, cultural and social. The term of time is instead linked to historical perspectives, but also to the ethical and moral implication of the preservation through time, across history. A preservation of this identity, which creates new issues and problems we have to consider. In the words of Jürgen Habermas, "For to guarantee survival would necessarily rob the members of the very freedom to say yes or no that is necessary if they are to appropriate and preserve their cultural heritage."[414] If we, as observed in the hypothesis above, are more inclined to consider both environment's influence on identity and identity's influence on the environment, we should open up the very perspective of the possible effect or relation (in some instances of current research mutually valid and intersected) of this interaction with the very concept of neuroplasticity.[415] This viewpoint will lead us back to the consideration of the validity of 'mind=brain', and yet we have to ask ourselves, whether we can apply this equation in general, that is to the single brain/mind within and across space and time, as well as the multitude of brains/minds in relation to and with themselves, one another and within context. To say that "a person's culture is a constitutive part of who this/the person is"[416] is to open up the discussion on the constitutive parts of individuality and

---

[412]   For instance, the conversion of Skip Hayward to a Pequot-Indian in the mid-1970s, within the discussion on the 'Revenge of the Pequots' presented in Gutmann, A. 2003 *Identity in Democracy*, Princeton University Press, Princeton, New Jersey, pp. 120–122.

[413]   Publius Vergilius Maro (Virgil), Georgica (The Georgics), III, 284.

[414]   Habermas, J. 1994. *Struggles for Recognition*, in: Gutmann, Amy, ed., *Multiculturalism*, Princeton University Press, Princeton, New Jersey 1994, p. 130.

[415]   To be more specific, we should investigate the ability of the brain to adjust and re-morph according to the stimuli coming from the environment, as previously defined combination of internal and external factors. Thus the very core of the concepts 'Individual' and 'Identity' takes on a new conceptual strength and differentiation, an exclusive (both in a passive and active sense) application whether we consider the identity between mind and brain as valid or, on the contrary, we base our consideration on the possible bias that such a principle would imply.

[416]   Gutmann, A. 2003 *Identity in Democracy*, Princeton University Press, Princeton, New Jersey, p. 39.

groups, and examine whether these parts and their relative influence are to be found in an external environment as well as in an internal environment. If there is a parallel between internal and external, we should be able to increase the focus of our analysis and draw considerations on the acceptance of these identities and their definition in cultural terms. Political theorists such as Avishai Margalit, Moshe Halbertal, Joseph Raz, and Will Kymlicka are more specific in defining cultural group as "a comprehensive, encompassing context in which its members make choices, and 'anchor for self-identification and the safety of effortless, secure belonging.'"[417] More specifically, Kymlicka's support of individual rights confronts more distant positions such as the ones by Moshe Abertal and Avishai Margalit: "protecting cultures out of the human right to culture may take the form of an obligation to support cultures that flout the rights of the individual in a liberal society."[418] From a social and political standpoint, they argue that the democratic state may protect one and one only basic right against claims of cultural groups, the right of individuals to exit cultural groups (we should add also the democratic state itself). Every other right of individuals becomes subordinate to the cultural group's right to culture. Gutmann argues that some of these principles might be based on the "special obligation view".[419] and include positive aspects like the defense of the ideal and character/tradition of the group,[420] which could also turn into negative aspects.[421] Let's remember for instance the statement by Rabbi Hillel, as quoted by Gutmann: "If we are not for ourselves, then who will be for us?"[422] This especially valid for religious groups, for which Gutmann does not consider a special status within identity groups. The author reconsiders the identification view: "an ideal theory of justice says that when people associate for political

---

[417]   Ibid., p. 38.

[418]   Ibid., pp. 58–60.

[419]   Including the personal responsibility of the members of a specific group toward other members of the same group, in terms of statement and protection; also "the fair share of more advantaged members of the groups is presumed to be greater than that of less advantaged members of the group." In: Ibid., p. 139.

[420]   "Expressing the idea that people should identify with their own kind for the sake of fighting against injustice; [...] it discourages people from pursuing broad egalitarian goals by focusing on the particular needs of particular identity groups rather than on the more universal cause of egalitarian justice." In: Ibid., p. 131.

[421]   Features of discriminatory exclusion: 1) based on false or statistical stereotyping; 2) exclusion occurs in a public realm and is connected to the distribution of public good; 3) the voluntary association is not primarily defined by its dedication to an expressive purpose, but on the discrimination against a group (like white or male supremacist). See Gutmann, A. 2003. *Identity in Democracy*, Princeton University Press, Princeton, New Jersey, p. 100.

[422]   Ibid., p. 128, see also Rosa Parks and Jackie Robinson.

purposes, they should do so on the basis of a general moral commitment to oppose injustice. They should not associate for political purposes on the basis of their identification with particular others."[423] In particular, the author analyzes the possible clash between identification view and special obligation view. We have to ask ourselves whether the contributions to combating injustice are in competition with the group members' own interests (=obligation view) or are a constitutive part of it (=identification view).[424] From a philosophical perspective,[425] religious identity is special in three ways, according to Gutmann: 1) because of the importance of publicly acknowledging religious truths; 2) because of religion's exceptional contribution to the public good; 3) because conscience is the ultimate force in the lives of the believers.[426] Furthermore, Religion itself is not good or bad from a political social perspective, especially in the sense of (modern) democracy, but the biggest danger comes from supporting (and legally subscribe to) public claims on the base of private truths. Arguments that are rationally based on the argumentative power of revelation, and not the revelation itself should be used in democracies, according to Gutmann.[427] Should we therefore include a more inclusive perspective on claims that are, contrary to the requirements above, below the realm of reason-based argumentation? How tolerant should we be in our attempt to achieve a more effective (from an ethical standpoint) democracy? Kymlicka argues that:

> "Liberalism and toleration are closely related, both historically and conceptually. The development of religious tolerance was one of the historical roots of liberalism. Religious tolerance in the West emerged out of the interminable Wars of Religion and the recognition by both Catholics and Protestants that a stable constitutional order cannot rest on a shared religious faith."[428]

---

[423]   Ibid., p. 144.

[424]   More specifically, the author raises the debate on *one-way* and *two-way* protection and policies.

[425]   Especially from a neurophilosphical perspective, encompassing the debate on the afterlife and NDE (Near Death Experiences). For further readings, see the works by Stanislav Grof, Karl L. R. Jansen, John Lilly and Raymond Moody.

[426]   Gutmann, A. 2003. *Identity in Democracy*, Princeton University Press, Princeton, New Jersey, p. 153.

[427]   "[...] The idea that god created humans cannot be proven true or false by empirical and logical means, the same applies to the kantian idea of human beings as end in themselves, or the democratic idea of free and equal citizenship." In: Ibid., p. 158.

[428]   Kymlicka, Will, *Multicultural Citizenship. A liberal theory of Minority Rights*, Clarendon Press, Oxford, 1995, p. 155.

This view seems to support the clear separation between state and church in policy and public matters. The content of a religious revelation might be proven usable and ethically good for the general public (with all the possible implications in terms of psychiatric evaluations), regardless of their religious, cultural and ethnical background, but only if the content is publicly debated, as seen above. At the same time, the identity of individuals and groups, as well as the identity of a governmental institution, state or country need to take into consideration aspects that go far beyond what is empirically proven or provable: "a purely empiricist position would yield no commitment to democratic justice or to treating people as equals, since evidence and logic alone are morally inconclusive. Empiricism alone is amoral (not necessarily immoral)."[429] Thus, in understanding the spiritual, philosophical and ethical needs of the individual and of the group, "Democratic governments should rule out faith as a sufficient basis for making mutually binding laws, but faith may still supplement otherwise good reasons for laws and public policies."[430] Amy Gutmann asks whether "all of the demands for recognition by particular groups, often made in the name of nationalism or multiculturalism, are *illiberal* demands."[431] The great point raised by Gutmann is that there is a relation between conscience, liberalism and public sphere, and that "the idea of conscience predates modern democracy, but conscience and democracy share a fundamental premise: persons are ethical subjects."[432] It is also true that conscience is ethically fallible, and that there is a need of ethical capacity in the public sphere. Democracies could not work without this ethical capacity, since the democratic group, state or country would not be able to command respect (thus being understood and obeyed to) without it.

Jürgen Habermas argues that "equal protection under the law is not enough to constitute a constitutional democracy. We must not only be equal under the law, we must also be able to understand ourselves as the authors of laws that bind us." He writes that "Once we take this internal connection between democracy and the constitutional state seriously, it becomes clear that the system of rights is blind neither to unequal social conditions nor to cultural

---

[429]   Gutmann, A. 2003. *Identity in Democracy*, Princeton University Press, Princeton, New Jersey, p. 158.

[430]   Ibid., p. 162.

[431]   Gutmann, A., ed. 1994 *Multiculturalism*, Princeton University Press, Princeton, New Jersey, p. 4.

[432]   Ibid., p. 168. The author also quotes De Toqueville: "nothing deserves more attention than associational life in democracy." In: Ibid., p. 99.

differences."[433] Habermas distinguishes between the first type of culture, understood from a general perspective and thus doesn't have to be shared by all members of society, and a second type of culture, which both common and political; marked by a shared (and mutual) respect for rights. According to the writer, there are individual rights of nondiscrimination and free association, which therefore do not guarantee survival for any culture. The very attempt to protect cultures in terms of their preservation deprives them of their intrinsic vitality. Furthermore, they prevent individuals of their freedom to modify, update and even reject their cultural inheritance, as part of their identity. K. Anthony Appiah agrees with Taylor in the statement according to which "[there are] legitimate collective goals whose pursuit will require giving up pure proceduralism," but indefinite cultural survival is not among those goals. Moreover, the author focuses on the mandatory expectations of a particular minority, whether we are talking about a sexual, ethnic, racial, national (etc.) one. These identification procedures "come with notions of how a proper person of that kind behaves: it is not that there is *one* way that gays or blacks should behave, but that there are gay and black modes of behavior." Personal dimensions of identity, as stated in the preface of this book, do not typically work in the same way as the collective dimensions. According to Appiah, these collective dimensions "provide what we might call scripts: narratives that people can use in shaping their life plans and in telling their life stories. In our societies (though not, perhaps, in the England of Addison and Steele) being witty does not in this way suggest the life-script of 'the wit'."[434] He continues: "The politics of recognition requires that one's skin color, one's sexual body, should be acknowledged politically in ways that make it hard for those who want to treat their skin and their sexual body as personal dimensions of the self. And personal means not secret, but not too tightly scripted."[435] We understand how the very elements shaping man's identity,[436] sense of belonging to a specific cul-

[433]   Gutmann, A., ed. 1994 *Multiculturalism*, Princeton University Press, Princeton, New Jersey, p. ix – for further readings, see the German edition of this volume, as presented in the *Preface* of the book.

[434]   Ibid., p. xi.

[435]   Ibid.

[436]   Amy Gutmann summarizes the various (political) reasons why individuals form and join identity groups: to publicly express what they consider an important aspect of their identity; to conserve their culture, which they identify with the group; to gain more material (and other) goods for themselves and their group (whether justified or not); to fight in a group for or against discrimination and other injustices; to receive mutual support from others who share some part of their social identity; and to express and act upon ethical commitments

ture, ethnicity, social and political organization, as well as the social and ethical implication of this sense of belonging (and the membership itself), are better framed and analyzed once we take into consideration not only the internal and external factors shaping these elements, but also the process itself. A metamorphosis, a re-creation of concepts and interpretation in which internal and external environment mutually influence each other and provide new keys of interpretation of man,[437] his role, choice, freedom, sense of belonging and of self, (his) conscience and identity, within himself and in the broader context of a group.

---

that they share with a group. See Gutmann, A. 2003. *Identity in Democracy*, Princeton University Press, Princeton, New Jersey, p. 210.

[437]   Taylor, Charles, cit. in: Gutmann, A. 2003. *Identity in Democracy*, Princeton University Press, Princeton, New Jersey, p. 42: "Free individuals can flourish only to the extent that [they] are [also politically] recognized. Each consciousness seeks recognition in another, and this is not a sign of a lack of virtue."

Chapter 6
Beyond the realms of this world

6.1 Camus, Sartre, and God: where are we now?

> *"Extraordinary claims require extraordinary experience"*
> Marcello Truzzi

A complete analysis of the philosophical debate on the belief and existence of God is beyond the scope of this writing, however we cannot complete avoid the issue, especially considering the impact of faith and personal beliefs within medical philosophy, in particular relation to medical outcomes, treatment process and meaning of suffering and healing. What is the role of hope in man's life, and how is it linked to the necessity of meaning in man's interpretation of life itself? According to Albert Camus, the fundamental thoughts and action which define our lives are built on the hope for tomorrow, yet tomorrow is the ultimate enemy and (or since?) it brings us closer to death. And yet, according to Zail Berry,[438] a societal/cultural denial of death is at the center of a problematic solution of advanced care planning in clinical settings. The 'death issue' is part of a series of obstacles to an open, fair, informative, and true communication between the physician and the patient. In this list we certainly find time:

> "[...] then, of course, there's the ticking clock. Physicians are famously, and almost universally, pressed for time. "Ten-to-fifteen-minute appointment slots are an insane system for helping people, especially those with complex chronic illnesses who need ongoing treatment. [...] No matter how highly skilled you are, it constrains you."[439]

Interestingly, the concept of a 'ticking clock', is appropriately used in reference to a complex substratum of emotions and general feelings of discomfort in

---

[438] Berry, Z.S. 2014. *Advanced Care Planning in Primary Care. A Patient-Centered Approach with Practical Strategies.* University of Vermont College of Medicine, Vermont Ethics Network Annual conference Advance Care Planning: It's Always Too soon...Until It's Too Late. Fairlee, VT.

[439] William Polonsky, founder and president of the Behavioral Diabetes Institute, as cited in Weir, K. 2012. *Improving patient-physician communication.* Monitor on Psychology, Vol. 43, N.10, Washington, DC: American Psychological Association, pp. 38–39.

facing unknown (future) perspectives, from both the patient and the physician's point of view; according to Marcum, "the trajectory of medical knowledge and practice is from the laboratory to the bedside. There is often little, if any, room in this model for the intuitive or emotional dimensions of either the physician or patient and medical knowledge is therefore generally impersonal."[440]

Alongside time and denial of death, Zail Berry lists discomfort with uncertainty, discomfort with emotional responses, experience with "boiler plate" documents that don't help, and competing medical issues.[441] Furthermore, the association with expected medical outcomes and unplanned, negative consequences can contribute to a generalized sense of loss of control, which could sometimes lead to harsh judgments of medicine as a whole. A very good example is the following extract from an article on "death by medicine" written by Dean, Null, and others, and analyzed in a confutation-based discussion[442] by Harriet Hall:

"A definitive review and close reading of medical peer-review journals, and government health statistics shows that American medicine frequently causes more harm than good. The number of people having in-hospital, adverse drug reactions (ADR) to prescribed medicine is 2.2 million. Dr. Richard Besser, of the CDC, in 1995, said the number of unnecessary antibiotics prescribed annually for viral infections was 20 million. Dr. Besser, in 2003, now refers to tens of millions of unnecessary antibiotics. The number of unnecessary medical and surgical procedures performed annually is 7.5 million. The number of people exposed to unnecessary hospitalization annually is 8.9 million. The total number of iatrogenic deaths shown in the following table is 783,936. It's evident that the American medical system is the

---

[440]   Marcum, J.A. 2008. *An introductory philosophy of medicine: humanizing modern medicine*. New York: Springer, p. 12.

[441]   Berry, Z.S. 2014. *Advanced Care Planning in Primary Care. A Patient-Centered Approach with Practical Strategies*. University of Vermont College of Medicine, Vermont Ethics Network Annual conference Advance Care Planning: It's Always Too soon... Until It's Too Late. Fairlee, VT.

[442]   "[Edward De Bono] argues that the West's tradition of settling disagreement by debate or argument is an example of *over*reliance on logic. In debate, the best debater wins. In argument, the person whose case best fits the rules of logic and the *current* evidence wins". Volk, S. 2011. *Fringe-ology: How I tried to Explain Away the Unexplainable—And Couldn't*, New York, NY: HarperCollins, pp. 125–126. Interestingly, this abstract talks about "anti*bio*tics prescribed annually for *viral* infections" (italics added), which is itself a quite problematic strategy, given that (as the definitions itself makes clear) antibiotics do not fight infections caused by viruses.

leading cause of death and injury in the United States. The 2001 heart disease annual death rate is 699,697; the annual cancer death rate, 553,251."[443]

Certainly, there is a lot of criticism of what is defined as "conventional medicine" in this article, and there are some very good points raised from both a theoretical as well as evidence-based perspective to support this claim. However, as we will see in future chapters, the complete and absolute condemnation of modern medicine is still partially reductivist, stereotyped, and imprecise. At the same time, the relationship between scientific (medical) method and certain expectation of a specific outcome, or sets of specific outcomes, and the very mystery of life, includes the unsolved problem of death: from an existential point of view, the absurd is a direct consequence of the absence of God.[444] Jean-Paul Sartre focuses on the concept of (human) death in order to further analyze its meaning, and in doing so he separates the two parts of the word as two concepts which allow multiple interpretations.[445] The word in English comes from the Old English *tō morgenne*, from the combination of *to* (at, on) + *morgenne*, dative of *morgen* (morning). Therefore, the etymology suggests different possible interpretations: as a noun "The day after (following) today" or "(in) the future"; as an adverb "on the day after (following) today or "at some time in the future"; the last also interpreted as "at some future time", which forces us to consider the temporal element, in terms of chronological value as well as applied extension in time. Thus, depending on our interpretation, the concept expressed by the word could lead us to a future *in atto* or *in divenire*; with the specific added value of "start", "new beginning". If we go to the Germanic root of the word, the confusion is even bigger. In fact, only the capital letter "M" helps us define the German word *morgen* (tomorrow) versus *Morgen* (morning). In this case, the etymology (same origin, dative singular) leads us back to the concept of "twilight", being the German word related to *Morgendämmerung*, from the Gothic *du maurgina* and the Germanic *murg(e)na*. These considerations could be of no value if we think of the origi-

---

[443]   Hall, H. 2008. *Death by Medicine*. Science-Based Medicine. Exploring issues & controversies in science & medicine. The complete discussion on the writing by Carolyn Dean, Gary Null, and others is available at http://www.sciencebasedmedicine.org/death-by-medicine/.

[444]   See Camus, A. in: West, D. 1996. *An Introduction to Continental Philosophy*, Polity Press Oxford, UK 1996, chapter 5: Beyond Theory: Kierkegaard, Nietzsche, Existentialism; 3rd Part: Jean-Paul Sartre and French Existentialism; pp. 151–153.

[445]   "To-morrow, after my death." In: Sartre, Jean-Paul, Existentialism and Humanism, translation and introduction by P. Mairet, Haskell House Publishers, Brooklyn, NY, 1997, p. 40.

nal language which Sartre used in writing his essay. It is also true that Sartre's mother, Anne-Marie Schweitzer, was of Alsatian origin, and therefore he might have been influenced, at least from a perspective of everyday basic conversation, by the German language, especially in its *Elsässerditsch* version, closely related to the Alemannic of the Upper German branch. If no influence or knowledge (even if subconscious) of the Alsatian dialect was in place at the time of Sartre's writing, we still have to take into consideration that the French word *demaine* (also divided in two parts in the original French edition) also leads us to a similar concept, because of the Latin origin *de mane* ("of morning").

Is tomorrow an expression of the present moment, a new beginning or an uncertain future? Where is man in all of that? How does man perceive time and future presence / essence / existence in relation to time and his own living at present time? As far as the future goes, Sartre is convinced that "things will be such as human beings have decided they shall be"[446]. In his view, the interpretation and meaning of man's current and future life is therefore linked to man's own actions: "there is no reality except in action."[447] Does that mean that there is no difference between the present moment and a future outcome? Certainly not, since man is the sum of his actions and therefore of his choices. Following this path we should be able to understand man's truth by analyzing his actions throughout his lifespan, even though in doing so we could already operate some sort of judgment. Thus, we have to find a way to indentify a universal principle. According to Sartre, the absolute truth is one's immediate sense of one's self, similar to the Cartesian *cogito ergo sum*, but applied to the whole humanity. Thus, we can define man's sense of self as deeply related to the sense of others' selves. In fact, "I cannot obtain any truth about myself, except through the mediation of another."[448] Therefore, other human beings are the key to understand oneself and one's meaning in this world. There is no such thing as a God or a prevenient design which can adapt the world to man's will. That is why we should act without hope. Is there room for feelings and emotions in this view? Camus states that people live as if they didn't know about the certainty of death and, without the embellishment or the added meaning (and value) of romanticism, the world itself is a strange and inhuman

---

[446]   Ibid.
[447]   Ibid., p. 48.
[448]   Ibid.

place.[449] Thus, Camus undertakes to answer what he considers to be the only question of philosophy that matters: Does the realization of the meaninglessness and absurdity of life necessarily require suicide? The term itself forces us to deal with the concept of self and self (one own's) slaughter, since the term is a new Latin coinage first used few years after Descartes' Death (in England, possibly around 1651). If I (as a human being) am the product of my actions, what does it mean "to kill myself"? Interestingly, Camus writes that it is exactly the moment when absurdity is recognized that life becomes full of passion, even more meaningful than before.[450] What looks like an oxymoron, is even better explained through Camus' analysis of man's perception: "A step lower and strangeness creeps in: perceiving that the world is 'dense', sensing to what degree a stone is foreign and irreducible to us, with what intensity nature or a landscape can negate us."[451]

These words could resonate the ones of Rudolf Steiner, when he describes "density" as a fundamental feature of human life on this realm of existence, a condition that human beings were subjected to after the passage from a pure etheric substance onto a more advanced, possibly non-symbolical form.[452] This statement echoes what Johann Wolfgang von Goethe and Helena Petrovna Blavastky already expressed, with regard to the etheric self-perception of being.[453] The perspective of a distant and remote condition is further described by Camus as "the primitive hostility of the world, (which) rises up to face us across millennia. For a second we cease to understand it because for centuries we have understood in it solely the images and designs that we had attributed to it beforehand, because henceforth we lack the power to make use of that artifice. The world evades us because it becomes itself again."[454] This concept

---

[449] Camus, A. 2000. *The Myth of Sisyphus*, Penguin Books London, translation by O'Brien, Justin, p. 22.

[450] Ibid., p. 24.

[451] Ibid., p. 20.

[452] Steiner, R. 1975. *Konferenzen mit den Lehrern der Freien Waldorfschule in Stuttgart*, Vol II, Rudolf Steiner- Nachlassverwaltung, Dornach, p. 15.

[453] For example, see: Von Goethe, J.W. 1947 ed., *Schriften zur Naturwissenschaft* mit Erläuterungen, versehene Ausgabe von Dorothea Kuhn. Weimar, D: Wolf von Engelhardt und Irmgard Müller, or the fundamental text on color theory Von Goethe, J.W. 1992 ed. *Beiträge zur Optik*, in: *Farbenlehre. Mit Einleitungen und Kommentaren von Rudolf Steiner. Herausgegeben von Gerhard Ott und Heinrich*, Stuttgart, D: Verlag Freies Geistesleben. For a more general reference to the concept of ether according to theosophy, see Blavatsky, H.P. 2007 Ed. *The key to Theosophy*. London, UK: The Theosophical Publishing Company. Theosophy Trust Books.

[454] Camus, A. 2000 ed. *The Myth of Sisyphus*, Penguin Books London, translation by O'Brien, Justin, p. 20.

is very interesting, especially if we compare to the position of Sartre, when he states that "man is all the time outside of himself, projecting and pursuing transcendent aims."[455] The 'self-surpassing' process seems to contradict what the French author said in previous pages, *id est* that: "existentialists don't believe in progress, because progress means amelioration; but man is always the same, facing a situation which is always changing, and choice remains a choice in the (that) situation."[456] Here Sartre seems to imply that, even though the human being is always subject to the same condition, and in this sense his is an absolute, universal truth; he is always facing *new* choices, totally dependent on himself, and for which he is completely responsible.

The French author continues onto a parallel between art and morality to further describe the process through which the human being is creator of his own destiny, thus seemingly quoting the Appivs Clavdivs Caecvs' famous phrase *homo faber fortunae suae*. Sartre adds that makes himself also by the choice of his morality. In this sense we have to do with creation and invention, thus leading the analysis of freedom, which is "the foundation of all Values."[457] This also implies that my freedom is mutually dependent on the freedom of others. By comparison, Camus writes in the Myth of Sisyphus that the question of human freedom in the metaphysical sense loses interest to the absurd man. He cannot explain the world: true knowledge is impossible and rationality or science provides only meaningless abstractions and metaphors. But the conclusion is pretty much the same we found in Sartre.[458] Man gains freedom in a very concrete sense: no longer bound by hope for a better future or eternity, without a need to pursue life's purpose or to create meaning, "he enjoys a freedom with regard to common rules."[459] Man realizes that the absurd arises when the human need to understand meets the unreasonableness of the

---

[455]   Sartre, J-P. 1997. *Existentialism and Humanism*, translation and introduction by P. Mairet, Brooklyn, NY: Haskell House Publishers, p. 53. Again, "men" intended as "human being" – this is a fundamental aspect we need to underline for appropriate comprehension throughout the text, and especially considering the broad range of the uses of the word "man" (not gender-defined/assumed) as translation of "human being", particularly in a philosophical context.

[456]   Ibid., p. 50.

[457]   Ibid. p. 52.

[458]   In this context, we would also like to refer to the work of the American author Joseph Heller, especially the emphasis on paradoxical situations from which an individual cannot escape because of contradictory rules, as evidenced (for instance) in his satirical novel *Catch-22*.

[459]   Camus, A. 2000 ed. *The Myth of Sisyphus*, Penguin Books London, translation by O'Brien, Justin, p. 32.

world, when "my appetite for the absolute and for unity" meets "the impossibility of reducing this world to a rational and reasonable principle." The possible mistake philosophers could do here, according both to Sartre and Camus, is reaching conclusions that contradict the original position (absurd for Camus, free from hope or illusion in Sartre) by abandoning reason (to some extent also the opposite, it is the case of the dry analytical statement of scientism or historicism) and committing "philosophical suicide." Heidegger and Jaspers are therefore guilty, and so is especially Kierkegaard, who didn't just abandon reason, but "turned himself to God" and Husserl, who elevated reason, ultimately arriving at ubiquitous Platonic forms and an abstract god. Camus also characterizes a number of philosophies that describe and attempt to deal with this feeling of the absurd, by Heidegger, Jaspers, Shestov, Kierkegaard, and Husserl. All of them, he claims, commit "philosophical suicide" by reaching conclusions that contradict the original absurd position, as we have seen. Thus, to embrace the absurd means acknowledging the contradiction between the desire of human reason and the unreasonable world. From the perspective of Medical Philosophy, this existential struggle is connected with the problem of death, and the impossibility for a perfect cure, able to heal very illness, disease and disorder. In this aspect lies perhaps the very mystery of the relationship with the (existence of a) divine power, especially in the form of grace, omnipotence, and goodness. Man struggles, man suffers. The only god who can help human beings is therefore a suffering god, a god who sacrifices himself (his own son in the Christian tradition) to redeem, save, and ultimately elevate and free humanity. It is the *God in Pain* by Žižek and Gunjević. [460] Furthermore, the existence (and essence) of this condition of suffering, of this struggle, of the absurd is possibly origin and cause, even reason/ing (in the sense of human need to find meaning, structure, sense, justification) of the ritualistic and esoteric aspects of the healing process. It is a translated form of magical thinking, and it represents the very mystery of human life in comparison with the alleged hard scientificity of modern science:

> "In high culture, religious medicine is something quite distinct from magic. The major religions reinforce resignation to misfortune and offer a rationale, a style, and a community setting in which suffering can become a dignified performance. The opportunities offered by the acceptance of suffering can be differently explained in each of the great traditions: as karma accumulated through past incarnations; as an invitation to Islam, the surrender to

---

[460] Žižek, S., and Gunjević, B. 2012. *God in Pain: Inversions of Apocalypse*. New York, NY: Seven Stories Press.

God; or as an opportunity for closer association with the Saviour on the Cross. High religion stimulates personal responsibility for healing, sends ministers for sometimes pompous and sometimes effective consolation, provides saints as models, and usually provides a framework for the practice of folk medicine. In our kind of secular society religious organizations are left with only a small part of their former ritual healing roles. One devout Catholic might derive intimate strength from personal prayer, some marginal groups of recent arrivals in Sao Paolo might routinely heal their ulcers in Afro-Latin dance cults, and Indians in the valley of the Ganges still seek health in the singing of the Vedas. But such things have only a remote parallel in societies beyond a certain per capita GNP. In these industrialized societies secular institutions run the major myth-making ceremonies."[461]

The very existence of myth and its human and/or artificial making is connected to the sense of meaning. And to be sure, without a meaning in life, there is no scale in values. This statement is almost identical in Sartre and Camus. Sartre thinks that there are no good or bad choices in life; what does exist is self-deception, which, again, is not a bad thing but an 'error'. A good example would be "to excuse oneself because one's passions." Camus writes that "What counts is not the best living but the most living." Thus, is the conclusion one and the same? Camus praises Sartre's descriptions of absurdity, the sense of anguish that arises as the ordinary structures imposed on existence, but also thinks that Sartre dwells on the repugnant features of humankind "instead of basing his reasons for despair on certain man's signs of greatness."[462] Sartre replies to this and other kinds of philosophical attacks by saying that what people (especially Christian Catholic critics) see as 'ugly' in his existentialist writing, is actually affirming the reality of every truth in a naturalistic manner, because it confronts man with the possibility of choice. He also adds that because man is responsible for what he is and at the same time he is responsible for other human beings, he always chooses the better for himself and therefore for humanity."[463] Turning directly to the context in The Myth of Sisyphus where this sentence occurs, and reading from this point forward, we are reminded of Nausea: "At any street corner the feeling of absurdity can strike a man in the face."[464] And on the next page of The Myth of Sisyphus is the Sartre-like passage about daily routine collapsing, which Sartre quotes in his re-

---

[461]   Illich, I. 1976. *Limits to Medicine; Medical Nemesis: The Expropriation of Health*. London, UK: Marion Boyars Publishers, pp. 108–109. Aspects which will encounter again in Chapter 5, *Complementary, Alternative, Traditional Medicine*.

[462]   Aronson, R. 2004. *Camus and Sartre. The story of a friendship and the quarrel that ended it*, University of Chicago Press, Chapter 1, p. 6.

[463]   Sartre, J-P. 1997. *Existentialism and Humanism*, translation and introduction by P. Mairet, Haskell House Publishers, Brooklyn, NY, p. 29.

[464]   Ibid., p. 31.

view. As we turn the page, Sartre's novel is mentioned explicitly: "This nausea, as a writer of today calls it, is also the absurd."[465] Whose voice, then, is heard in the original quotation above? In a stunning reflection of kinship, Sartre enthusiastically quoted Camus, whose analysis he actually drew upon Sartre himself. It is both of their voices at one and the same time.[466] The concept of Absurdity and Meaninglessness is well discussed in the previously mentioned book by Naylor, Willimon and Naylor.[467] The authors propose a scheme of interpretation of human values and key processes and development in the search of human life's meaning. This scheme is the *Life Matrix:*[468]

States of Meaning → Effects ↓	Meaning- lessness	Separation	Having	Being
Spiritual	Despair	Detachment	Orthodoxy	Quest
Intellectual	Nihilism	Alienation	Hedonism	Growth
Emotional	Depression	Anxiety	Narcissism	Balance
Physiological	Death	Somatization	Health fetish- ism	Homeostasis

Table 2.   The "Life Matrix" scheme as proposed by Naylor, T.H., Willimon, W.H., and Naylor, M.R. in *The Search for Meaning* (1994).

The authors clarify that "On a given day one may encounter all four of these states of meaning-moving from one state to another in response to mood shifts or changes in the external environment."[469] Is it therefore anything absolute and universal about these categories? Can we identify a character, a personality that is shaped by one (or more) of these concepts in a definite way? How are these values created? For Sartre, meanings and values are created the same way in the field of art and in morality, that is through creation and invention. For Camus, creation of meaning is not a viable alternative but a logical leap and an evasion of the problem. The philosopher gives examples of how others would seem to make this kind of leap. The option we saw above, namely suicide, would entail another kind of leap, where one attempts to kill absurdity by destroying one of its terms (the human being). Camus points out, however, that

[465]   Ibid., p. 32.
[466]   Aronson, R. 20004. *Camus and Sartre. The story of a friendship and the quarrel that ended it*, University of Chicago Press, 2004, Chapter 1, p. 10.
[467]   Naylor, T.H, Willimon, W.H., and Naylor, M.R. 1994. *The Search for Meaning*. Nashville, TN: Abingdon Press.
[468]   Naylor, T.H, Willimon, W.H., and Naylor, M.R. 1994. *The Search for Meaning*. Nashville, TN: Abingdon Press, pp. 16–19.
[469]   Ibid., p. 16.

there is no more meaning in death than there is in life, and that it simply evades the problem yet again. Camus concludes, that we must instead "entertain" both death and the absurd, while never agreeing to their terms. Camus arrives at three consequences from the full acknowledging of the absurd: revolt, freedom and ultimately, passion; as in revolt, both intimate as well as social, political. In regard to this position, Sartre shares in *Existentialism and Humanism* that the communist critics define his existentialism as a philosophy of contemplation and pure subjectivity, therefore bourgeois. He replies that we (existentialists and philosophers in general) must begin from the subjective because "man is nothing else but that which he makes of himself."[470] Human beings are indeed free to choose, but we as human beings cannot base our confidence in people we don't know. Therefore he criticizes movement and revolutions from the perspective of future meaning; no man can predict where a revolution will lead us to. At the same time he, as a human being is able to value (and validate) a revolution at the present moment, without expectations, hopes or illusions for the future. Thus, both rejected religion and determinism, but Camus adopted a more humanistic point of view, not willing to sacrifice morality as a fundamental concept. The French-Algerian philosopher believed that the absence of religious belief can simultaneously be accompanied by a longing for "salvation and meaning". Without religion, the discrepancy between human aspirations and the world is acute. This line of thinking presented an ostensible paradox and became a major thread in defining the idea of absurdism in Camus's writings. According to the philosopher, only the 'lucid' recognition of the absurdity of existence liberates us from believing in another life. Thus, acknowledging the absurd permits us to live for the instant. This is the real revolution. In regard to the political application of these views, Camus also maintained his pacifism, spoke out against and actively opposed totalitarianism in its many forms and resisted capital punishment anywhere in the world.[471] Therefore, Camus philosophical break up with Sartre is rooted in his opposition to totalitarianism. Camus detected a reflexive totalitarianism in the mass politics espoused by Sartre in the name of radical Marxism.

---

[470]   Sartre, J-P. 1997. *Existentialism and Humanism*, translation and introduction by P. Mairet, Haskell House Publishers, Brooklyn, NY, p. 28.

[471]   Camus also wrote an essay against capital punishment in collaboration with Arthur Koestler, the writer, intellectual and founder of the League Against Capital Punishment.

Politics aside, and apart from Camus' rejecting any ideological associations with existentialism[472] the other main difference in the viewpoints of the two philosophers, and the quarrel that put an end onto their friendship originated as we saw, in that Sartre believed human beings have complete control over their actions, while Camus believed there was also the possibility for random acts of absurdity. Certainly, Camus regretted the continued reference to himself as a "philosopher of the absurd," especially after the publication of *The Myth of Sisyphus*. We have to keep in mind, that Camus analyses the absurd in man as an alienating and real condition, not as necessity or only way. He focuses on the existential problem through a diagnosis which asks for human solidarity as main therapy. Thus, absurdity is an intellectual stimulus, yet frustrating and painful. The problem presented in *The Myth of* Sisyphus is only overcome in his 1945 novel *The Plague*. Therefore, the plague represents an evolution and final overcoming of the tragic and absurd sense and meaning of human existence. Still, the theme of human solidarity is a thesis that does not carry the convincing weight of other previous statement, especially by comparison with the cultural, social and existential torment at the beginning of the 1940s, a possible derivation of the unstable environment of the Post-Weimar Berlin culture, which gave birth to a series of reactionary and extremist movement culmination in the totalitarian regime of National Socialist Germany. This torment expresses itself in the existential atheism of Camus, who writes: "The absurd world more than others derives its nobility from that abject birth."[473] And how can we judge this nobility? Carrying the absurd logic to its conclusion, Camus has to admit that that struggle implies a total absence of hope, which he defines as a completely separate thing from despair.[474] He continues with this analysis and states that:

> "The immediate consequence is also a rule of method. The odd trinity brought to light in this way is certainly not a startling discovery. But it resembles the data of experience in that it is both infinitely simple and infinitely complicated. Its first distinguishing feature in this regard is that it cannot be divided. To destroy one of it terms is to destroy the whole."[475]

---

[472]   Albert Camus stated in *Les Nouvelles Litéraries*, an interview published in 1945, that "No, I am not an existentialist. Sartre and I are always surprised to see our names linked."

[473]   Camus, A. 2000 ed. *The Myth of Sisyphus*, Penguin Books London, translation by O'Brien, Justin, p. 19.

[474]   Ibid., p. 34.

[475]   Ibid.

This concept of destruction and violence, whether we are talking about metaphysical, libertarian or terrorist violence, is further discussed in the 1951 book *The Rebel*, a socio-psychological analysis of the reasons and motivations leading to violent rebellion and homicide, which again contributed to the intellectual and personal break-up with Sartre. While the war opened Sartre's eyes to a political reality he had not yet understood until forced into continual engagement with it, also through the group "Socialism and Liberty", which he founded in Paris and "Writers' Resistance Group" he joined in 1943, Camus continued his philosophical and political action, and was in this sense still an atheist existentialist very similar to Sartre, although he chose to abandon philosophical, existential (and personal) pessimism, to open up more to previously distant and controversial concepts, such as hope, interpreted as a sense of fight against evil. This parallel between the two authors continued throughout the years, and Sartre continued to be an active writer both in terms of political awareness as well as philosophical debate, and it was due to this life changing experience of war and captivity that Sartre began to try to build up a positive moral system and to express it through literature. From this perspective, both philosophers deal not only with social issues, but certainly also with metaphysical research, even though the definition wasn't openly accepted, especially by Sartre. In this regard, Heidegger wrote that:

> "Existentialism says existence precedes essence. In this statement he is taking existentia and essentia according to their metaphysical meaning, which, from Plato's time on, has said that essentia precedes existentia. Sartre reverses this statement. But the reversal of a metaphysical statement remains a metaphysical statement. With it, he stays with metaphysics, in oblivion of the truth of Being."[476]

The problem of free will itself is a metaphysical issue, as well as a moral one. It is the problem of whether rational agents exercise control over their own actions and decisions. For Camus, as we saw, the road to understand himself and the world around him is for the thinking man the active fight against absurd and the plague. What is very interesting, especially from a psychoanalytical point of view, as well as from an ontological one, is that the plague and the absurd are often interpreted as a metaphor of totalitarian regimes, which paradoxically should prevent society from a complete annihilation caused by the lack of rules, morality and the plague *of* the absurd. That is why, according to

---

[476]   Heidegger, M. 1978. *Letter on Humanism,* in Basic Writings: Nine Key Essays, plus the Introduction to Being and Time , translation by David Farrell Krell, London, UK: Routledge.

Camus, the plague/dictatorial regime can be destroyed only by solidarity and collaboration between human beings. Here we see how the two philosophers come together and define personal responsibility as deeply interconnected with social responsibility. Human beings, if united by positive ideals, which they follow with determination, will and strength, always have to be alert and ready. All this preparation needs to take into consideration the personal (individual) level of activity, especially in terms of personal limits and limitations. Does this mean that there is an element of individuality, departure, separation we need to be more focused on? Naylor, Willimon and Naylor argue that "although it may be possible to find meaning in life, meaning often eludes those who are separated from themselves, from others, and from the center of their being."[477] The authors stress the importance of the connection between a political, social (even activist) sphere and human beings' physical, medical and spiritual well-being. In fact, they compare the capitalistic "fake liberty and freedom" of modern USA to the lack of meaning which ultimately leads to those very issues we discussed at the beginning of this analysis of Medical Philosophy, in particular to disorders related to psychiatric intervention:

> "We are exhorted by radio, television, newspaper, politicians, educators, business leaders, and the clergy that to be a good American is to be a rugged individual. We are repeatedly encouraged to "do your own thing". "Freedom of Choice Makes America Great", so say the Chevrolet advertisements. [Note: the volume was published in 1994] Yet in our family life, work, play, religion, and politics, most Americans behave as mindless conformists. Freedom is uninteresting if buying a Chevrolet is the most significant thing we can do with it. While recognizing that our very existence depends on our uniqueness and separateness, most people fear the loneliness and existential emptiness of being isolated from other people. Whether or not we achieve a sense of meaning depends on how we confront our conflicting needs for separation and togetherness."[478]

Are we all "mindless conformists" or is there some hope of finding a differentiation without complete separation? For Sartre, but especially for Camus, the artist is a metaphor of the common man, and he is always trying to balance solidarity with loneliness.[479] Camus here seems to take a different road and states that man can face defeat and fall, unless he learns the lesson of the

---

[477]   Naylor, T.H, Willimon, W.H., and Naylor, M.R. 1994. *The Search for Meaning*. Nashville, TN: Abingdon Press, p. 55.

[478]   Ibid.

[479]   Better expressed in the French *Solidaire ou Solitaire*.

past.[480] This concept of past can therefore be interpreted as a combination of internal and external factors, ultimately presenting a view distant from Sartre's, a view which takes into account the impact and role of social, cultural, personal, as well as historical and geographic background.

Man's struggle against evil is ultimately a fight for freedom. And this very freedom reveals itself in anguish and despair, but can also be characterized and defined through the existence of that nothing which we find between reasons and action. Thus Sartre also deals with humanity's limits and ideas; more specifically he believed that our ideas are the product of experiences of real-life situations, and that novels and plays can well describe such fundamental experiences, having equal value to discursive essays for the elaboration of philosophical theories such as existentialism. This is especially true in his early writings, such as the 1938 novel *La Nausée*, but also in the *The Roads to Freedom* trilogy which charts the progression of how World War II affected Sartre's ideas. In this way, *The Roads to Freedom* presents a less theoretical and more practical approach to existentialism. During and after the war, this struggle for Sartre was against the monopolizing corporations who were beginning to take over the media and destroy the role of the intellectual. His attempts to reach a public were mediated by these powers, and it was often these powers he had to campaign against. Thus his ferocious and restless writing activity, both as a novelist as well as a philosopher (if not openly working as a journalist against colonialism), was the core of his skilled interactive approach to the various forms of media. In synthesis, history plays a major role in comparing these two authors. It is indeed from a pure political viewpoint that the two philosophers cannot find a common ground. Here we are talking about the value of tyranny. The concept of a "just fight" against totalitarianism because of the meaning and manifestation of totalitarian regime itself is defined as a struggle against a "government without laws". The opposite view sees tyranny as a necessary step (or stage) toward a much brighter and better future. The social factors play here a huge role in putting history (and its interpretation) into practical application. The awareness of a future *in divenire,* as we saw at the beginning of this essay is core and *hope* for a better world, in which all human beings could work toward the same goal, whether through a revolution –personal or social– or human solidarity. In this sense we can interpret the self-perception of man within a social system. Thus both Sartre and Camus shed

---

[480]   See *The fall*, in Camus, A. 2004 ed. *The Plague, The Fall, Exile and the Kingdom, and Selected Essays*, New York: Everyman's Library.

light on the eternal quest for freedom and search of meaning in man's life. Views that create and dissipate opinion and bias, writing strength and social responsibility. There is also the need of finding guidance, whether through pure analysis, freedom of choice or rule from above, structure and certainty of meaning, a desperate need to find answers coming from a shared, universal and absolute interest. Thus awareness is raised of the illusion of freedom given not only by the Stalinist communist dictatorship of the time (fought *in primis* by Camus), but also the struggle against the corporative, capitalistic and oppressive media brainwash of the self-called free governments, core and cradle of crypto-fascist intolerance (in the case of Sartre). Years of struggle and of oppression, but also years of intense and passionate analysis of true wisdom, if such thing can ever be attained by philosophy. A battle of man within and often against himself, as a being in constant unpredictable balancing activity between self-perception as belonging and belonged, as separate and absolute, as free and prisoner. A human being which creates himself every single day, through an imagination which is more certain and yet less rich than perception, which, in turn, presents an inexhaustible infinite series of profiles.[481] A man trying to understand and at the same time create his own values, his own morality, who transcends and exhausts himself (just like absolute knowledge) in order to reach an object, the object, himself.

This is the analysis of truth and meaning of philosophy itself; it is the trial of personal responsibility in comparison to the statements of psychoanalysis and the epistemological definition of knowledge. A balancing act that deals with philosophical, and to some extent, philological statements and the necessity of scientific proof, especially after the most current outcomes of analysis and clinical trial in neuroscience. Are we human beings really free to choose? What is the impact of this statement in the practical application of our morality?

6.2 Alfa et Omega, Diagnosis et Prognosis:

a) The time of our life

When we talk about time, we necessarily talk about a point of reference to which time is related. *Man* counts. Furthermore, man keeps track of the succession and mutation of e-vents, which, as the word explain, "came" from

---

[481]   See Sartre, J-P. 1984 ed. Being and Nothingness: An Essay on Phenomenological Ontology, New York, NY: Washington Square Press.

somewhere, this somewhere being a specific, countable place in space and time. And yet, grasping the ultimate significance, the absolute meaning of time is a very complicated task, especially from a human perspective, constrained by what appears to be a somewhat stable, and yet finite structure in which we life our earthly existence. Certainly, things began to shift after the debate around Einstein's relativity theory, in particular with the recent analysis in quantum string theories and quantum physics and mechanics in the recent years. Scientist such as Michio Kaku, Gerald Schroeder, as well as other academics like Roger Penrose and Stuart Hameroff, shed some light on our quest for understanding time and space in a deeper and more scientifically accurate way. Certainly, it is very hard to make a distinction between personal attitude, and somewhat childish reaction to claims to fitting our own worldview, when we are forced to compare the scientific version of the fact with a more religious, spiritual, transcendental, even metaphysical point of view.[482] In the case of Schroeder for instance we are talking about a culturally-religiously orthodox Jewish filter in analyzing some scientific analysis, such as the theory of the Big Bang, which concludes that the very existence of a Universe created *ex nihilo*, from a set of forces, or laws of nature, which are non-physical, yet acting on the physical, and which predate (the birth of) the universe is a sufficient proof of the existence of God. Although this claim might not be supported by hardliners in the agnostic and atheistic environment division of the scientific community, another claim, the one according to which any religious tradition serves as an obscurantist force against the advancement of "pure", "true" science is, from a purely scientific, as well as from a precise and accurate historical perspective, simply wrong. Just to follow the example, first of all the very theory of the Big Bang has to be rightfully credited to Georges Lemaître, who himself was a Catholic priest. Secondly, the very birth of the first (Western) Universities in Italy, and following the XII century throughout Europe, was promoted by the Church, as a way to advance culture in general, especially scientific theory and evidence-based practice.[483] To go back to our discussion on the concept of time, Aristotle argued that we should ask ourselves whether

---

[482]   For further reference, see Steinpach, R. 2006 (Aufl.; Schönemann, D., Red.). *Wieso wir nach dem Tode leben und welchen Sinn das Leben hat*. In: *Der Tod, ein Übergang; das Jenseits, eine andere Realität*. NOI International, Jahrgang 41, N. 154. Klagenfurt, A: NOI-Verlag, pp. 8–43.

[483]   The same of course applies also to institutions beyond Christianity, since the Moroccan al-Qarawiyyin mosque founded by Fatima al-Fihri in 859 was indeed first created as an Islamic religious school, but was further transformed into a university.

time would exist without the soul, given that there wouldn't be anything to count if there was nobody actively engaging in the action of counting. The order of events counted by man is succession and secession, ultimately a *separation*, a di-vision. The Greek *temneim*, as prime origin of the Latin term *Tempus* illustrates this *actio* of separating, dividing, ordering in units, thus requiring a counting actor. Even in the less common etymological explanation of the concept, related to the Sanskrit *Tàpas* (warmth), the focus is on space/time environmental elements connected to the duration, the extension (Latin *extensio / tensio*, Lithuanian *tempiti/tampyti* = to transport, to pull, to distend), and the atmosphere. Where and how do human beings exist, act and interact, relate to each other and one another (the distinction is fundamental in viewing the specific feature of *the Other* and *the Third* in Emmanuel Levinas), communicate, and finally perceive themselves within the structure (perhaps bonds, boundaries, limits) of time, their story and history, through the categories of past, present and future? Levinas writes:

> "The future that death gives, the future of the event, is not yet time. In order for this future, which nobody's and which a human being cannot assume, to become an element of time, it must also enter into relationship with the present. What is the tie between two instants that have between them the whole interval, the whole abyss, that separates the present and death, this margin at once both insignificant and infinite, where there is always room enough for hope? It is certainly not a relationship of pure contiguity, which would transform time into space, but neither is it the *élan* of dynamism and duration, since for the present this power to be beyond itself and to encroach upon the future seems to me precisely excluded by the very mystery of death. Relationship with the future, the presence of the future in the present, seems all the same accomplished in the face-to-face with the Other. The situation of the face-to-face would be the very accomplishment of time; the encroachment of the present on the future is not the feat of the subject alone, but the intersubjective relationship. The condition of time lies in the relationship between humans, or in history."[484]

The relation of contiguity between past, present and future, and the possible solution of continuity between them is fundamental in this extract. This consideration is immediately (both from a temporal/chronological as well as conceptual perspective) close (for the scope of this analysis, which is both comparative and dialectical, certainly not in terms of identical value) to the notion of infinite, of eternal. According to Plato's cosmology, time is in fact a "moving image of eternity". A similar position is the pre-Socratic philosophy of Parmenides. The philosopher thought that the (metaphysical) essence of reality

---

[484]   Levinas, E. 1947. *Time and The Other*, Duquesne University Press, Pittsburg, PA, English Translation by Richard A, Cohen, 1987, p. 79

was *a*chronical, *e*ternal. In particular, the very concept of time equals to an opinion, *id est* a position of the (Way of the) *Doxa*. Furthermore, Parmenides applied the law of noncontradiction to define "That which does exist" (the Parmenidean One) as timeless, uniform, and unchanging. It is immobile and unchanging because if it did indeed move, than he would be subjected to becoming, thus he would be now (at this very moment) and he would not be then (at that/another moment). That which does exist is One because there cannot be two (separate, different) Being(-s).[485] In fact, if (the) one is being (the one which exists), (the) other could not be the same as (the) one, thus it (the other) would be non-being, non-existing, that which does not exist.[486] That which does exist is eternal because there cannot be a moment in which it is not. It cannot cease to exist, it cannot be in a stage in which it is not yet. The contradiction lies in the fact that if it did exist only for a limited (period of) time, there would be another (period of) time in which it did not exist. It follows that it cannot be generated/born and cannot die. Also, that which does exist is indivisible (atom), because of the impossible existence of a non-being (non-existing) as a separating (dividing, defining) element.

Aristotle position is different, and presents time as measuring a movement from what is (has happened) 'before' and what is (will happen) 'after'. Thus, time is linked to change. And change is fundamental in medicine, especially in the continuous dance between therapy and diagnosis/reevaluation. In other terms, there is time if there is change, and there can be change if there is time. At first, we could view the Aristotelian position as stating that time can also be perceived as identical with change and movement, as well as described by its essence in the "hic et nunc" of the present moment, of the "now". There is a difference, and therefore a movement, a succession, an order, a quantitative measure, in the words of Aristotle, a "number of changes" (*arithmos kineseos*, which expresses a potentiality of coming-into-being of that-which-is-(cap)able-of coming-to-be, also defined, respectively, as *energeia* and *dynamis*) between the time (which is) not yet and/to the time (which is) no longer. This movement can happen only if there is change, the change that allows time to elapse. Thus, space becomes necessary to define time. To be more precise in this analysis and move onto a more specific definition of the term, we need to

---

485   We could also talk about "those which do exist" in a risky, perhaps imprecise translation.
486   "[What exists] is now, all at once, one and continuous... Nor is it divisible, since it is all alike; nor is there any more or less of it in one place which might prevent it from holding together, but all is full of what is." Parmenides, B 8.5-6, 8.22-24.

realize that time is not completely identical to change because change presupposes movement in space, and time has no physical space, or location. Heidegger presented the succession, ordering and movement of time in *The Basic Problems of Phenomenology*: "The now also is never the same and never a single one, but another, a not-the-same and not-one, a manifold."[487] More specifically, the very concept of time is linked, in Heidegger, to the historical essence or "historicality" of Dasein. The process, which is also a progression, in which the German philosopher focuses on the existential aspects of Dasein leads to the statement according to which the ontological constitution of Dasein (or, better said, the totality of Dasein) is to be found (and thus rooted, grounded, structured) in temporality. In this sense, Heidegger defines as *Gewesenheit* (past[488]) the *Schon-sein-in-der-Welt*; *Gegenwart* (present) as *Sein-bei*,[489] and *Zukunft* (Future) as *Sich-vorweg-sein*.[490] Thus, we can view the Dasein as an element in between birth and death, able to choose among its possibilities (and also forced to, as it is thrown into the world, which is also its world). Furthermore, the very ability to choose, the access to these possibilities is closely linked to its historicity, to the tradition. Dasein's potential and very essence has to do with the concept of *Sorge*, the care, the meaning of concern, whose temporality is defined by the above mentioned three historical moments of past, present and future. The focus on this historical, existential aspect of Dasein, and in general of human life, si very well described by Rüdiger Safranski:

> "In *Being and Time* Heidegger develops the philosophical proof that human existence, *Dasein*, has no other support that this *da*, this there-ness. In a sense he continues Nietzsche's work: to think the death of God and criticize the "last humans" (Nietzsche) who make do with pitiful substitute gods and do not even permit appalled horror over the disappearance of

---

[487]   Heidegger, M. 1927. *Die Grundprobleme der Phänomenologie*. Frankfurt am Main, D: Klostermann, 2005 ed., p. 233. See also the description on pp. 247–248: Also: The now is the same with respect to what it always already was —that is, in each now it is now; *its essentia*, its "what is always the same' (*tauto*)— and nevertheless every now is, by its nature, different in each now, *to d'einai auto heteron*; nowness, being-now, is always otherness, being-other; being how or *howness—existentia—heteron* ... the now is in a certain way always the same and in a certain way never the same."

[488]   Also in relation to the German term "*Vergangenheit*".

[489]   Better described by the concept of "*dem momentan zu Besorgendem*", in Heidegger. In the definition of the *Duden* Dictionary of German Language, the term is the "*Bezeichnung für einen nicht genau bestimmten Zeitraum zwischen vergangener Zeit (Vergangenheit) und kommender, künftiger Zeit (Zukunft)."*

[490]   Also "im Entwurf".

God. In *Being and Time* the formula for the capacity to experience horror is "Courage for anxiety."[491]

Dasein becomes human life, or human life is defined by and through this Dasein. Therefore, its potentiality for authenticity lies in revitalizing an element of tragedy, in choosing a hero. We see here how humanity is addressed through the calling of its transformative meaning and the possibility of transformation. Human beings exist and perceive their existence: "Dasein always understands itself in terms of its existence – in terms of a possibility of itself: to be itself or not itself."[492] This is fundamental to understand the conceptual and historical perspective created by Heidegger's Dasein, a mode of being that makes us aware of our potential and also forces us to accept this potential, by showing us that we indeed are what we become. This process of becoming is the coming-to-oneself of the existential future, which is more of a dimension rather than a sequence of single not-yet-present moments. The very stretching of the Being is in this sense reminding us of the openness and the "towardness" to *the Other* in Levinas, though in Heidegger we are talking about "standing outside oneself", as expressed by the Greek term ἔκστασις. The ontological and ethical aspects of this viewpoint are further expresses in Heidegger critique of the objectification[493] in philosophical, social and cultural terms, making him a "virtuoso interpreter of philosophical tradition."[494] Furthermore he addresses the problem of the relationship between time, existence and technology, also in metaphysical terms:[495]

[491]   Safranski, R. 1999. *Martin Heidegger – Between Good and Evil*, Cambridge, MA: Harvard University Press, p. 147.
[492]   Heidegger, M. *The Ontical Priority of the question of Being*, from the Introduction to *Being and Time*, in Richard Kearney and Mara Rainwater, eds. (1996). *The Continental Philosophy Reader*, London & New York: Routledge, p. 33.
[493]   In Heidegger's definition "*Vergegenständlichung.*"
[494]   Safranski, R. 1999. *Martin Heidegger – Between Good and Evil*, Cambridge, MA: Harvard University Press, pp. 147–149.
[495]   According to David West, "For Heidegger, the very character of western metaphysical thought is responsible for the all-pervasive influence of scientific reason and technology, which, in common with Husserl, he regards as an ultimately destructive influence on western culture. Specifically, Heidegger indentifies a pathological distortion in the predominance of what he calls an 'ontotheological' conception of substance as something absolutely unconditional, something which depends on nothing else for its existence". See David West (1997). *An Introduction to Continental Philosophy*, Cambridge: Polity Press, p. 97.

"For contemporary man, who no longer has time for anything, the time, if he has free time, becomes immediately too long. He must drive away the long time, in shortening it through a pastime. The amusing pastime is supposed to eliminate or at least cover up and let him forget the boredom."[496]

Human life is to be experienced in a non-objectivized, better in a beyond-objectivized manner, since the objective attitude "de-experiences the experience and "de-worlds" the world we encounter."[497] That is also why, in our philosophical analysis, which becomes perception in this process, we need to focus on the ecstatic-horizontal temporality of existence:

"Now, because the *ecstasies* are interconnected under the primacy of the future, because they belong together intrinsically, temporality is an ecstatic unity of future, past and present. Such unity has itself a horizon which is the condition of possibility of the world as existential and of *Dasein*'s transcendence."[498]

This transcendence is also transformation, of the tradition in relation to temporality, a tradition which is history, thus implying the de-struction (we could argue that, from this perspective, the term could also indicate a deconstruction)[499] of the history of philosophy. This destruction is the temporal dimension of Being and its towardness to death. Being "is" within time, acts within time, becomes within time. Thus, Being not only "is" but "gives itself" in its happening, in its becoming-in-time. This process happens on (within) the horizon of history, and towards its potentiality-for-Being. This *propensio* is linked to the above mentioned freedom of choosing itself, becoming, taking hold of itself, and lead its (one own's) life. Thus, we understand how, in Heideggerian terms, Anxiety brings Being face to face with its Being-free for and towards. More specifically, Dasein is truly contextualized in the *there* of Being-there, the "temporal horizon of intelligibility for Being-in-general,"[500] the ecstatic project of being-in-general. From this perspective, Heidegger shows us how "becoming" (the becoming Being, Being in becoming, but not

---

[496]   Heidegger, M. *Reden. Gesamtausgabe,* vol. 16, Vittorio Klostermann, Frankfurt, 2000, p. 579, cit. In Wrathall M. 2006. *How to Read Heidegger,* W. W. Norton, p. 111.

[497]   Ibid., p. 146.

[498]   Taminiaux, J. 1994. *Philosophy of existence I: Heidegger.* In: Kearney, Richard (Ed.) *Continental Philosophy in the 20th Century.* Routledge History of Philosophy, New York, NY: Routledge, 2003 edition, Vol. 8., p. 52.

[499]   But certainly not a deconstruct*ivist* de-construction.

[500]   Richard K, Rainwater, M. 1996. *The Continental Philosophy Reader,* London & New York: Routledge, p. 24

becoming being) is the true origin of history. The beginning *is* still (here),[501] it is not behind us or (historically) beyond us (beyond Being and beyond us beings) but right here/there in front of us. It *is*, and it *is becoming*. The difficulties in understanding the deeper meanings of Heideggerian philosophy and the impossibility to deliver those meanings in a clear and precise manner are due to the linguistic challenges represented by the conceptual terms and relative concepts formulated by the German philosopher. Those very terms, in many stances true neologisms created by Heidegger tend to lose their meaning and contextual significance in the process of translation, itself a process of tradition, and (re)interpretation. For instance, the very consideration of the juxtaposition-contradiction between the being of Dasein as becoming project and process and death and *towardness* to death is hard to define within the lexical, syntactical and grammatical realm of modern English language, especially in a philosophical context, and particularly in the form of (traditional, Western) metaphysics.[502]

This contradiction expresses the modality of being when this being also contains (or becomes that in totality when we add that to it) the concept (which, again, is a meaning, a signifying significance, not a restricted, structured, closed-up, term) of "being-dead", a form of being which, in historical-temporal terms of impossibility of existence is a "*there*-is-which-is-not-*there*-anymore". Almost a paradox, and yet absolutely evident in its essence, it is often defined by the very impossibility to grasp it, sometimes masked in non-awareness or "existential procrastination", also in Western medicine, as Naylor writes:

> "After reading the passages on death in Ecclesiastes to our undergraduate students at Duke [University] each semester, we ask them what comes to mind when they contemplate their own death. Their responses usually include separation, powerlessness, loss of control, meaninglessness, and nothingness. Magdalena [Naylor, MD] once replicated this exercise with first-year medical students at the Medical College of Virginia. Their overall response was, "We don't think about dying. Death is for the very old, not the young." The undergraduates openly acknowledged their fear of death. The medical students, who were preparing to spend their entire careers confronting death, were engaged in utter denial of an integral part of their work"[503].

---

[501]   With an obvious temporal/special contextualization, in terms of reference, to the "there" of Dasein.

[502]   For reference, see Heidegger's *Letter on Humanism*, 1949.

[503]   Naylor, T.H, Willimon, W.H., and Naylor, M.R. 1994. *The Search for Meaning*. Nashville, TN: Abingdon Press, p. 69

The anticipation of death in its becoming makes it (death, becoming death, Dasein in becoming) more apparent, thus making Dasein more aware (of itself and of its being / being there / "Being-there-ness"). In this sense, death becomes the historical term *par excellence*: it represents the unconditional possibility, since it belongs to the individual, as isolated/absolute man/human-being. Death isolates man, thus making him aware of himself and his self as being. This perspective throws us back into the world but not as totally captured[504] within the world, except in its historical-contextually environmental terms.[505] In Heideggerian terms, the "mundane" being-here represents the vanity of a hidden death, it is a form of life which is not living, not anticipating, not living-with, not being-toward (death). Thus it hides death, it tries to escape death, it flees from it and from the true essence of human existence (of Being) which is being-for(toward)-death. This type of being is true (philosophical) comprehension, an understanding which does indeed include *Angst*. Thus, time is possibility, it is being-towards, being-for, an authentic form of being, which "chooses the choice," thus opening (itself) up to possibility, to destiny. The historical-temporal component of these considerations makes us compare the perspectives of other definitions of a (temporal) reality. For instance, Zeno of Elea thought the metaphysical essence (use, inner structure, ontological anchorage) of reality as eternal (beyond time in the classical Greek etymology). Thus, time was itself an opinion, a position (an imprecise, incomplete, truth) of the *doxa*. According to Heidegger, the metaphysical tradition failed to understand the problem of Being because it leaves behind its relationship with time, a time configured in its temporality, in its history, through the process/progression of past, present and future. In metaphysical tradition, being-in-general is "just" a (one) being, therefore understood as "being-there" only as translation for "being-present" (not in Heideggerian terms, but in the "nowness" of the present time-moment). Past-present-future add dimension to (the understanding of) being, understood and explored through its temporality. Time is no more a "moving image of eternity" as in Plato, and it is even beyond the "before" and "after" of Aristotle. Space is not added as requirement or added para-concept to time, space is understood through the *there* of Dasein. In the words of Hegel "Human life is in its everyday doing oriented towards

---

[504]   In the etymological sense of the Lat. *Captivus*.

[505]   We could draw here some similarities to the "*In* the world but not *of* it" as expressed by Jesus: "My prayer is not that you take them out of the world, but that you protect them from the evil one. They are not of the world, even as I am not of it" (John, 17: 15–16).

Time."[506] Being means therefore "being-in-the-world", contextually, historically, fully present in the "being-together" of *Miteinandersein*, which shares the same origin of being, its character and structure (*gleichursprünglicher Seincharakter*) with the Being-in-general. Thus, Heidegger focuses and presents two fundamental elements of this "being-in-the-world", namely the world, also understood in its contextual historicity of environment surrounding and conceptually (in the same way, from the perspective of the *Umgang*) "embracing" man, and man itself. The focus on time from the perspective of man and/in the world has been at the center of philosophical speculation since ancient times. According to Saint Augustine of Hippo, time has been created by God together with the universe, this "togetherness" to be interpreted from conceptual, historical/temporal and chronological point of view. In his *Confessiones*, time is an "extension of the soul", which is also a dis-tention linked to the perception of the individual. Thus, man has perception (conscience, awareness) of the past only thanks to memory and of the future because of expectancy. Man lives in the present moment, with attention/conscience. The Christian perspective on time becomes therefore linear and progressive (toward a spiritual eternity), not circular-cyclic as in pagan times. We encounter the debate between circularity and linear unfolding of time with Georg Wilhelm Friedrich Hegel, who indentified the "end of history" with the times linked to the upcoming revolution brought by Napoleon. Alexandre Kojève states that "[...] with Hegel a new, closed circle comes in existence, an absolute knowledge representing a contin-

---

[506]   Heidegger, M. 2004 ed. *Der Begriff der Zeit.* In: *Martin Heidegger Gesamtausgabe, III. Abteilung: Unveröffentlichte Abhandlungen, Vorträge, Gedichte,* Band 64, Ln., Klostermann, Frankfurt, p. 134 ss. The complete description: "Das menschliche Leben ist in seinem alltäglichsten Tun und Lassen nach der Zeit orientiert. Wenn es als forschendes der Zeit selbst nachgeht, um zu erkunden, was sie sei, sieht es sich auf die „Seele"oder den „Geist" verwiesen. Sie wird umso mehr in den Blick gebracht werden können, je ursprünglicher das menschliche Dasein selbst hinsichtlich seiner Seinscharaktere sichtbar gemacht ist. Die Analyse der Zeit schafft sich das Fundament in einer ontologischen Charakteristik des menschlichen Daseins. Dasein besagt: „In der Welt sein." Die Welt ist das Worin solchen Seins. Das „In der Welt sein" hat den Charakter des Besorgens, des besorgenden Umgangs. Damit meint Heidegger Vorgänge wie etwas herstellen, etwas in Verwahrung halten oder etwas betrachten. Die Umgebung, in der sich dieses Besorgen aufhält, hat den Charakter der Vertrautheit. Hinzu kommen die Eigenschaften des Vorscheins und der Vorhandenheit. Sie sind die Strukturmomente des Grundcharakters der „Welt", nämlich der Bedeutsamkeit: die Weise des Anwesendseins des Werkzeugs an seinem Platz gründet in dem, worauf es in seiner Dienlichkeit verweist. Dieses Wozu und Worum trägt sich in den weiteren Verwendungszusammenhängen, in denen das Besorgen sich bewegt. In diesem nutzenden und gebrauchenden Besorgen begegnet die Natur. Das Besorgen kennt sich in seiner Umwelt aus."

uum of time and concept, in which relationship becomes identification and then identity."[507] In particular, human history is understood through human *actions*, a totality, a series of human creations. These actions are the creation of a series of *worlds* which are specifically and originally human, thus completely different from the natural world.[508] In the relationship between Master and Slave, Hegel explores the evolution of time from the antiquity, onto the Christian World (which ends with the French Revolution) and finally to what Kojève has described as the "third historical world."[509] This evolution of the Christian World leads to a form of edification (*Bildung*) with several layers of significance, especially from the perspective of education, intellectual work. But what is the criterion of significance of time according to Hegel? In analyzing time and its relationship with history we saw how not only the facts, the event we encounter represent the core of the problem, but also man as the main element experiencing those facts. Hegel helps us understand this relation, which is obviously also difference, between what has happened, is happening, will happen and all the meta-conceptual structure of the becoming of the concept, what emerges (what effectuates) in the historical sphere of the concept, and the concept itself. Conceptually speaking "Time, as the negative unity of being outside of itself, is just as thoroughly abstract, ideal being: being which, since it is, is not, and since it is not, is."[510] Hegel continues:

> "In time, it is said, everything arises and passes away, or rather, there appears precisely the abstraction of rising and falling away. If abstractions are made from everything, namely, from the fullness of time just as much as from the fullness of space, then there remains both empty time and empty space left over; that is, there are then posited these abstractions of exteriority. But time itself is this becoming, this existing abstraction, the *Chronos* who gives birth to everything and destroys his offspring. That which is real, however, is just as identical to as distinct from time. Everything is transitory that is temporal, that is, exists only in time or, like the concept, is not in itself pure negativity. To be sure, this negativity is in everything as its immanent, universal essence, but the temporal is not adequate to this essence, and therefore relates to this negativity in terms of its power. Time itself is eternal, for it is neither just any time, nor the moment now, but time as time is its concept. [...] Time, is not, therefore, the power of the concept, nor is the concept in time and temporal; on the contrary,

507   Kojève, A. 1969. *Introduction to the Reading of Hegel*, Basic Books, p. 131.

508   Ibid., p. 32: "[...] This substructure which supports both Religion and philosophy, is nothing but the totality of human Actions realized during the course of universal history, that History in and by which Man has created a series of specifically human Worlds, essentially different from the natural World."

509   Kojève, A. 1969. *Introduction to the Reading of Hegel*, Basic Books, p. 57.

510   Hegel, G.W.F. 1817. *Werke. Zweiter Teil: Die Naturphilosophie*, Band 8, Frankfurt a. M., 1979 ed., § 201.

the concept is the power of time, which is only this negativity as externality. The natural is therefore subordinate to time, insofar as it is finite; that which is true, by contrast, the idea, the spirit, is eternal. Thus the concept of eternity must not be grasped as if it were suspended time, or in any case not in the sense that eternity would come after time, for this would turn eternity into the future, in other words into a moment of time. And the concept of eternity must also not be understood in the sense of a negation of time, so that it would be merely an abstraction of time. For time in its concept is, like the concept itself generally, eternal, and therefore also absolute presence."[511]

The very structure of Hegelian thought presents the concept in complete identity with itself. The concept is time, more specifically the modification, the progressive change of the valuation constituting history; it is the "empirically existing Concept itself". In the words of Kojève, "an absolute knowledge representing a continuum of time and concept, in which relationship becomes identification and then identity."[512] Understanding Hegel's perspectives on time requires indeed a very attentive analysis of his work, but if we really wanted to answer the question "what is time for Hegel?" we could try to summarize an answer, using his own words: "*die Zeit is der Begriff selbst, der da ist*"[513] or "Time is the concept itself, which is there". We should also note that in translating the above quotation, we could choose "notion" instead of *concept* and "here" instead of *there*, to take into account specific Hegelian problems as well as pots-Hegelian philosophical debate, such as the one in Heidegger's *Da*sein. In detail, this notion knows itself as notion and the moments of time appear before (earlier) than the one-complete, the whole, the *ful*filled. According to Hegel, there is a strong connection between spirit/mind (Geist), time and destiny: "Time appears as the destiny and necessity of spirit that is not yet complete within itself [...] For this reason it must be said that nothing is known that is not in experience, or, as it is also expressed, that it is not felt to be true."[514] We understand how time presents itself to (human) consciousness as intuition, before notion, thus as an *empty* intuition: "for this reason, Spirit necessarily appears in Time, and it appears in Time just so long as it has not grasped its pure Notion, i.e. has not annulled Time."[515] In Hegel, Time is something that exists empirically in space, and it is also the negation of space. Time is History, and Nature is Space; we see the succession of facts within history, and their

[511]   Ibid., § 201 ss.
[512]   Kojève, A. 1969. *Introduction to the Reading of Hegel*, Basic Books, p. 131.
[513]   Hegel, G.W.F. 1807. *Phänomenologie des Geistes*, Frankfurt am Main, D: Suhrkamp Verlag, I. Auflage (edition) 1986, § 801–802.
[514]   Ibid.
[515]   Ibid.

significance from the perspective of time, as these events unfold. More specifically, Hegel focuses on the *Akkusativ* and *Dativ/Modal/Instrumental* of these unfolding events: the objective "what" is not exactly the same as the "how" or "in which way" history unfolds. Thus, we understand how time is not something totally separated from the concept, is not something that happens "outside", "beyond" the unfolding of the (sum of the) facts. The understanding of time cannot be complete without the understanding of negation and relation with space. Space is, according to Hegel, the inner negation of itself, the "self-sublating" (*Aufheben*) of its moments in its truth, while time—being beyond, outside this unfolding—is the existence of this perpetual "self-sublation". The relation is thus understood in the following statement: "time is the truth of space, [...] the abstract multiplicity of points distinguishable in it."[516] Thus, time provides meaning, time *is* the meaning, a meaning which is not indifferent to (the content of) history. But where does this meaning come from? Since we saw how time is the concept itself, we must understand the very meaning of Hegelian Geist, a mind/spirit which has fallen "into" Time, thus providing (being) content, which, in turn, is the "imminent differentiation of Spirit."[517] Furthermore, Spirit does not annul time, but appears in it just "so long as it has not grasped its pure concept."[518] We see here how, from this time-history perspective which carries (or has been permeated by) content, points of space express an actual difference, not just and no longer *possible* differentiations. In this sense, Hegel presuppose the present-moment, the "now" as the condition of the "self-positing" of the point(-s). In Hegel, time becomes "history" in the very process of "coming about itself" of history. In Heidegger instead, the historical moment is indeed a single moment, or better expressed, the "world-time" originates from *each* moment of time, from its structure, its meaning, its relevance (and structural value), its significance, its regular recurrence (as perceived by the *Dasein*). We should also focus here on the concept of "regularity" in dealing with the succession of recurrent events, and examine the history of philosophy regarding these terms.

b) Multiple perspectives

For instance, in understanding the philosophical basis to the scientific debate on time during the Industrial Revolution, we could go back to Isaac Newton

---

[516]   Ibid., p. 428.
[517]   Ibid., §802.
[518]   Ibid., §801. We need to stress again the importance of the term *Begriff* in defining the "grasping process" of the (towards the) concept.

and his definition of time and space as *sensorium Dei*, eternally and immutably, always the same and the same-to-itself, in its own image. According to Newton, time is completely distinct from the world-space, and it passes uniformly regardless of the succession of (historical) events in the world. Thus, Newton does not consider time and space as true, genuine substances, but talks about absolute space and absolute time.[519] These concepts are different from the human perception of time/space, or more specifically, from the way human beings measure time/space. These types of time/space he called relative space and relative time. What is important to note here, is that the main view toward space and time until the XVIII century presented the idea of empty space as a conceptual impossibility. Thus, while space is abstraction, time is the measure of succession, series, cycles of change in the world. Aside from the debate between substantivalism versus relationism from the perspective of the ontology of time and space, we see here that for Newton (and for Galileo Galilei), time is not an internal/interior intuition of conscience, but an objective dimension of reality, which (together with space) represents a measurable parameter of motion.

One difference can be traced between the position of Newton and the one of Leibniz (not to mention the controversial debate on calculus between them, John Keill and others). According to Newton, as we saw above, time is a "container of events" (similarly to the function of space); while according to Leibniz, time and space are a conceptual "apparatus" describing the interrelations between events. For Newton, the existence (its way, structure and manner) of time (and space) is necessitated by God's eternality and omnipresence, while for Leibniz time has three levels. The first level is the atemporality or eternality of God, similarly to what is encoded in the Greek concept (and Hellenistic deity) of *Aἰών*. The second level is drawn from the Aristotelian concept of *ἐντελέχεια*, which describes the condition of a thing whose essence is fully actualized. Now, it is important to notice that in Leibniz the concept is more related to the "continuous immanent becoming-itself" of the point, the word, the idea represented by the *monad*. Finally, the third level is the chronological structure of the (sequence of) present moments, or "nows". In terms of perception of time and space, one of the best examples of the idea that time and

---

[519]   This is very important in considering the relationship between time and space, since Newton defined the true motion of a body to be its motion through absolute space. See: Rynasiewicz, R. 2011. *Newton's Views on Space, Time, and Motion*. Stanford, CA: Stanford Encyclopedia of Philosophy.

changes within time are complete illusions is possibly the work by John Ellis McTaggart, in particular *The Unreality of Time*, published in 1908. In particular, McTaggart argues for the unreality because our descriptions of time are either circular, contradictory, or insufficient. We see how, according to Hegel, time is closely connected with the *Geist*. Thus, time becomes the core of being, the medium of subjectivity (and the mediating power of the negative), attached to its perception by being. A (human) being perceives time, *thinks* time; therefore time is linked to the development of the subjectivity ("I" think) of the spirit. This development is the potential-being-actualized. Furthermore, this development is also the arising of significance, thus the process in which history becomes actualized, establishing meaning, values and evaluation, which is also de-valuation, interpretation, tradition, transmission. This is fundamental in understanding not only what history is, but also its role, and the role of being *in* history. Through the facts, the events, the happenings (what is/that which is/those which/who are happening) more specifically through the actions of (human) beings, history becomes the process (the significance) justifying the existence *of* being from the perspective of valuation. That is precisely why history represents the very structure of interpretation; while time embodies the possibility of significance becoming, arising, as well as making this very significance arise.

The close link between being and time is well described (in different ways) both by Hegel and Heidegger, and the same could be said about the view of time according to Immanuel Kant. However, there is a very important distinction to make. Both Hegel and Kant see "subjective" in time, but for Hegel time is completely attached, bound up with the "I think", in Kant time stands "beside" it, passes "along with" it. In Kantian terms (and through his first, second and third argument),[520] time possesses both empirical reality and transcendental ideality. Since time stands beside the subjectivity of being, time can determine it without emptying itself into this subjectivity, thus losing its (independent) character as time. At the center of Kantian philosophy is the

---

[520]   Mainly: 1) The claim that human representations of simultaneity and succession have to be driven or originated in human mind, since they are presupposed in our (human) experience of simultaneous and successive moments in time. 2) The argument is based on (the possibility of) considering time without any appearances of objects—but not vice versa—shows time to be an *a priori* structure which makes experience possible. 3) Our necessary principles about time show that the representation of time must be a priori rather than a posteriori. For further reading, see Mertz Hsieh, D. 2004. *Kant on Time*, Phil 5010, Hanna – Kant, available on http://www.philosophyinaction.com/.

subject, not the object; and time becomes an a priori form of sensation, it is not an empirical concept drawn from experience. If the subject (the human being) could not perceive the passing of time, he would not be able to perceive the sensible world and its elements (objects), which exist in space. This is called "external sense" in analogy with time, which is the "internal sense". Thus, the subject is at the center of kantian analysis, since everything that exists can only be perceived (both in terms of value and structure, order) by and through the *a priori* structures of the subject. In Hegel, time is not just focused through the process of a subjective perception,[521] but it is the development of the criterion of significance. Time is the *Begriff* in which (and in how) this criterion of significance may develop within a particular fact, event, act.

The relation between subject, time and perception is fundamental in the work of Emmanuel Levinas. In particular, the focus on subjective particularity is well explored through the lenses of the subject, the time and the main element of Levinas' philosophy, *the Other*. The Other is a concept (or rather a non-concept)[522] which is at the center of an investigation towards a deeper understanding Levinas' thought on time. The relationship between Time and the Other is at the center of the philosophical investigation of the world, of life, of existence as a whole. Moreover, it is the very correlation, intimate, subjective, phenomenological (in terms of method, perspective and structure beyond a correlation which is both noetic as well as noematic), and in a very particular way "conversational" (in the higher sense describing the ability to connect on different levels) of the subject with the other: "while the First speaks the Second is listening."[523] This is a true relationship, a relationship which moves beyond the subject-centric view of Kant, a relationship which is not the achievement of subject alone, but lies in the very *encounter* with the other. This is not just a mere metaphorical, symbolical, synonymical way to describe a link, a relation or correlation between these two terms; it is instead a deep analysis, cognitive as well as phenomenological, rooted in the essence and existence of life and living being of the otherness and the perception of this otherness from the perspective of the whole. In the words of Dimitrova:

---

[521]   Always taking into consideration the connection of time with/to the development of the subjectivity ("I" think) of the spirit.

[522]   In the sense of "towardness beyond", "continuous progressive striving towards" that-which-is-not-yet-grasped, the moment (immediately, and yet atemporally) before the active action of be-*greifen*, the con*cipĕre*, cum*capĕre*, cum*prehendĕre*.

[523]   Dimitrova, M. 2008. *Emmanuel Levinas: Time and Responsibility*, Sofia Philosophical Review, Vol. II, n. 1, p. 25.

"For Levinas, the notion of totality (understood ontologically by a traditional philosophy as the sum of all possible elements and their relationships identical with the Being or existence as a Whole) is derived analytically from thinking, which is viewed as the highest instance of synthesis of knowledge. Levinas opposes this philosophy with the idea of ethics prior to ontology."[524]

The greatness of Levinas lies, among many other contributions, in the movement from myself, the I (the *personal I*, the *I-think*, the observed/observable/perceived/perceivable *me*) towards the Other. From the cognitive perspective of the inescapable, and absolutely founding experience of this encounter with the Other, we need to observe the psychological implications of this connection, interaction, and existential struggle. The Other is also Other-from-me, and yet, it represents, it is, a "face", another and the same, in the consequential relationship with the (conceptual and spiritual) *image/presentation/epiphany* of "the (my) Neighbor". The neighbor is "the other me", my correlative, my peer. I rely on *him* for support and meaning.[525] In Levinas' philosophy I am not everything, I don't possess everything, not everything moves around me, though it does concern me, and my consciousness does not encompass everything. But this is certainly not absence of interest, relativist(ic) morality, indifferentiation. Furthermore, it is not even the possible ability, capacity, strive for an absolute perspective, concept and interpretation/structure/re-structuralization of totality: "Levinas' ethics never engages in a more or less coherent systematization of the entirety of regulations concerning the behavior of a human group. Neither does he found the possibility of a rational justification of moral norms through or under a unifying principle."[526] As human beings, as subjects, we understand this through "the face of the other". Beneath all the possible layer of interpretation of Levinas' thought, and I

---

[524]   Dimitrova, M. 2011. *In Levinas' Trace*, Newcastle upon Tyne, UK: Cambridge Scholars Publishing, Foreword, p. viii.

[525]   The psychological implication is evident in researches such as the one by Randy Auerbach, a Harvard Medical School instructor in psychology at McLean Hospital. Elizabeth Dougherty writes: "Auerbach recently examined the relationship between social support and stress and the development of depression among adolescents. He found that young people with little support from parents and classmates are more likely to experience depressive symptoms in the face of stress. A lack of friends and supportive peers, however, did not contribute to risk for depression." See Dougherty, E. 2011. *The Path to Sadness. The roots of depression can be uncovered*. In: Byron, P.B. (Ed.) 2011. *The Science of Emotion*, Boston, MA: Harvard Medicine. We will discover the loci for this and other mental health disorders in the following chapters.

[526]   Bensussan, J. 2011. *Ethics in an Extra-moral Sense*. In: Dimitrova, M. 2011. In Levinas' Trace, Newcastle upon Tyne, UK: Cambridge Scholars Publishing, p. 3.

would suggest[527] also beneath a broad spectrum of the history of philosophical investigation in general, is this encounter with the (personal) Other. This encounter helps me understand not only myself, my world, my position and role (we could argue *my mission*[528]) in my world, but also all the considerations around these elements when the possessive "my" is eliminated. Thus, the other does not limit my freedom, my ability to grasp, my cognitive "dominion". On the contrary, the other "invests" my freedom, my knowledge (and "cognitive awe"), setting me free from the reduction in terms through the consideration of the very action of time: "Time that separates Ego from death, that is, existential time, gets thinner in the course of life."[529] And this very separation between us in the form of ego and the supreme concept of Death is at the center of the problem, as we previously discussed:

> "Although many of us spend our lives denying that we are going to die, some like Albert Camus have discovered that death is an important source of meaning. The fact that life is finite makes every remaining moment precious and beautiful. In a very real sense, life without death would not be worthwhile. Death liberates us from the present and grants us the wisdom to sort out our priorities as to how best to use our remaining time on earth."[530]

In the midst of this struggle, as a human being I realize the existence of something totally, absolutely and irreducibly other-than-myself. This is pure, true, effective dialectics between me and the other: "While monological philosophy deals with cognition and activity, dialogical philosophy pays attention to communication and its various forms."[531] This communication is also *com-*

---

[527]   I dare to affirm this position, in thinking about all the possible connection of this very topic to the most important questions of philosophical debate, questions of existence, questions of meaning, questions of method, questions of truth, questions of perception etc., whenever we are interested in understanding and exploring (the process of, the understanding of, the didactic and teaching of) knowledge. Furthermore, Levinas states (in *Totality and Infinity: An Essay on Exteriority*) that "[...] The relation with the Other, or Conversation, is a non-allergic relation, an ethical relation; but inasmuch as it is welcomed this conversation is a teaching." The teaching is indeed *einsegnement*; it shares, it leaves a *sign in* me, who is in connection, communion, correlation, communication, encounter, embrace with the other.

[528]   Especially in the sense (ontological, cognitive, practical, etymological, possibly messianic) of "being sent (to, for towards)", as in Lat. *missio, missa, mitto* It. *missiva, mettere, ammettere, emettere, omettere* etc.

[529]   Dimitrova, M. 2008. *Emmanuel Levinas: Time and Responsibility*, Sofia Philosophical Review, Vol. II, n. 1, p. 16.

[530]   Naylor, T.H, Willimon, W.H., and Naylor, M.R. 1994. *The Search for Meaning*. Nashville, TN: Abingdon Press, p. 69.

[531]   Dimitrova, M. 2011. *In response to Jeffrey Andrew Barash: The immemorial time*. In: Dimitrova, Maria 2011. *In Levinas' Trace*. Cambridge Scholars Publishing, Newcastle upon Tyne, UK, p. 40.

munion, and here is where we need to focus on in our debate on time and history. How can there possibly a communion, if there is a separation between me and the other? Indeed, mine is an encounter with the Other, a moment-in-time where my perception, my opportunity and possibility for openness toward the Other becomes a *momentum*-toward-moment. It pushes me toward the Other, who is not only other-than-me, but also other-than-myself (in terms of value and perception, thus judgment) but also other-in-me, which is in turn-me-in-the-other, but in an incomplete sense, way and time. The other doesn't simply push me in this towardness, it *"invites* me in *investing* me;" right here where the time opens, not by splitting in two moments, two halves, between me (myself) and the other, but by becoming "infinity". In particular, "the *face* is present in its refusal to be contained."[532] Thus, since I cannot grasp (in terms of possessive containment) the Other or reduce the Other to a finite concept (that is why it is a non-concept) or image, the Other is "infinity", that is, it is identified (not just by the author, Levinas, but by me as subject) with infinity, it produces in me "the idea of Infinity." How can we understand this infinity from the perspective of time? In the words of Dimitrova, "The difference between the Other and me is similar to the one between Infinity and finitude."[533] In Levinas, time is not strictly duration or measure of movement, but is something beyond this frame of understanding, something with a different level of transcendental-synthetical value. It is indeed a new dimension, both spatial and temporal: "The being that presents himself in the face comes from a dimension of height, a dimension of transcendence whereby he can present himself as a stranger without opposing me as obstacle or enemy."[534] This transcendence is related to existence itself, and it is exactly a "moment beyond" a point in time and beyond time: "Postponing the death moment, no matter whether by heroic, nostalgic, or well calculated behavior—this delay, in which life of the finite being is lived, is existential time."[535] Furthermore, it is a suspension, an interruption, which leads us to the considerations on the ethical debate on being:

---

[532]   Levinas, E. 1961. *Totality and Infinity. An Essay on Exteriority*, Duquesne University Press, 3rd ed. 1969, p. 194.

[533]   Dimitrova, M. 2008. *Emmanuel Levinas: Time and Responsibility*, Sofia Philosophical Review, Vol. II, n. 1, p. 22.

[534]   Levinas, E. 1961. *Totality and Infinity. An Essay on Exteriority*, Duquesne University Press, 3rd ed. 1969,, pp. 214–215.

[535]   Dimitrova, M. 2008. *Emmanuel Levinas: Time and Responsibility*, Sofia Philosophical Review, Vol. II, n. 1, p. 15.

"[...] by interpreting the Good as distinction between the Good and essence, by interpreting the Good as "otherwise than being", [Levinas] calls for a dissociation of the Good from the objects of any possible reminiscence. The Good is identified, in other words, with the im-memorial which no reminiscence is able to recall. "*The Good which reigns in its goodness*", as Levinas writes, "*cannot enter into the present of consciousness, even were it to be re-membered.*"[536]

This moment of transcendence is a relational moment,[537] that is exactly why it is hard to define this type of time or interruption of it in Levinasian terms. It is certainly a break in the flowing of historicality or, better formulated, it is a wave, a bending act (or non-act), an in-flection, a trace, a sign in history. The encounter with the Other is certainly an event, since it does happen in the frame of time and in the sequence of "nows", but it flows through a movement. This is the movement toward the other, is the calling upon felt, perceived by the subject in being (becoming)[538] face to face with the other: "In the face the Other expresses his eminence, the dimension of height and divinity from which he descends."[539] This dimension of transcendence, of divine, is central to Levinas' philosophy. The very idea of sainthood, of holiness is derived from this encounter with the Other, in changing priorities, in putting the Other before myself. This is very well understood from the perspective of time, and by comparing the space of physical pain with the "moral pain": "While in moral pain one can preserve an attitude of dignity and compunction, and consequently already be free; physical suffering in all its degrees entails the impossibility of detaching oneself from the instant of existence. It is the very irremissibility of being."[540] This detachment is at the centre of Levinas' discussion on the absurdity of hate; in particular, the logical impossibility (it is the case of the extermination camps) of the reduction of the subject to an object-thing and the expectation/will of having the subject assisting his reduction to object/thing.

---

[536]   Barash, J.A. 2011 *Memory and the Immemorial in the Philosophy of Emmanuel Levinas.* In: Dimitrova, M. 2011. In Levinas' Trace, Newcastle upon Tyne, UK: Cambridge Scholars Publishing, *I. Memory and the Immemorial*, p. 28.

[537]   In this sense, we also understand the analysis of dichotomy provided by Dimitrova: "[...] in addition to these meanings gained through reference to the illuminating totality, they take on meanings in dialogue." Ref. in Dimitrova, M. 2011. *In response to Jeffrey Andrew Barash: The immemorial time.* In: Dimitrova, M. 2011. In Levinas' Trace, Newcastle upon Tyne, UK: Cambridge Scholars Publishing, p. 37.

[538]   Again, the notion of being versus becoming is quite hazardous, considering the importance and value of this transcendental interruption in the sequence of now-moments.

[539]   Levinas, E. 1961. *Totality and Infinity. An Essay on Exteriority*, Pittsburg, PA: Duquesne University Press, 3rd ed. 1969, p. 262.

[540]   Levinas, E. 1947. *Time and The Other*, Pittsburg, PA: Duquesne University Press, English Translation by Richard A, Cohen, 1987, p. 43.

The other is simply not reducible, and transcendence is not conceptualizable, and is understood, from the perspective of time and history, through and as the face-to-face and I-the other relation. This relation is at the basis of Levinas' discourse on morality and justice, it is not a new series of rules and dogmas, nor a new philosophical ethics, it is truly an encounter. Thus, we understand Levinas' problematic criticism of the justification of human rights, "the limitation of rights for the maintenance of justice [as] a way of treating the other as means rather than ad end alone [...]"[541] This analysis of human rights and morality from the perspective of time and the Other is especially important in considering the momentum of interruption *par excellence*, the moment of death. We saw how in Heidegger *Sein-zum-Tode* is a true way of being, a towardness rather than an orientation, a revelation of the process of Dasein as a threefold condition of Being. Levinas writes: "Death in Heidegger is an event of freedom, whereas for me the subject seems to reach the limit of the possible in suffering. It finds itself enchained, overwhelmed, and in some way passive. Death is in this sense the limit of idealism."[542] In Heidegger, Time, the present and the eternal are all related to the notion of temporality, or the way human beings perceive time.

The problem of (human) perception is also taken into account by Henri Bergson. In particular, he makes a distinction between the time of physics and the time of consciousness, which do not coincide. In fact, time as the unit of measurement of the physical phenomena is en-coded through *spatialization*, in a process in which every moment is represented objectively and qualitatively identical to all the others. However, the original time is known by (individual, subjective) intuition, in and through our consciousness. The issue of the differentiation, in terms of value and modality, represents a core problem in understanding the work of Bergson, but also of Heidegger and Levinas. Heidegger's (notion, concepts of) present and eternal are modes of temporality, in an ecstat-

---

[541] Wolff, E. 2011. The *Quest for Justice versus the Rights of the Other?* in: Dimitrova, M. 2011. In Levinas' Trace, Newcastle upon Tyne, UK: Cambridge Scholars Publishing, *I. Memory and the Immemorial*, p. 78.

[542] Levinas, E. 1947. *Time and The Other*, Duquesne University Press, Pittsburg, PA, English Translation by Richard A, Cohen, 1987, p. 36. In the words by Dimitrova: "However, the awareness of my transience, which I can see in the eyes of the Other, dispels the illusion that I am an infinite and imperishable being or an eternal origin; [...] There is a future which does not belong to me, in which other people will be living without me [...]" Ref. Dimitrova, M. 2011. *In response to Jeffrey Andrew Barash: The immemorial time*. In: Dimitrova, M. 2011. In Levinas' Trace, Newcastle upon Tyne, UK: Cambridge Scholars Publishing, p. 46.

ic sense of projection and possibility which determine man's place and role in the world, in the historical moment. It is historicity (or, "futurity" in the sense of direction toward the future) rather than a sequence or linear unfolding of the three moments of past, present and future. The existence as possibility (or sum of possibilities, towardness, direction toward the future) in Heidegger is the true meaning of Being, thus stressing the importance of this Being from the historical (active) perspective. Levinas instead argued that there is something far beyond ourselves as Being and our *proprio*ception in terms of the "mine" (my world, my story, which becomes history, etc.) when we analyze time. This is the (transcendental, personal, even mysterious) encounter with the Other versus the Heideggerian version of this encounter, in which Dasein is able to meet other beings only on the basis of its own (self) perception and (self) understanding. In Levinas the core is the Other, in Heidegger is the objectivation of "this" other. Given these premises, we might ask ourselves what is the meaning of the subject in terms of knowledge or possibility for knowledge, in terms of awareness, perception. Levinas writes:

> "The living per se, then, is not without consciousness, but has a consciousness without problems, that is, without exteriority, an interior world whose center it occupies, a consciousness not concerned with situating itself in relation to an exteriority, which does not comprehend itself as part of a whole (for it precedes all comprehension), consciousness without consciousness to which the term unconscious (which hides no fewer contradictions) or instinct corresponds. The interiority that, to thinking being, is opposed to exteriority, plays itself out in the living being as an absence of exteriority. The identity of a living being is essentially the Same, the Same determining every Other, without the Other even determining the Same. If the Other did determine it – if exteriority collided with that lives – it would kill instinctive being. The living being lives beneath the sign of liberty or death."[543]

The spiritual dimension of time is clearly identified in the relation (which is dichotomy) between interiority and exteriority, and between freedom of life (liberty) and death. In this sense we also understand how "fear of death is the fear of violence of the other exercised on the Ego—fear of the absolutely unpredictable,"[544] as well as the spiritual crisis in modern, especially Western (American) society:

---

[543]   Levinas, E. 1998 ed. *Entre Nous: Thinking of the Other*. Translation by Simith, Michael B., and Reynolds, Martha, New York, NY: Columbia University Press, *The I and Totality*, p. 12.

[544]   Dimitrova, M. 2008. *Emmanuel Levinas: Time and Responsibility*, Sofia Philosophical Review, Vol. II, n. 1, p. 16.

"Our popular culture celebrates the material and largely ignores the spiritual. Greed is the order of the day in a society preoccupied at all levels with the pursuit of bottom lines, a society which celebrates consumption, careerism and winning [...] We have become a numbers-oriented culture that puts more faith in what we can see, touch, and hear, and is suspicious of the unquantifiable, the intuitive, and the mysterious."[545]

The problem of a "number-oriented culture is especially true in the realization that "what life is all about for most Americans is "looking out for number one."[546] What is missing here is the Other, as essential different from myself, and yet not a number, but a deeper connection to me, on a much higher level. In fact, understanding this problem is facing the human personal and political problem (including ethical debates on value and worth of life in medical, theological and social audiences) of this century, in a day and age post-world war II, post-Cold War, postmodernist, post-communist, but certainly not post-capitalist: "Eastern Europeans have been easily seduced by Western consumerism. [...] Isn't it interesting that the current debate over abortion pits "Freedom of Choice" against "Rights to Life"? This makes abortion sound like a consumer issue. Life becomes a right to be had; abortion becomes another lifestyle choice."[547] Certainly, the core of our discussion on the understanding and the value of the Other, whether other-than-myself in general, "neighbor" in the theological, especially Christian conception of the term, or patient in Medical Philosophy, rests on the belief, for some on the awareness on a spiritual dimension, a spiritual link with the divine sphere, which can be attained through a conceptual and yet para-rational (which, let us repeat that, it is absolutely not antirational) "jump", as the famous quote by Heisenberg states: "The first gulp from the glass of natural sciences will turn you into an atheist, but at the bottom of the glass God is waiting for you.[548]"

Over a half century ago, while I was still a child, I recall hearing a number of old people offer the following explanation for the great disasters that had befallen Russia: "Men have forgotten God; that's why all this has happened." Since then I have spent well-nigh 50 years working on the history of our revolution. [...] But if I were asked today to formulate as con-

[545]   Norman Lear, as quoted in: Naylor, T.H, Willimon, W.H., and Naylor, M.R. 1994. *The Search for Meaning*. Nashville, TN: Abingdon Press, p. 72.
[546]   Naylor, T.H, Willimon, W.H., and Naylor, M.R. 1994. *The Search for Meaning*. Nashville, TN: Abingdon Press, p. 72.
[547]   Naylor, T.H, Willimon, W.H., and Naylor, M.R. 1994. *The Search for Meaning*. Nashville, TN: Abingdon Press, pp. 76–77
[548]   "Der erste Trunk aus dem Becher der Naturwissenschaft macht atheistisch, aber auf dem Grund des Bechers wartet Gott." As quoted in Thürkauf, M. *1987. Endzeit des Marxismus. Mit einem Nachwort von Anatolij Korjagin*. Stein am Rhein, D: Christiana-Verlag.

cisely as possible the main cause of the ruinous revolution that swallowed up some 60 million of our people, I could not put it more accurately than to repeat: "Men have forgotten God; that's why all this has happened."[549]

In Levinas, the focus is on the divine dimension of the Other, which calls us to (personal) responsibility (toward, in a movement outside ourselves, an e-motion) and service to him who is calling us. This is the dimension of God, who does not act directly, but through the face of the Other. It is the command for exteriority, the "very search for justice, without which justice is impossible [...], inspired by charity."[550] This command-commitment, and its relation with the transcendental sphere (certainly not in terms of transcendent superiority, as disconnected from the human sphere) is further examined by Dimitrova:

> "As it is known, Descartes says that God has implanted in us a spark of Reason and no matter how much we try to step on and extinguish it, that is impossible. The human mind, according to Descartes, contains something divine where the first seeds of thought have been sown, and even when we prevent them from being developed and distort them, nevertheless, they bear fruits, which ripen by themselves. In a similar way, Levinas thinks about a "sociality" whereby human reason is manifested first of all. For Levinas something divine is contained in the relation of the One to the Other, which cannot be destroyed and stamped upon. God has created us in such a way that no matter how we pretend to be deaf and blind to the other, the Other is present, although as the one ignored, unnoticed, and neglected. The Other is present even in its absence."[551]

Dimitrova explores the depth of this relationship, and in particular the complex dynamism between the *incontro—scontro* with the otherness in and of the Other:

> "From that moment on, the intrigue with the otherness of the Other, which is love to the fellow human beings—love with no union, with no voluptuousness, with no flirt and self-interest, degenerates into a plot, a calculation of interests, a struggle for recognition and more power, on into war or peace, which is only a temporary cease fire until the next battle. However, the question stands not about this compromised peace, achieved at the battlefield

---

[549]   Ericson, E.E. Jr.; Mahoney, D.J. (eds.) 2009. *The Solzhenitsyn Reader: New and Essential Writings, 1947–2005*. Wilmington, DE: ISI Books. Of note, in the translation "men" indicates "human beings" as in the Russian люди.

[550]   Dimitrova, M. 2011. *In response to Ernst Wolff: There is Justice and Justice*. In: Dimitrova, M. 2011. In Levinas' Trace, Newcastle upon Tyne, UK: Cambridge Scholars Publishing, p. 89.

[551]   Dimitrova, M. 2008. *Emmanuel Levinas: Time and Responsibility*, Sofia Philosophical Review, Vol. II, n. 1, p. 24.

as a result of temporary agreements and hostilities, but about Messianic peace, which is a saving and supra-historical one."[552]

This dynamic relationship, this mystery behind the connection between me (the Ego) and the Other, acts through, lies in, even is defined *as* time and history, more specifically a deeper connection beyond the natural process of cause and effect. The logical sequence here (logical in the higher sense of λόγος which again is both the link and the action of saying λέγω) is the word. From the Hegelian *die Zeit is der Begriff selbst* we have to understand the meaning, which becomes purpose, of the Heideggerian Being-in-the-world through Levinas' Other: not a simple survival, not mere existence, and not even coexistence, but full commitment.

c) Near Death Experience and a Mindful Awareness

What are the implications and the outcomes, both from a clinical as well as more philosophical perspective, of the application of mindfulness to Cognitive Behavioral Therapy (CBT)? In the study by Dr. Daniel J. Moran,[553] the relationship between CBT and Mindfulness is closely linked to the very history of this type of therapeutic practice; in particular, we are investigating and asking ourselves whether we, as human beings, can learn how to *change* our thought patterns. One of the methodological elements analyzed in this context is the ability of meditation to influence language, and control/check for mirroring images, effects, structures as formulated in what we define, often misleadingly,[554] as 'internal stimuli'. Thus, we can check the patient's behavior at baseline and then apply statistical and epidemiological methods of interpretation of the data. For instance, Moran suggests we count the frequency of a determined-specific element.[555] We can measure the rate and then try to change it by applying this combination of CBT and mindfulness. As general example we could focus on latency in behavior, perseverance and duration of a certain behavior or behavioral pattern. Hans Jürgen Eysenck defined behavior therapy as "the attempt to alter human behavior and emotion in a beneficial manner ac-

---

[552]   Ibid., p. 27.

[553]   Moran, D.J. 2013. *Cognitive Behavioral Therapy & Mindfulness – An Integrative Evidence-Based Approach*, CMI Education Institute, Eau Claire, Wisconsin. Note: lecture presented in Burlington, Vermont, 2013.

[554]   To the extent in which we all can respond to internal stimuli in the shape and conceptual meaning of non-more specifically and exclusively defined 'thoughts'.

[555]   Moran, D.J., *Cognitive Behavioral Therapy & Mindfulness – An Integrative Evidence-Based Approach*, CMI Education Institute, Eau Claire, Wisconsin, 2013, s. 3–4.

cording to the laws of modern learning theory."[556] The mutual correspondence, in terms of conceptual relation as well as therapeutic practice, between the terms behavior and emotion is the main element of the application of meditation in the clinical setting following this theory. More specifically, we can give a first definition of mindfulness as "paying attention in a particular way; on purpose, in the present moment, and nonjudgmentally."[557] We cannot proceed with our analysis if we don't take into account the implication of the concept of 'mind'. Etymologically speaking, the term is related to similar terms in Latin (*mens*) and Greek (*μένος*, which also includes concepts such as desire, courage and even anger). At the same time, the proto-Indo-European root **mén-* is also related to the Sanskrit term *manas*.[558] This word has a wider range of possible translations and interpretations, one in particular is of interest in the specific frame of this analysis. In this conceptual meaning, the word translates a concept closely related to the physiological activity of breathing,[559] as well as the more philosophical interpretation of a "living soul which escapes from the body at death."[560] At the same time, the term is linked, also in its English version, to the concept of 'memory'.[561] Beyond the distinction between short-term and long-term memory, we could look at the concept as the process in which a specific (single or combined) information is encoded, stored, and retrieved, similarly to what happens in modern English with the expressions 'call to mind', 'come to mind', '(to) have mind of' and 'keep in mind'. Thus, focusing on meditation in a therapeutic setting is to work[562] on mnemic/mnemonic con-

---

[556]   Eysenck, H. J., cit. in Moran, D.J. 2013. *Cognitive Behavioral Therapy & Mindfulness – An Integrative Evidence-Based Approach*, CMI Education Institute, Eau Claire, Wisconsin, s. 2.

[557]   Moran, D.J. 2013. *Cognitive Behavioral Therapy & Mindfulness – An Integrative Evidence-Based Approach*, CMI Education Institute, Eau Claire, Wisconsin, s. 4.

[558]   A term that generally includes intellect, intelligence, perception, sense-conscience, understanding, as well as a more figurative – conceptual interpretations such as the (power of the) will, the spirit or spiritual principle, etc.

[559]   Similarly to what happens in the German verb *Atmen*.

[560]   Thus opening up more defined considerations on the specific historical aspects of the psychological and psychiatric practice, especially the related term *ψυχή*.

[561]   From the Proto-Germanic *gamundiz-* through Old English *gemynd* (Subs. Part. Perf.) and Old Norse (Nominative) *munr* (both terms closely related to the Germanic *Huginn* and *Muninn*). In particular, the verb 'to remember' as combined or opposed to 'to think' is an interesting consideration, once we compare Germanic linguistics with Latin and Neolatin languages, especially in their Italo-Romance branches. For instance, *ri-membr-are* versus *ri-cord-are*.

[562]   First of all by being aware and raise awareness in the subject, moving through isolative and (omni)comprehensive features, attitudes and (conscious and subconscious) thought processes.

struction and associative process while (for instance) being aware of the creative (codifying, code-producing and hierarchizing) process of the *central executive system*.[563] Furthermore, whenever we want to focus on these models and applications of 'mind' in the clinical practice, especially if we are to focus on cognitive aspects, we need to remember the historical (psychological and philosophical) legacy of this type of therapy. From the perspective of mind, it is impossible not to mention Stoicism and Hedonism in the ancient philosophical tradition, and Descartes, Kant, Hegel and Heidegger in more recent times.[564] The very thought that man is disturbed not by things (internal and external environment) but by the view he takes of them is to be found in Epictetus, while consideration on the term of *phronesis* of Aristotelian legacy is well applied within the debate on the very purpose of the 'genuine life of pleasure' according to Epicurus, thus being a life of prudence, honor, and justice.[565] A stoic perspective on this theme can be drawn from the thoughts of Marcus Aurelius on the transformative nature of the universe, which in turn leads to acknowledging life as a (conceptual) product of our thoughts.[566] In this relativistic (in terms of applicability of thoughts to a behavioral-ethic standpoint) structure, we see the work by Albert Ellis and the legacy of the *Rational Emotive Behavior Therapy* (REBT), defined by the author as "a comprehensive, active-directive, philosophically and empirically based psychotherapy which focuses on resolving emotional and behavioral problems and disturbances and enabling people to lead happier and more fulfilling lives."[567] In comparison to Ellis' Model, Beck's Cognitive Therapy is "based on the cognitive model, which is, simply that the way we perceive situations influences how we feel

---

[563] As a mere example of the short-term memory analysis according to the working model by Alan Baddeley and Graham Hitch.

[564] The very debate on *die Philosophie des Geistes* and the very translation of *Geist* as 'mind' or 'spirit' (versus 'ghost') is fundamental in this debate, and further readings are necessary to further expand considerations, which are not possible here due to the size and scope of this essay. We suggest in particular, the analysis by Marco Filoni, Alexandre Kojève, and Donald Philipp Verene for Hegel and Rüdiger Safranski, David West, and Mark Wrathall for Heidegger.

[565] As stated in the 40 *Sovran Maxims*, as quoted here in: Moran, D.J. 2013. *Cognitive Behavioral Therapy & Mindfulness – An Integrative Evidence-Based Approach*, Eau Claire, WI: CMI Education Institute, s.11.

[566] "Everything that happens as it should, and if you observe carefully, you will find this to be so", from Τὰ εἰς ἑαυτόν, as quoted in Ibid., ss. 15–16. The author also quotes Shakespeare: "There is nothing either good or bad but thinking makes it so." From *Hamlet*, Act 2, Scene 2, cit. in Ibid., s. 15.

[567] Ellis, A., *Reason and Emotion in Psychotherapy: Comprehensive Method of Treating Human Disturbances: Revised and Updated*, New York, NY: Citadel Press, 1994.

emotionally."[568] In order to better understand the concept we need to focus on the concept of perception and on the three levels of cognition, in Beck's model: Schema, Maladaptive Assumptions, and Automatic Thoughts. Perception involves the (conceptually *active*) *action* of the identific*ation*, interpret*ation* and organiz*ation* of sensory information, by involving signals in the nervous system. Therefore, perception helps represent and understand the environment. What is the result of the perception, from the perspective of imagination and creative process, as well as from the relativistic consideration of individuality and originality of thought? We could focus on a specific trauma (or perception of it) in our analysis, perhaps the very quest for meaning and purpose in relation to the end of the world, or afterlife. In dealing with the concept of an imminent, postmodern image and imaginative process of Apocalypse, also intended as an end of the world as previously known, Martin Jay and Agnes Heller address a reality beyond good and evil. This very apocalyptic imagination can also be understood through the lenses of psychoanalysis, which provides, according to Jay, a better insight, especially in comparison to a mere cultural analysis. At the same time, quoting figures such as Bois, Conrad, Kermode, Lawrence and Yeats, he adds that "what makes the postmodern version [of the apocalyptic myth related to the debate] somewhat different is its suppression of one of the traditional faces of the janiform visage of apocalypse."[569] How can we as human beings, patients and health care providers, contribute in a positive way to the debate on (this type of) perception? How can we relate to our thoughts, positive or negative, understand them and our position and role towards them? Are there certain stages, perhaps certain *truths* (*a priori*, in comparison to the empirical evidence-based features of the *a posteriori* methodology) accessible directly to the mind, this time also intended as (individual) soul, perhaps related to a (universal) spirit? Trying to answer this last question is certainly beyond the capacity (in terms of scope, focus and ability within certain limits of space) of our analysis, but we need to understand how the possible response might influence our relation with the patient and with ourselves, from a therapeutic standpoint. In regard to this topic, I would like to focus here on what have been called 'Near Death Experiences' (NDE), phenomena "of considerable importance to medicine, neuroscience, neurology,

---

[568]   Beck, J. S., *Cognitive therapy: Basics and beyond*, quoted in Moran, D.J. 2013. *Cognitive Behavioral Therapy & Mindfulness – An Integrative Evidence-Based Approach*, Eau Claire, WI: CMI Education Institute, ss. 19–24.

[569]   Robinson, Gillian, Rundell, John; eds. 1994. *Rethinking Imagination. Culture and Creativity*, London, UK: Routledge, p. 33

psychiatry, philosophy and religion."[570] An interesting study which considers the philosophical and medical implication of a specific *attitude* toward NDEs has been conducted by Karl L. R. Jansen,[571] who describes the effects of ketamine on brain receptors, resulting in modifications of the state of consciousness:

> "Near-death experiences (NDE's) can be reproduced by ketamine via blockade of receptors in the brain (the N-methyl-D-aspartate, NMDA receptors) for the neurotransmitter glutamate. Conditions which precipitate NDE's (hypoxia, ischaemia, hypoglycaemia, temporal lobe epilepsy etc.) have been shown to release a flood of glutamate, overactivating NMDA receptors resulting in neuro ('excito') toxicity. Ketamine prevents this neurotoxicity. There are substances in the brain which bind to the same receptor site as ketamine. Conditions which trigger a glutamate flood may also trigger a flood of neuroprotective agents which bind to NMDA receptors to protect cells, leading to an altered state of consciousness like that produced by ketamine."[572]

Beyond the definition of NDE, we are forced to reconsider the way we define our perception in terms of self and (its/our) relationship with the mind and the related (produced? producing?) 'states of mind' which we are focusing on in terms of the combination of Cognitive Behavioral Therapy and Mindfulness. Every term we use in our therapy session is thus fundamental in order to better relate to the above mentioned consideration, from the concept of thought, to affection, desire, excogitation, imagination, inclination, intention, invention, mood, reflection, opinion, soul, spirit, and temper. If we postulate a standard baseline level of perception and relative thought process, what are the possible cognitive distortions? According to the model of Beck, we can have Arbitrary Inference, Overgeneralization, Minimization or Maximization, Selective Abstraction, Dichotomous Thinking, and Personalization.[573] Thus, in a therapy

[570]   Greyson, B. and Stevenson, I. 1980. *The phenomenology of near-death experiences.*, American Journal of Psychiatry, 1980, 137, 1193–1200; Ring, K. 1980. *Life at death: a scientific investigation of the near death experience*, New York, NY: Coward, McCann, Goeghegan; Sabom, M. B. 1992. *Recollections of death: a medical investigation*, New York, NY: Harper and Row; Jansen, K.L.R. 1991, *Transcendental explanations and the near-death experience.* Lancet, 337, 207–243.

[571]   Jansen, K.L.R. 1998. *The Ketamine Model of the Near Death Experience: A Central Role for the NMDA Receptor*, Journal Article, The Maudsley Hospital, Denmark Hill, London [direct web link: http://www.mindspring.com/~scottr/nde/jansen1.html]. For a more detailed analysis, see Jansen, K.L.R, 2000. *Ketamine: Dreams and Realities*, Sarasota, Fl: MAPS.

[572]   Jansen, K.L.R. 1998. *The Ketamine Model of the Near Death Experience: A Central Role for the NMDA Receptor*, Journal Article, The Maudsley Hospital, Denmark Hill, London.

[573]   Beck, J. S., *Cognitive therapy: Basics and beyond*, quoted in Moran, D.J., 2013.*Cognitive Behavioral Therapy & Mindfulness – An Integrative Evidence-Based Approach*, CMI Education Institute, Eau Claire, Wisconsin, ss. 25–27

session is fundamental to share the model with the patient, and explain our willingness to offer alternative ways of thinking. In this sense, REBT model agrees with the cognitive model, but focuses on other (types of) cognition(-s) as well. In particular, and in relation to what we examined on the topic of meaning of life, apocalypse and NDE, we are focusing also on (moral, religious, social, cultural, personal) expectations, as well as philosophy and ethics. We need to incorporate these elements in our basic understanding, not only of the medical/mental conditions of the patient, but of the patient himself. In particular, the Cognitive Model according to Ellis includes: Activating Event, Belief (Irrational / Rational), Consequence, Disputation (in which our philosophical and therapeutic-psychological effort plays a major role), and finally Effective Emotion/Action.[574] As direct outcome, we can see how a change in beliefs, from irrational to rational, is followed by an emotional change: "What is considered central to emotional disturbance are the *evaluative beliefs*, which in RET parlance are known as the core irrational Beliefs."[575] That is actually the very goal of REBT, which aims for "transforming suffering into appropriate, adaptive, albeit negative emotions."[576] To go back to our example, it is difficult to justify, from a scientific, empirical and evidence-based perspective, the claim according to which NDEs *must* have a *single* explanation, or that "a scientific theory must explain all of the experiences ever given the name of NDE.[577] The same could be said for a variety of mental and emotional phenomena, which could have multiple causes and variable expressions.[578] In regard to this concept, Dr. Jansen states that "The glutamate hypothesis of the NDE is not intended to apply to every NDE"[579] and proposes a multi-leveled interpretation of the data. This viewpoint is fundamental for our analysis of the relation and application of CBT and Mindfulness.

The very concept of mindfulness forces us to reconsider our attitude toward the term 'mind', and whether or system of beliefs draws elements from a reli-

---

[574]   In short, defined by the sequence A-B-C , or Activating Event, Belief, Consequence. Consequence in particular can be emotional/affective on baseline, disturbed/dysfunctional with Irrational Belief and appropriate/functional with Rational Belief.

[575]   Walen, Di Giuseppe, Dryden, 1992, cit. in Moran, D.J., *Cognitive Behavioral Therapy & Mindfulness – An Integrative Evidence-Based Approach*, CMI Education Institute, Eau Claire, Wisconsin, 2013, s. 39.

[576]   Ibid., s. 39.

[577]   Gabbard, G. O. and Twemlow, S. T. 1989. *Comments on 'A neurobiological model or near-death experiences'*, Journal of Near-Death Studies, 7, 261–26.

[578]   Jansen, K.L.R. 1998. *The Ketamine Model of the Near Death Experience: A Central Role for the NMDA Receptor*, Journal Article, The Maudsley Hospital, Denmark Hill, London .

[579]   Ibid.

gious, spiritual, agnostic or atheistic perspective, ultimately we are working with a specific (single, singular, particular) individual (but the same applies to group therapies as well), a human being, a patient with a specific life story (and history), system of belief, mental/medical condition etc., and we need to consider these elements in our practice, from initial assessment to therapy. Claiming that 'alternate states' do exist, does not prove the existence of (an) afterlife; a quest far beyond the scope of this analysis. At the same time, scientific research has demonstrated that chemical components (pharmacological interventions and drugs), psychological practices as well as meditation may render certain 'states' more accessible. We need to be careful not to mix or invert cause and effect, and starting a debate on what we mean by 'states', whether they are product of the mind (in this sense, mind as brain) and whether *we* are taking part in this production (again, whether the equation mind=brain=*I, myself* still holds its validity). Saying that pharmacological, psychological or meditative interventions and practices help reach a certain state *does not mean* that these practices *create* this state.[580] From this example we can see why paying special attention to mindfulness and system of belief is so important in the therapy with the patient, especially from the viewpoint of CBT and REBT. The core process is this (psychological and philosophical) cognitive, behavioral, imaginative *disputing*, "a debate or challenge to the patient's irrational belief system and can be of a *cognitive, imaginal*, and/or *behavioral* nature."[581] Furthermore, the very style of this disputation can vary from didactic, to Socratic (as in the *Socratic* or *Maieutic* method), metaphorical or humorous. A cognitive disputation presents the following elements, according to Moran:[582]

Logical Disputation: "Is that true?"

Reality Testing Disputation: "Where is the evidence?"

"Can you stand it?" "Haven't you stood it already?"

Pragmatic Disputation: "When you think that way, how does it feel?"

"Where does thinking this get you?"

580 See for instance the work by John C. Lily and Stanislav Groff.
581 Walen, Di Giuseppe, Dryden 1992, cit. in Moran, D.J. 2013. *Cognitive Behavioral Therapy & Mindfulness – An Integrative Evidence-Based Approach*, CMI Education Institute, Eau Claire, Wisconsin, s. 44.
582 Moran, D.J., *Cognitive Behavioral Therapy & Mindfulness – An Integrative Evidence-Based Approach*, CMI Education Institute, Eau Claire, Wisconsin, 2013, ss. 46–47.

Rational Alternative: Offer substitute thoughts that help

Unconditional Self-acceptance (USA)

Unconditional Others acceptance (UOA)

Moving on to Imaginal Disputation, we see how this practice encourages relaxation; helps examine the problematic situation in an imaginative and vivid way; encourages changing the feeling attached to the issue and examine "how it was done"; encourages further use of that solution. In a Behavioral Dispute instead, a rational role playing, in-vivo exposure, 'shame' attacks and 'anger barbs' are all part of the practice. Moran also suggest we combine the terms 'disputing' and 'defusing' to create a third, hybrid term: *Disfusing*.[583] This concept identifies the attempt to uproot the word from its meaning, thus changing the form/function of language and the belief in a particular, word, statement, thought. One of the best methods to achieve this goal is, according to Moran, practicing Mindfulness. With Mindfulness we focus on the *hic et nunc* of a situation (and of no situation at all), we also pay "attention in a particular way; on purpose, in the present moment, and nonjudgmentally."[584] Moran gives another, more extended definition of Mindfulness, as a: "Purposeful, present focused committed responses, maximally influenced by relevant stimulus events, and unimpeded by self-judgment, other judgment, or private events."[585] Now, the question of the very personalization of judgment in terms of self-perception and perception of (the) other(-ness) is at the center of the most recent research in the fields of cognitive science, neuroscience, neurophilosophy and philosophy of mind, which in turn has further developed into several categories, including eliminative materialism and reductionism. The work by Paul and Patricia Churchland is well known in this regard, especially in the focus on the possible ethical and moral application of the above disputed equation *mind=brain*: "My brain and I are inseparable. I am who I am because my brain is what it is."[586] In regard to the philosophical method and the ability of our mind to discover truth, particularly pertaining the very analysis of our own

---

[583] A neologism-creative process similar to the work by Derrida on the concept of *Différance*.

[584] Kabat-Zinn, J., cit. in: Moran, D.J. 2013. *Cognitive Behavioral Therapy & Mindfulness – An Integrative Evidence-Based Approach*, CMI Education Institute, Eau Claire, Wisconsin, s. 59.

[585] Moran, D.J. 2013. *Cognitive Behavioral Therapy & Mindfulness – An Integrative Evidence-Based Approach*, CMI Education Institute, Eau Claire, Wisconsin, s. 60.

[586] Churchland, P. S. 2013. *Touching a nerve. The self as brain*, W.W. Norton & Company, New York, NY, p. 11.

mind, Churchland suggests we would "do best to resign ourselves to the probability that there is no special faculty whose exercise yields the Absolute, Error-Free, Beyond-Science Truths of the Universe."[587] The assumption that localization and functional specialization of certain mental phenomena, for instance through fMRI observation, is according to some one of the proofs and verified/verifiable examples needed to defend the reductionist position for which there is absolute no need for specific spiritual, metaphysical or religious basis to define, explain or justify those phenomena. From the perspective of eliminative materialism, the so-called 'folk-psychology' should also be subjected to this *treatment*. On the other side of the spectrum, the criticism to this position bases its observation on multiple elements, such as the presence of *qualia* in relation to a specific or a group of mental states,[588] the controversy on intuition, introspection, appearance versus essence and perception,[589] and epistemological self-refutation. Again, the core problem is our epistemological understanding of what (medical) science is, produces, is applied to, and ought to be, especially in the realm of psychiatry and psychology:

> "Harman notes, "There was, many felt, something unnatural about a science that denied consciousness as a causal reality when everyday experience seemed to confirm again that any decision to act causes action". According to the dualism between mind and body, not only is this not possible but in a dualistic science, it's not possible to study it. Harman does point out that there have been attempts to bring in self-reports of subjective experience as primary data (e.g., introspection, phenomenalized approaches, and Gestalt psychology), and they have tended to be considered failures."[590]

The above discussed perspectives, though not representing a *condition sine qua non* for the applicability of disciplines such as mindfulness and meditation to Cognitive Behavioral therapy, are fundamental in our attempt to understand the patient and his internal and external environment, first of all in the focus of the therapy itself and by extension throughout the therapeutic relation with the mental health professional. Thus, we can look at the variety of interventions incorporating mindfulness training under a different light. Among these inter-

---

587   Churchland, P. S. 2002. *Brain-Wise: Studies in Neurophilosophy*, Cambridge, MA: MIT Press, p. 41.

588   Though we should again agree on what can be defined as a mental 'state'.

589   Let us focus at the dichotomies in etymological-conceptual terms of *Scio –Scheinen / Shine / Show* and *Monere/Monstrum – Monster -Mirror, Speculum – Spectrum* etc.

590   Harman, W. 1987. *The Postmodern Heresy*. Conference Paper: *Toward a Post-modern World*, January 16–20, 1987, Santa Barbara, CA, USA, pp. 119, 123 as quoted and commented in: Schaef, A.W. 1992. *Beyond Therapy, Beyond Science*. New York, NY: HarperCollins, pp. 223–224.

ventions, according to Moran,[591] we find Mindfulness-based Stress Reduction, Mindfulness-based Cognitive Therapy, Dialectical Behavioral Therapy, Acceptance and Commitment Therapy, Cognitive Behavioral Therapy, Gestalt Therapy, and Relapse Prevention. In 1979 Jon Kabat-Zinn presented the *Eight-week Mindfulness-based Stress Reduction (MSBR) course*, in the words by Moran a "Vehicle for the integration of Eastern meditative dharma practices and the Western paradigm of behavioral intervention, [...] clinically proven effective for depression and anxiety disorders."[592] The focus on MCBT went from an attempt to change the patients' degree of belief in attitudes and thoughts to change the modalities in which patients relate to content, thus focusing more on the process. In practice, the combination of CBT and mindfulness helps broaden the perspective on thoughts and thought processes, also using repetitive function to foster a decentered relationship to mental contents. At the base of the need of combining these two therapeutic methodologies is the focus on helping the patient disengage (or *decenter*) from negative thought patterns, as well as the need to notice stressors and triggers earlier. More specifically, the Eight Sessions of MCBT include automatic pilot, dealing with barriers, mindfulness of the breath[593] and full body relaxation, staying present, allowing and letting be (also, 'go of'/'off'), awareness of the disparity thoughts vs. facts, learning how to take better care of oneself, and practical application of what has been learned. Research has shown that a Mindfulness-based Cognitive Therapy reduces rates of relapse by 50% among patients who suffer from recurrent depression,[594] and was found useful, despite "methodological weakness,"[595] in the treatment of pain, stress, anxiety, depressive relapse, eating disorders, and addiction,[596] with a reduction in depressive symptoms and suicidal ideation in Bipolar Disorder.[597] How could we better define Mindful-

---

[592]   Moran, D.J., *Cognitive Behavioral Therapy & Mindfulness – An Integrative Evidence-Based Approach*, CMI Education Institute, Eau Claire, Wisconsin, 2013, s. 68.

[593]   Again, a reference to Buddhist meditative disciplines (*sati* or 'mindfulness') as related to the Sanskrit *smrti* (to remember).

[594]   Teasdale J. D., Williams, G. M. G., Soulsby, J. M., Segal, Z. V., Ridgeway, V. A., Lau, M. A., *Prevention of Relapse/Recurrence in Major Depression by Mindfulness-Based Cognitive Therapy*, Journal of Consulting and Clinical Psychology , Vol. 68, No. 4, 615–623, American Psychological Association, 2000 [direct link: http://www-psych.stanford.e du/~pgoldin/Buddhism/MBCTrelapsedepressionTeasdale2000JCCP.pdf].

[595]   Moran, D.J., *Cognitive Behavioral Therapy & Mindfulness – An Integrative Evidence-Based Approach*, CMI Education Institute, Eau Claire, Wisconsin, 2013, s. 76.

[596]   Ibid.

[597]   Miklowitz, D. J., Alatiq Y., Goodwin, G. M., Geddes J. R., Fennel, M. J. V., Dimidjian, S., Hauser, M., Williams, J. M. G., *A Pilot Study of Mindfulness-Based Cognitive Therapy for*

ness-based Cognitive Therapy? We partially identified methods and structures, especially the patient's recognition of negative, self-devaluative and hopeless thinking, but how could be better define cognition, in this context? The term is closely linked to the English verb 'to know' through its Latin equivalent *cognoscere*, from the Greek γνώσκω, similarly to the translation 'knowledge' for γνώσις. Thus, cognition and knowledge are two parts of the same concept, with the first term focusing more on mental processes, human skills and abilities linked to the mind, including attention and memory, awareness, reasoning and problem solving, learning, comprehending and producing (language in particular), as well as decision making and further applied to planning, imagining, ordering, etc. According to Denise Dellarosa Cummings:

> "Cognition is a biological function, not a cultural invention. Our nervous systems detect, encode, and process information, not because someone invented these capacities in antiquity, but because evolutionary forces shaped the organs that instantiate these biological functions. Cognition is the function that ensures a nonarbitrary relation between perception and action. Historically, psychologists have tended to overlook or downplay the role of biology and evolution when developing theories of cognitive functions, with the inevitable result that our theories have often provided inadequate predictions and explanations of cognitive phenomena, from basic inductive processes to higher cognition."[598]

It is evident how the physical-physiological component of this biological-evolutionary base for the above definition represents a fundamental statement in regard to the structure and the possible application of cognition, in particular the sentence "Cognition is the function that ensures a nonarbitrary relation between perception and action." These biological bases are, in a figurative way, the theater of our therapeutic action (perhaps the term 'play' is not totally inappropriate in this sense);[599] a space in which these physical *nonarbitrary* elements can be subject of our analysis, cross- and self-analysis and attempt to modify, from the perspective of neuroplasticity the links between thought process, their perception and behavioral outcome.[600] Furthermore, considering the

Bipolar Disorder, International Journal of Cognitive Therapy: Vol. 2, Special Section: Cognition in Bipolar Disorders, 2009, pp. 373–382.

[598] Cummins, D. D., *The Evolution of Reasoning*, in: Sternberg, R. J. and Leighton, J. P. ed., *The Nature of Reasoning*, Cambridge University Press, Cambridge, UK, 2004 pp. 339.

[599] Especially in relation to the Old English *plēon*, which could be translated as 'to risk', 'endanger' corresponding, in a morphed/translated (opposite) conceptual structure to the German *pflegen*.

[600] See also Davidson, R. J., and Lutz, A. 2008. *Buddha's Brain: Neuroplasticity and Meditation*, US National Library of Medicine, National Institutes of Health, IEEE Signal Process Mag. 2008 January 1; 25(1): 176–174.

specific features of the patient's personal (life- *as a whole*) experience,[601] in order to compare and verify the possibility of therapeutic generalization of treatment on empirically based principles is the core of another therapeutic method, developed by Steven C. Hayes, Kelly G. Wilson, and Kirk Strosahl under the name 'Acceptance and Commitment Therapy' (ACT). This therapy uses the previously discussed mindfulness-based approach (within *functional contextualism*) with behavior change strategies (including applied behavior analysis and traditional behavior therapy strategies) built on evidence-based[602] studies, and with the aim to increase psychological flexibility. With the latter, we express "[...] contacting the present moment fully, [...] as conscious, historical human being, [...] and based on what the situation affords, [...] changing or persisting in behavior [...] in the service of chosen values."[603] The focus on 'chosen values' is again a fundamental component of this type of therapy, which includes all the biological, behavioral, emotional, rational and cognitive components with a specific aim (similarly to what we said in regard to REBT) to work on the interrelation and interconnectedness between therapist and patient and within the core processes of the ACT model: Acceptance, Contact with the present moment, Values, Committed action, Self as context, and Defusion. In synthesis, the combination of mindfulness-based CBT (as expressed in the examples offered above and in the work by John D. Teasdale on MBCT, designed to aid in preventing the relapse of depression, specifically in individuals with MDD) and the therapeutic relation between patient and therapist, as presented through the philosophical and psychological (cognitive, imaginal, behavioral, etc.) dispute, as the core of this analysis, wants to provide further explanation of the applicability and clinical effectiveness of such practices, while addressing more specific neurophilosphical issues linked to the 'states' of mind' and their perception within the clinical setting, as well as a guidance, value and direction in everyday life.

---

[601]   In particular, in the person-centered, humanistic approach of Carl Rogers.

[602]   Used to address test anxiety, mathematics anxiety, public speaking anxiety in college students, enhancing psychological health of students abroad, and eating and weight concerns. See Moran, D.J., *Cognitive Behavioral Therapy & Mindfulness – An Integrative Evidence-Based Approach*, CMI Education Institute, Eau Claire, Wisconsin, 2013, s. 82–84.

[603]   Ibid., s. 94.

Chapter 7
Translational science

7.1 Taxonomic considerations

Reaching the end of this volume, we want to address the further continuation and applicability of the research in Medical Philosophy. This is a form of translational research, in the sense that what we propose and support here, is a paradigm of scientific investigation which is by its very nature alternative to the dichotomy of basic research and applied research and integrative to the relationship between evidence-based medicine and patient-centered medicine. Translational research is usually divided between the T1 research domain, which focuses on the so-called "bench-to-bedside," and the T2 research domain, which translates the findings from the laboratory into social applicability. More specifically, T1 translates the knowledge apparatus of basic sciences into the developments of new therapeutic strategies; and T2 translates the data collected in clinical trials into clinical practice. In this sense, we argue that Medical Philosophy is a form of Translational Science, in that it helps bridge the theoretical gap between fundamental science and applied science, in particular when at the center of the scientific investigation is the human being, in his medical, mental, and philosophical complexity.

As we previously discussed, in dealing with mental illness, the psychiatric/psychological approach in conventional medicine sometimes forgets an important part, perhaps the fundamental core, of therapy, *id est* the sense of meaning and purpose in life. Medical Philosophy does not portray itself as a new branch of scientific enquiry or as a subfield of this or that therapeutic school. On the contrary, Medical Philosophy represents the core of a philosophical analysis as basis for medical/scientific practice, especially in the fields of psychiatry and psychology. Certainly, we praise and value very highly the most current research in neuroscience and neurology. To complete the picture, especially considering the complexity of human beings, we want to help medicine by making sure that the theoretical basis of our understanding of human nature is not forgotten, but continuously employed in out therapeutic efforts. But is this focus on the meaning of life baring fruits in this scientific context? In other words, is this type of knowledge attainable at all? Heintzelman and King write:

"[...] we noted the paradox that characterizes psychological approaches to meaning in life: it is portrayed simultaneously as a necessity of life and as something that is next to impossible to obtain. It simply cannot be both of these things. If meaning in life is essential to our survival "in about the same sense" as sunlight, or calcium, then it must be available to us. Otherwise, human beings would have long since been rendered extinct. If we take seriously the notion that meaning in life is a human necessity, then we must tolerate an understanding of meaning in life as a relatively common experience. Large-scale representative surveys and numerous studies of meaning in life suggest that meaning in life is widespread and relatively high."[604]

The authors present as a conclusion of cause-effect typology in addressing the *conditio-sine-qua-non* for the validity of the impossibility of simultaneous presence of necessity and unattainability of life's meaning. However, it is not sure how the authors can move from an empirical, observational, evidence-based categorization of data based on patients' response to an ontological claim of mutual exclusion of the above mentioned terms. Furthermore, the cited studies show the highest percentage of the *belief* in the meaning of life, not the meaning of life itself. In fact, the authors conclude their article by stating that "Life is pretty meaningful. If we truly need meaning in life to survive, it cannot be otherwise."[605] Certainly, there is still a very important value in such studies, but we need to be careful in avoiding confusion between belief and "real" existence. This is not to discredit the useful data gathered in this type of research; in fact this type of analysis is presented in this study as well. However, the biggest difference lies in the conceptual understanding of the questions asked, and the following interpretation of the answers collected. As with the God question, we cannot honestly claim that the scientific research, in any field, has yielded a definitive answer, whether positive or negative, yet. The approach in this study is to question our perception of the very meaning of "scientific method" and open up the discussion on possible differences in conditions determining the scientific validity of thesis, studies, examinations, observations, analysis etc. The understanding of these differences should not lead to a possible discrediting of modern Western science, on the contrary. The parallel, and analogy, between the successes of science in medical fields such as psychiatry should give us the opportunity to praise the biologically-based claims in neuroscience, and realize that the missing part for a complete, or at least closer to completeness (perhaps to completion), understanding of human nature, life, and health lies in Philosophy.

---

[604]   Heintzelman, S.J. and King L.A. 2014. *Life is pretty meaningful.* Vol. 69 N.6, p. 570.
[605]   Ibid.

Medical Philosophy thus brings together all these elements to present a much more complex, and yet accurate, picture of man. In fact, to use a term often charged with a wide range of *emotional* response, Medical Philosophy presents a *holistic* picture of man and of nature, an image of wholeness in which all the aspects of existence *and* essence are combined in a omnicomprehensive whole that focuses on the interactions between the material physical/organic/biochemical levels and the psychological/behavioral perceptual, as well as the transcendental/spiritual/religious (or non) elements of man.

This approach is finally *re*discovered, at least in part and thanks to both medical research as well as CAM disciplines, by modern, western, conventional medicine and science in general.[606] We need to open up to a more encompassing form of Science, a Translational Science, which 1) understands its limits and successes, and makes sure that, whenever the scientific method is applied in Evidence-Based practice is not compromised by pseudoscientific claims; and 2) does not close itself up to different forms of cognitive processes, possibly leading to different forms of knowledge, especially in realms (such as meaning and purpose of life) which are still not completely understood by means of Western empirical science, so that we don't risk to *throw the baby out with the bath water*. Furthermore, the search for mechanisms underlying diseases, disorders and their healing process also support a more open (and open-minded) viewpoint regarding the possible connection of human health to elements often perceived as "foreign" to classical (used here in the sense of modern Western) medicine. A good example is the connection between cognitive ability, and mental health in general, and the environment. For instance, many studies have shown that air pollution takes a toll on our well-being, due to fine particulate matter,[607] a type of pollutant. Research has shown that beside cardiovascular effects, this pollutant also affects our mental abilities in a sensitive manner.[608]

---

[606]   For further reference, see for instance Carpenter, S. 2012. *That gut feeling. With a sophisticated neural network transmitting messages from trillions of bacteria, the brain in your gut exerts a powerful influence over the one in your head, new research suggests*. Monitor on Psychology, Vol 43, No. 8, Washington, DC: American Psychological Association, pp. 50–55.

[607]   The size of which amounts about a 1/30th the width of a human hair. Those particles are found in the emission of vehicles, power plants, and factories.

[608]   "Jennifer Weuve, MPH, ScD, an assistant professor of internal medicine at Rush Medical College, found that older women who had been exposed to high levels of the pollutant experienced greater cognitive decline compared with other women their age (Archives of Internal Medicine, 2012) [...]. Shakira Franco Suglia, ScD, an assistant professor at Boston Univer-

"Modern psychology has tried hard to be a science and to be accepted among the sciences. To be accepted as a science, as modernist science is defined, a field must [...] accept that reality is only what can be proved empirically, use the methodology of mechanistic science with which to experiment and define truth, and deny or ignore any information that does not match the scientific paradigm. [...] There is no question but that psychology has seen itself, and has been seen, as the bastard child of the sciences. All the social sciences have suffered under this inferiority complex, and like all codependent hero children (a role in which psychology might easily see itself in the "family" of the sciences), it tires harder and harder to be accepted. When a person or a discipline needs acceptance, it becomes progressively rigid and rigorous in trying to do the right thing while becoming increasingly aware of its inadequacies. [...] Psychology has confused understanding and knowing. [...] We do this in the laboratory, and we do it in the therapy session. The basis for this understanding is always linear thinking and logic – no real knowing is involved. Knowing is never just logical, rational, and linear. Knowing requires much more brain functioning and interaction with experience."[609]

7.2 Applied Medical Philosophy

a) The Third Way

Medical Philosophy has certainly the features of scientific targeted applicability, in the sense that it provides the necessary links between scientist, clinicians and the general public, by investigating and promoting multidisciplinary interactions and resources and implementing the theoretical analysis of medicine as a whole. Furthermore, the translational aspects of Medical Philosophy help us identifying and reducing errors[610] in clinical judgement, medical epistemology (and "scientific" assumptions as well as assumptions of scientificity), and ther-

sity's School of Public Health, and colleagues followed more than 200 Boston children from birth to an average age of 10. They found that kids exposed to greater levels of black carbon scored worse on tests of memory and verbal and nonverbal IQ (American Journal of Epidemiology, 2008). Frederica Perera, DrPH, at the Columbia University Mailman School of Public Health, and colleagues [...] discovered that children who had been exposed to higher levels of urban air pollutants known as polycyclic aromatic hydrocarbons while in utero were more likely to experience attention problems and symptoms of anxiety and depression (Environmental Health Perspectives, 2012) [...]. A study by Portuguese researchers explored the relationship between psychological health and living in industrial areas. They found that people who lived in areas associated with greater levels of air pollution scored higher on tests of anxiety and depression (Journal of Environmental Psychology, 2011)." See Weir, K. 2012. *Smog in our brains. Researchers are identifying startling connections between air pollution and decreased cognition and well-being.* Monitor on Psychology, Vol 43, No. 7, Washington, DC.: American Psychological Association, p. 32.

[609]   Schaef, A.W. 1992. *Beyond Therapy, Beyond Science.* New York, NY: HarperCollins, pp. 214–219.

[610]   As in the definition by Reason: "an error is a failure of achieving the intended outcome in a planned sequence of mental or physical activities when that failure is not due to chance." See Reason J. 1992. *Human error.* Cambridge, UK: Cambridge University Press.

apeutic method and practice. According to Zhang, Patel, Johnson, and Shortliffe, a cognitive taxonomy of errors can "(1) categorize major types of medical errors along cognitive dimensions, (2) associate each type of medical errors to a specific underlying cognitive mechanism, (3) describe how and explain why a specific error occurs, and (4) generate intervention strategies for each type of error."[611] This cognitive perspective is especially useful in the comparison between the fundamental science and applied science perspectives on the application of medicine. At the same time, translational science in Medical Philosophy brings this analysis further, and literally throws back the question on the scientific nature in/of medicine, while providing useful resources to society and the medical community. This activity not only bridges the gaps between fundamental and applied science in medicine but opens up a third option, a *third way* which focuses on the narrative aspects of medicine. This third way is the theoretical basis of the empirical research in this study, and is included in the previously mentioned concept of Central Medicine. By opening up the investigation to the patient's own perspective on (his/her) diagnostics and therapy, we are aiming at the very core of the problem: if medicine is not just a science, but much more, we need to incorporate those scientific bases in our investigation. However, our evidence goes beyond the conventionally accepted laboratory and clinical trial evidence, because it focuses on those elements that, by their very nature appear to be opaque and unintelligible to the general (conventional, modern, Western, etc.) scientific methods. To be sure, our target is also not completely identical to the focus of EBM research and it is absolutely not intended to replace the methods and practices of modern medicine in areas such as pharmacological testing. Our target is the nature of human being within the healing process, a complex and fascinating path drawn on the relationship between the individual and the environment (provider, medical practice and research, society as a whole and the infinite list of *translated parameters* e.g. personal beliefs, culture, ethnicity, tradition, philosophy, interpretation, etc.) and vice versa:

> "[...] "The patient walks in" is a Levinasian moment. Emmanuel Levinas, the Lithuanian-French Jewish philosopher, held that before knowing, even before consciousness of being, human beings are confronted with the ethical. We are face to face with another whom we are compelled to recognize and acknowledge. We are constituted as persons, he believed, by our response to that other. It is our ethical duty and it precedes our own existence. Here is a

---

[611] Zhang, J., Patel, V.L., Johnson, T.R., and Shortliffe, E.H. 2004. *A cognitive taxonomy of medical errors*. Journal of Biomedical Informatics 37 (2004) 193–204, p. 202.

post-Heideggerian philosophy very well suited to a service profession, and it bears an ele-
mental truth for physicians. A physician becomes a physician only by taking care of patients. Medical education confers a social identity and a way of looking at the world that
lasts beyond a clinical career, but a physician without a patient is not a clinician any more
than a sick person without medical attention is a patient. Levinas captures this dyadic relationship. The patient's presentation to medical attention is just such an en face encounter. It
is the moral claim at the heart of the medical encounter. This inseparability of the moral
from the diagnostic and therapeutic in clinical medicine is the germ of the clinical imperative."[612]

*Medical Philosophy. Philosophical Analysis of Patient Self-Perception in Di-
agnostics and Therapy* is aimed at investigating all these aspects, to honor and
respect medicine in its entire and whole complexity (which is related-caused,
although not in a linear fashion such as cause-effect relation), as well as to
reframe, reshape, reconstruct its very structure on the basis of the theoretical
elements we have discussed so far, to make sure that medicine is aware of the
uncertainty and mystery (in the highest possible sense of the terms, certainly
not associated with reductivist/imprecise/superstitious impressions) which lies
within its practice, a thick layer of interpretation, emotion, technique and technology, ultimately an art which has far too often, especially in Western geographical areas and especially in the United States,[613] been subjected to institu-
tionalization and professional ritualization in ways that not only impoverish its
very nature, but present increasing difficulties associated with diagnosis and
therapy of a wide range of health disorders. In fact, this approach does not take
anything *away* from the evidence-based science, but incorporates a broader
theoretical approach (in this sense, an approach similar to the one proposed by
Bunge and Pagnini) and a narrative-interpretative-hermeneutic dimension to
diagnostics. This is medical science, this is medical philosophy: a translational
science incorporating all these elements.

b) Finding Balance

The translational approach of Medical Philosophy is particularly helpful when
discussing the best therapeutic approaches to use in specific cases, as well as to
investigate the individual response to them. As we previously discussed, there

---

[612]   Montgomery, K. 2006. *How doctors think: clinical judgment and the practice of medicine.*
New York, NY: Oxford University Press, p. 161. In regard to medical education, especially
in the United States, Montgomery adds: "[...] medical education is a moral as well as an intellectual education: experiential, behavioral, and in important ways covert [...] it is also hi-
erarchical, ritualized, and characterized by paradoxes and contradictions that foster habits of
skepticism and thoroughness." Ibid., p. 4.
[613]   Ibid.

are many aprioristic and even biased assumptions on the definition, role, structure, methods and applicability of science in (modern) medicine. These assumptions are better understood under the accurate and precise lenses of theoretical and translational investigation, which not only challenge them on the field of laboratory research, but also in their purpose and usefulness in everyday clinical practice. A good example is the challenges that the modern pharmaceutical industry presents to the needs of patients suffering from mental disorders. As we previously discussed, data suggests that in the United States (from this point of view the best example) physicians tend to overprescribe medications[614] in a way that is not only ineffective, but also very harmful for the whole well-being of the patient. This is even more important when we understand the balance and direct effect between physical health and his/her well-being in mental, as well as psychological, philosophical and spiritual areas. Medical Philosophy challenges the status quo of modern, *hypermedicating* medicine, a medicine which is controlled by power and money, more specifically by an extremely capitalist-oriented pharmaceutical corporations and insurance companies,[615] which ultimately strongly influence decision-making processes in scientific/medical research and academia. Medical Philosophy sheds light on the interactions between patient and provider, as well as be-

---

[614] Especially in comparing pharmacological interventions versus psychotherapy in psychiatry, as Smith writes: "Most antidepressants are prescribed by primary-care physicians who may have limited training in treating mental health disorders. In the United States, almost four out of five prescriptions for psychotropic drugs are written by physicians who aren't psychiatrists (Psychiatric Services, 2009). And fewer of their patients receive psychotherapy than in the past. In 1996, one-third of patients taking antidepressants also received therapy. By 2005, only one-fifth of patients did, according to a study of more than 50,000 medical surveys that was co-authored by Mark Olfson, MD, professor of clinical psychiatry at Columbia University (Archives of General Psychiatry, 2009)." See Smith, B.L. 2012. *Inappropriate prescribing. Research shows that all too often, Americans are taking medications that may not work or may be inappropriate for their mental health problems*. Monitor on Psychology, Vol 43, No. 4. Washington, DC: American Psychological Association, Vol 43, No. 6, p. 38.

[615] In fact, in the United States, where a universal health care policy is still neither applied, nor popular (especially by members of certain areas within the political spectrum), it is much easier to get health insurance reimbursement for pharmacological intervention than psychotherapy. Daniel Carlat observes: "Psychiatrists have settled for treating symptoms rather than causes, embracing the apparent medical rigor of DSM diagnoses and prescription in place of learning the more challenging craft of therapeutic counseling, gaining only limited understanding of their patients' lives. Talk therapy takes time, whereas the fifteen-minute "med check" allows for more patients and more insurance company reimbursement. Yet DSM diagnoses, he shows, are premised on a good deal less science than we would think." See Carlat, D. 2010. *Unhinged: The Trouble with Psychiatry. A Doctor's Revelations about a Profession in Crisis*. New York, NY: Simon & Schuster.

tween provider and the system as a whole, and fights its battle on several grounds: the theoretical-scientific-philosophical (with the analysis of concepts, structure, method, etc.), the social-translational (including the applicability of the findings in therapeutic/clinical practice), and the ethical-moral (the debate on universal health care, patient's and provider's rights, etc.). Moreover, Medical Philosophy also challenges those claims in evidence-based science which are generally and widely assumed to be accurate and true (again, evidence-based). The best example is again the research on the effectiveness of psychotropic medications vs. placebo effect, whose results are far too often influenced by the aforementioned powers in charge:

"An analysis of all FDA clinical trials for four SSRI antidepressants found that the drugs didn't perform significantly better than placebos in treating mild or moderate depression, and the benefits of the drugs were relatively small even for severely depressed patients."[616]

"[A study] examined 74 FDA-registered studies for a dozen antidepressants and found that most studies with negative results were not published in scientific literature or were published in a way that conveyed a positive outcome. The FDA studies showed that half of the drug trials had positive results, but 94 percent of the trials cited in published literature were positive."[617]

"The use of second-generation antipsychotics nearly tripled from 1995 to 2008 in the United States, ballooning to more than 16 million prescriptions for drugs such as aripiprazole (Abilify), clozapinel (Clozaril) and quetiapine (Seroquel). More than half of those prescriptions in 2008 were for uses with uncertain scientific evidence."[618]

All the aforementioned considerations provide elements supporting the idea of a deeper connection, perhaps one of mutual correspondence or systemic inter-

---

[616]   PLoS Medicine, 2008, as quoted in: Smith, B.L. 2012. *Inappropriate prescribing. Research shows that all too often, Americans are taking medications that may not work or may be inappropriate for their mental health problems.* Monitor on Psychology, Vol 43, No. 4. Washington, DC: American Psychological Association, Vol 43, No. 6, p. 38.

[617]   Study led by researchers at the Portland Veterans Affairs Medical Center and published in 2008 by the *New England Journal of Medicine* and cited in: Smith, B.L. 2012. *Inappropriate prescribing. Research shows that all too often, Americans are taking medications that may not work or may be inappropriate for their mental health problems.* Monitor on Psychology, Vol 43, No. 4. Washington, DC: American Psychological Association, Vol 43, No. 6, p. 38.

[618]   According to a study, published in *Pharmacoepidemiology and Drug Safety*, in 2011 from Stanford University and the University of Chicago based on more than 1,700 physician surveys, and cited by Smith, B.L. 2012. *Inappropriate prescribing. Research shows that all too often, Americans are taking medications that may not work or may be inappropriate for their mental health problems.* Monitor on Psychology, Vol 43, No. 4. Washington, DC: American Psychological Association, Vol 43, No. 6, p. 39.

sect between Medical Philosophy and translational science. However, we also need to be aware that, since our focus is on medicine and medical science, we are using the term "translational science" in a specific, field-related sense. Certainly, a widespread use of the definition has to do with transporting the information collected in a laboratory to the bedside, thus translating biological knowledge into medical practice. In the process, translational science helps bridge the gap between further areas of investigation and applicability, such as public health and public policy. To be sure, since in this sense "translating" means to transfer, morph, and/or change information into action, translational science means to connect scientific knowledge to its applicability in several areas—therefore not only in medicine, from an epistemological perspective.

We could hence argue that translational science follows a functional understanding of knowledge, and is in this sense akin to applied science. At the same time, by its very (translational) nature, it also includes other criteria which go beyond analysis and prediction as the only parameters to defines was "real" (as compared to "hard") science is. Thus, a target of translational science is to define, characterize, structure a specific investigation, intervention, analysis with the goal of obtaining/attaining a desired (medical, clinical in this sense) end. We could certainly argue that based on these considerations, the demarcation line between science in general and translational science is very, very thin. In fact we also need to include in our discussion terms such as Translational Research and Translative Research. Perhaps, we could frame the problem by defining the first as focused on gaining information about the (natural) world, and the latter as focused on applying (positive) changes to the status quo.

Furthermore, this combining, complementing, relating, completing approach to science is the base of our investigation under the lenses of Medical Philosophy in the sense that it helps us avoid falling prey to an excessive emphasis on mere data collection. In fact, the theory behind the data plays a bigger role in this understanding and application of science. For example, increasing the amount of data we can collect doesn't necessarily mean that we will find a specific pattern or structure. Moreover, if this inconsistency of data is observed, we could infer that our theoretical model might not be appropriate for understanding and analyzing the great amount of information we could gather from outliers. On the other side, our theoretical model should also contemplate a possible incompleteness beyond inconsistency and beyond size. It should certainly push us to possibly implement or, in some cases even reconsider or reformulate our theories. Thus, we need to make sure that a strong philosophical discussion is put in place to formulate the correct answers if we want to obtain meaningful answers (this is after all, what the principle of falsifiability is based upon). In scientific terms, formulating these questions means 1) understanding the complexity of the issue, and 2) applying a model. The first aspect is related to the progressively increasing level of abstraction needed in modern science. In other terms, due to the refined specialization of areas, fields, and subfields, it is becoming very difficult for a single scientist to master enough knowledge *and* information in every area of analysis (for instance biomedical science, clinical intervention, policy making, sociological analysis, etc.) to guarantee, alone, translational success in the form of efficient applicability of appropriate theoretical investigation, and previously verified hypotheses. Therefore, a more cooperative approach is needed. Specialists in different fields should come together to work on a project and understand enough of each other (scientific) language to be able to communicate and share their inputs and observation to the rest. From this perspective, science is indeed a shared effort. Certainly, among the roles of the (medical) philosopher is to make sure that this happens, and possibly monitor the ways in which it happens, for example through observations, suggestions, dialogue, and debate. The second aspect is about creating a model that would allow all the collected data to *make sense* in a translational context. One or more systems of variables connected in mathematical-statistical relations allow our theories to be translated (this time, also in a linguistic way) into a deeper (and predictive) understanding of substructures relating measurements and judgments. Philosophy is again in the background (or as a base), monitoring the measurable outcomes (operational correlations, consequences, definitions) of our theories and the related model through logical analysis. As it turns out, this model is the hard core of our knowledge; it is the object[619] at the center of our investigation, and which will allow for a *translation* to take place.

c) Research and beyond

The aforementioned considerations force us to reconsider the role of Medical Philosophy in translational research and its scientific, social, and ethic outcomes. To be sure, this role is even more important in consideration of our choice to focus on those subfields of medicine, psychology and psychiatry, in which the complexity of human mind is especially challenging our scientific

---

[619]   Also in Kantian terms.

methods and therapeutic strategies. This choice is not only theoretical in nature, but also justified by cutting-edge research in epidemiology and current statistical data:

> "The majority of people in the United States seeks and receives care for mental disorders, substance use disorders, and health behavior problems in the primary care setting. They present with the need for health behavior change for better management of their chronic diseases, with freestanding mental disorders, and with psychological symptoms and disorders comorbid with other medical illnesses. It turns out that about one third of the patients seen for care in primary care settings meet criteria for a mental disorder, and another one third, while not meeting those criteria, nevertheless [has] psychosocial symptoms or problems that impair their function."[620]

Health issues are therefore correlated, in terms of statistical presence, to philosophical and psychological elements which we need to take into account in the attempt to solve them or at least alleviate them. Thus, in order to have better chances in achieving our goal, the previously discussed focus on provider-patient communication and perception plays a key role. From the perspective of the doctor, we already examined how communication and understanding are determinant factors in therapeutic effectiveness and medical success, together with what Atul Gawande defines as "diligence, doing right, and ingenuity."[621]

The very mystery underlying the science and practice of medicine is at the center of Gawande's writing efforts, and it opens up new perspectives on the very connection between laboratory investigation, clinical practice (especially palliative care), public policy and society as a whole, including very important philosophical considerations regarding life's meaning and purpose. In this sense, it represents one of the best examples of philosophy in and *within* translational science.[622] We can therefore understand how translational science helps researchers, policy makers, and practitioners focus on the core ethical values in medicine, which also address social and political issues, as we have seen in Chapter 4, *The patient at the center of therapy*, in part 1. "Patient's

---

[620]   See McDaniel, S.H., and deGruy III, F.V. 2014. *An Introduction to Primary Care and Psychology.* American Psychologist, Vol. 69, No. 4, 325–331. Washington, DC: American Psychological Association, p. 327. Cited research by Kessler, R.C., Berglund, P., Demler, O., Jin, R., Merikangas, K.R., and Walters, E.E. 2005. *Lifetime prevalence and age-of-onset distributions of DSM-IV disorders in the National Comorbidity Survey Replication.* Archives of General Psychiatry, 62(6), 593–602.

[621]   Gawande, A. 2007. *Better: A Surgeon's Notes on Performance*, New York, NY: Picador, pp. 56–72.

[622]   A very interesting documentary has been recently published by Frontline on PBS, starring Atul Gawande and available at: http://www.pbs.org/wgbh/pages/frontline/being-mortal/.

communication, perception and self-perception", and in Chapter 5, *Complementary, Alternative, Traditional Medicine*, in Subchapter c -"Culture and Identity". To summarize those values, we need to remember these principles:

- Respect for autonomy; important because the patient has the right to refuse or choose a specific treatment, intervention or procedure— *Voluntas aegroti suprema lex*;
- Beneficence; patient's best interest should be at the center of medical practice—*Salus aegroti suprema lex*;
- Non-maleficence; the "first do no harm" of Hippocratic heritage— *Primum non nocere*;
- Double effect (including conflict); the principle according to which the combined effect of beneficence and non-maleficence may be produced by a single medical action, for instance in the case of pharmacological intervention. In the case of conflict, a sociocultural dimension is opened in understanding the parameters societies use in prioritizing beneficence over autonomy or vice versa.
- Justice; a concept that is truly translational, in the sense that it covers the whole spectrum of laboratory-to-bedside approach, including distribution of scientific research, economic, and health resources, as well decision-making policies related to the equality and fairness and of treatment, intervention or procedure;
- Respect for people; every person in the medical equation, starting from the patient and the provider have the right to be treated with dignity. This includes debates on important concepts such as human rights, abortion, sexual preference and expression, euthanasia, as well as those problematic aspects in medical practice related to disciplines such as eugenics[623], etc.
- Honesty and Truthfulness; in other words the focus on the concept of informed consent and confidentiality both in the laboratory (experimentation, testing, clinical trials) and in the hospital bedroom (treatment, therapy, procedure, standard of care, and again clinical trial).

Certainly, making sure that these principles are applied in everyday clinical practice depends as much from appropriate philosophical debates in contexts such as clinical ethics committees, as from the quality of interpersonal communication, in our case with a special attention to patient-provider communication. Medical Philosophy is a form of translational science in the sense that it

---

[623]   Let us not forget that the very expression "nature and nurture", so important in psychological and philosophical debates, was popularized by the British eugenicist Francis Galton.

brings all those values together in an effort to improve this communication and thereby guarantee an overall better quality of care. To be sure, an improved quality of care may also produce better treatment outcomes, and therefore ameliorate the general health of the patient. However, the great message of this approach is that, although we cannot completely, with a 100% accurate forecast, predict the *medical future* of a specific patient, we can better understand ways to improve his/her well-being by focusing on all those elements brought us by this translational debate. In particular, the focus on patient's perception and sense of meaning plays an important part in *feeling better*. Research has shown over and over again that a positive attitude, a positive thought process, and a positive self-talk are the cognitive-behavioral strongholds for therapeutic success.[624] As we have seen, if these strategies seem to work on an individual/self-actualized level, this might not necessarily be the case from a broader, generalized perspective, especially when the provider is the one providing this type of positive talk, as some studies have suggested.[625] Again, more and more research is needed to identify the parameters of interactions and the level of perceptual effectiveness (e.g. the cognitive, emotional, and ultimately physical reception by the patient, throughout the conversation and onto the healing process) in the patient-provider relationship, but all the aforementioned consideration point to a solution which takes into account all these different realms of investigation. Addressing patient perception and self-perception in diagnostics and therapy is the theoretical pathway that appears to present the best approach to add to the more conventional ones, to answer the questions asked in this study. While approaching the end of our study, we also need to treasure the

---

[624] See for instance the article by Barker, J. (Smith, M.W., review) 2013. *Express Yourself: Your Mouth, Your Life. The Power of Positive Talking*. New York, NY: WebMD. Available at: http://www.webmd.com/balance/express-yourself-13/positive-self-talk.

[625] For example, the 2006 study by Pahal, and Li, which showed that medicine residents asked 80% of the total questions, and patients asked 20% of the questions; while in the physician-only sample, physicians asked 89% of the questions and patient 11%. Interestingly, "patients' overall satisfaction and communication satisfaction were negatively correlated with residents' positive talk, which constitutes 31.5% of a given resident's total utterances. In the physician-only sample, physician positive talk was 26% of a given physician's total utterances and physician positive talk was not correlated with patient satisfaction." See Pahal, J.S., and Li, H.Z. 2006. *The dynamics of resident-patient communication: Data from Canada*. Communication & Medicine 3(2) (2006), pp. 161–170. New York, NY: Mouton de Gruyter. Certainly, there are several aspects we should analyze in this context, for example the very understanding of a concept such as "patient's satisfaction", which is quite problematic –especially in subfields such as psychology and psychiatry, but not only- because it might depend on the willingness to cooperate and support certain life (in a very board sense, including behavioral, physical, etc.) choices.

very nature of the types of relations and relationships we examined in our discussion. To be sure, whenever we mentioned conceptual pairs such as patient-provider, patient-environment, patient-perception or life-meaning, and life-purpose, we realize that we are integral part of these equations. There is a level of presence, of existence, of permanence and even of historicity in our role as investigators. Starting from a purely anthropological consideration, as well as by monitoring the differences in research methods, we have to be aware that our presence has potential for influence, effect/affect and bias, and might ultimately influence *our* perception of the interactions and the results. Furthermore, our presence is to be intended in a translational sense, too. Thus, through our role (-s) and action/effect (-s) in different stages and on different levels of translation, such as in theoretical work, laboratory experiment, statistical and epidemiological analysis, bedside care and everyday clinical interaction, all the way to social work in terms of popular science discussions, public policy (making) and ethical considerations (it is the case of universal health care, for instance), we are constantly changing these parameters. Therefore, we are again *actors and prisoners, masters and slaves* of this *traduzione-tradizione* at the center of our therapeutic and scientific efforts. To be sure, these considerations should not prevent us for engaging in translational science and translational research. On the contrary, the realization of the philosophical weight of all these parameters should spur us to fully embrace our nature, essence, existence and identity as human beings, in relation to other human beings. In fact, these mutual relation, which is ultimately an attempt for mutual understanding helps us expand and redefine science as a whole, in a translational way. This is especially true when we are talking about medical science, since at the center of the connection (also in historical, economic and political terms) between evidence-based science and scientific medicine is, once again, a human being, with his wonderful complexity far beyond all the possible data and information collected through descriptive, field, laboratory, empirical, experimental, epidemiological studies and meta-analysis.

Conclusion

"There is a tendency to ignore everything published before the personal computer."[626]

We are finally reaching the end of our study. We postulated several hypothesis and ideas related to the assumption that man's complexity can be investigated and better understood if we are willing to consider the multilayered structure of being in our clinical assessment (diagnostics) and treatment efforts (therapy). In this sense, we proposed the analysis of a specific subfield of medicine, namely psychiatry, and its connection with the broader scientific field of psychology,[627] as a basis for inference of value and meaning onto others branches of the medical field. Furthermore, we also wanted to analyze the impact, both in qualitative and in quantitative terms, of patient's perception in regard to the aforementioned concepts. Certainly, the choice of a combination of these two approaches is also rooted in our view of philosophy as an all-encompassing "mother field" for the theoretical and practical, hard and applied, sciences. To be sure, the ultimate focus on understanding and linking correlation such as cause and effect in our analysis is absolutely complementary (and even founded, in some areas of our discussion) in the search of meaning, of (ultimate) purpose, of mechanism, of truth. The latter in particular has been approached as "direction", "inclination", and "tendency". In other words we attempted to come as close as possible to an approximation of *the* absolute truth of *the* patient. If, in purely conceptual terms, associating "absolute" with the "absolutely relative" component of patient's individuality seems to be an oxymoron, it is also true that the term served us in a non (overtly strict) comparative conception. Thus, the absolute truth we aimed for is, in this context, intrinsic (to the patient, as well as to his/her perception *mechanisms*, and to patient-provider relationships), and free from limitations and constrictions. We can definitely argue that this truth *had to be* approached as direction, inclination, and tendency exactly because of these considerations, which made us more aware of met-

---

[626] Bunge, M. 2013. *Medical Philosophy. Conceptual Issues in Medicine*, Singapore: World Scientific Publishing, p. 156. We might add that a similar tendency is found in discarding paper/printed versions of texts, images and data in favor of internet/web-based resources.

[627] To be sure, the line drawn to separate these disciplines is often very thin, such as in behavioral medicine v. clinical/health psychology.

aphysical considerations. We had to embrace the differences between *certain certainties* of the sciences following the logical-linear-inductive model and a more comprehensive, and yet more targeted, focused, even sensitive approach that is aimed at moving beyond the realm of the above mentioned cause-effect relation and investigate theoretical aspects of hidden mechanisms and intermediate links.[628] Moreover, our attempt to investigate what is a often referred to as "what makes us *thick*", as well as "what makes us *tick*", a common contemporary American idiomatic expression,[629] has helped us examining each layer of this complexity separately, but with the consistency, which is also plausibility, connection, association, relation and correlation of the realization and awareness of the existence, first postulated, then examined, of a "higher", or better "deeper"[630] meaning or purpose. In this sense, connecting our theoretical investigation with an empirical survey directly focused at –and administered to– patients, had a teleological component which addressed, though investigation, perception, awareness, understanding, explanation, etc., the aforementioned questions. As we have examined, our physical health depends on our sense of connectedness with others, or, in other terms, our perception of (our) selves in relation to others, including health providers. In statistical terms, our empirical research provided ulterior evidence of the importance of such perspectives, as examined in the Appendix at the end of this volume. In particular, data has indicated that the way patient relate to themselves, the medical environment, and a sense of meaning and purpose in life plays a fundamental part in their well-being. Furthermore, our research has been both qualitative and quantitative due to the very complexity of the *issues* (in medical and philosophical terms) addressed, as well as because we *think and believe* that even our assumption of rational strength of human cognitive abilities needs to be understood as such[631] and investigate enough to avoid jumping to conclusion. We certainly refrained from completely embracing philosophical positions which discourage any attempt of understanding (human nature) due to the (perceived, declared) absolute impossibility to achieve knowledge. Thus, some postmodernist, and especially some post-structuralist positions are not discussed in this study. However, we also refrained from accusing these positions

---

628   See in particular the Vichian perspective, as examined in Gungov, A.L. 2012. *Logic in Medicine: Approaches to Patient Safety*. Sofia: Avangard.

629   Which is ultimately very appropriate in a medical-biological context focused on investigating diagnostic criteria such as the principles defined by Robert Koch and Friedrich Loeffler.

630   Since, once more, it is "what makes us *thick*."

631   *Id est* assumption.

to be "obscurantist", "esoteric" or even "elitist". We might agree with Chomsky in that some philosophical speculations belonging to the above mentioned "movements" are not on the forefront, the avant-garde of analytical-empirical knowledge; but we are also aware of the fact that throughout this study we embraced a perspective that goes beyond these parameters. There is no doubt a strong empirical component in our surveys, and also a well-grounded analytical element in our statistical examination. However, we stressed many times that "good epidemiology"[632] goes far beyond that. We do believe that theoretical and empirical research is a founding basis of experimental philosophy in the sense we discussed through this volume. We stressed the importance of humility in analyzing the data collected. First and foremost because, let us repeat that once more, "numbers don't lie, nor they tell the truth." It is in the interpretative, epidemiological analysis that we find meaning and possible application of the data. This is especially important when we observed the relation between perception and meaning in life, in particular when this connection is filtered through a spiritual lens. Furthermore, our study also carried an ethical dimension, in the sense that our focus has been truly philosophical, *id est* it has not only examined several theoretical positions, hypotheses, ideas and assumption, but also proposed a paradigm which embraces the question of "what should and ought to be", instead of only focusing on the "what is". This is not a study on religion or spirituality, but religion and spirituality cannot be avoided in discussing life's meaning and purpose, especially in the framework of medicine, due to its very nature of "trying to heal, cure, treat, and ease (human) suffering, pain, and sorrow." For all these reasons we decided not to propose yet another study on, let say, the links between depression and religion or depression and spirituality. There are over 450 studies done in the last 60 years investigating these links[633]. At the same time, we recognized the importance of understanding these connections, whether purely correlational or causational, in attempting a description of "patient self-perception in diagnostics and therapy." This is why we decided not to work on a meta-analysis of the combined data of all these studies -something which is widely available in scientific ar-

---

[632]   Again, as mentioned before, "good" in the sense brought us by Greco-Latin heritage, thus "pleasing", but also "appropriate", "beneficial", "benevolent", "skilled, "apt", "adapt", "adaptive", etc.

[633]   From 1962 to 2011 only, at least 444 studies have now quantitatively examined these relationships. See Bonelli, R., Dew, R.E., Koenig, H.G.; Rosmarin, D.H.; and Vasegh, S. 2012. *Religious and Spiritual Factors in Depression: Review and Integration of the Research*. Depression Research and Treatment. Cairo, EG: Hindawi Publishing Corporation.

chives and bibliographies- but to include a *new* survey to *new* patients as a starting point, a dialogue, and a conversation for our philosophical debate. Certainly, we asked ourselves some very basic, and yet important, questions such as "is it really worth it?" or, in a slightly different form "will our investigation provide new knowledge to the existing studies?" To be sure, throughout our investigation we wanted to keep in mind the ethical weight of our assumption, in the attempt to provide better explanations of the complexity of (for instance) patient-provider relationship. The focus of medicine is to help heal the patient. Our focus is to help understand those hidden elements which can positively or negatively affect this medical effort. We postulated that human beings are true organisms, and that an investigation of those layers that deal with existential questions and questions of perception is fundamental to achieve our goal.

A good direction in this sense is offered by the examination of the above mentioned study on depression and religion/spirituality, in a purely quantitative sense (religion and spiritually do play a very important role in dealing with depression) and qualitative[634] (the combined data yielded over 60% of less depression ad faster remission from it in those more religious or spiritual, or a reduction in depression severity in response to an religious or spiritual intervention).[635] Generally speaking, the vast majority of studies found a positive relation between religious and spiritual practices in order to help with depression. However, certain studies seem to disprove this statement, by yielding opposite data. Some argue that most of these studies were conducted in Western countries, especially in the US, where there is a high percentage of people reporting religious affiliation of some sort. Others indicate that religious beliefs are often associated with strict dogmas, which negatively impact self-perception in the struggle to "live up" to these rules, thereby increasing sense of guilt and depression. Among the most recent studies, the University of London created a survey[636] (nearly ten thousand people from Great Britain, Chile, Estonia, the Netherlands, Portugal, Slovenia, and Spain) focused on the analy-

---

[634] The terms are here philosophically intended, thus providing an emphasis on the ethical value of such findings, versus the more common statistical definitions of correlation v. causation.

[635] "Of the 178 most methodologically rigorous studies, 119 (67%) find inverse relationships between R/S and depression". Bonelli, R., Dew, R.E., Koenig, H.G.; Rosmarin, D.H.; and Vasegh, S. 2012. *Religious and Spiritual Factors in Depression: Review and Integration of the Research*. Depression Research and Treatment.

[636] Leurent, B., Nazareth, I., Bellón-Saameño, j., Geerlings, M.I., Maaroos, H., Saldivia, S., Švab, I., Torres-González, F., Xavier, M., and Kin, M. 2013. *Spiritual and religious beliefs as risk factors for the onset of major depression: an international cohort study*. Psychological Medicine. London, UK: Cambridge University Press.

sis of the ability of family doctors to predict depression from their patients' worldview. The data in this study indicated that 10.3 % of religious people had had at least one severe episode of depression during the year; 10.5 % of people with a spiritual worldview fell into deep depression, and only 7% for secularists, with $p < 0.001$. Furthermore, it appeared that the more people viewed themselves as strongly religious or to have a strong religious faith, the greater the risk of severe depression. Although the results varied depending on the country, the study had found a very strong link between depression and religiosity. We should point out that, based on the results and the very focus of this research, the notion that religious and spiritual life views enhance psychological well-being was not supported. This does not mean that, in this study, a direct causal effect between religion and depression was found. In fact, as the researchers discuss, it is not clear whether people with depression are more prone to become more religious or at least find some relief in spiritual practices, or if those practices are the cause of depression. Once again, even if in the vast majority of studies, everything else being equal, religious or spiritual practices and beliefs are related to less depression, especially in the context of life stress, it is important to notice that our health is strongly influenced by the interaction between behavioral, cultural, developmental, environmental, genetic, social (etc.) factors. Thus, our very perspective and perception on ourselves as related to all the above indicated concepts is a key to investigate our well-being and possibly provide a better cure for our physical, mental, emotional, social, spiritual (etc.) problems.

As we have seen, Medical Philosophy addresses all these concept in combining subfields such as theoretical medicine, epistemology, medical and bioethics, ontology and metaphysics. Moreover, although the name is often used as a synonym for philosophical medicine, and other definitions, it represents the theoretical base for disciplines like metaethics, philosophy of healthcare, public health and public policy, and healthcare practice. In this volume we provided a very brief excursus on the history of the discipline, especially within the geographical and cultural apparatus of what is now considered Europe and its connected cultural spheres of influence, especially in regard to philosophical roots found in ancient Greece. From this perspective, the Apollonian *philosophia divina* is the conceptual cradle of the so-called *medicus* who observes, examines, discusses, diagnoses, and treats. More specifically, he treats not just the disorder, but the whole patient (or the patient as a whole, in a philosophical viewpoint very similar to the now defined complementary and alternative practices). Therefore, he understands, knows, comprehends and measures symptoms and therapeutic outcomes. Medical Philosophy starts and goes beyond translational science;[637] a synthesis of interaction, from the laboratory and the scientific analysis to the bedside, thus connecting the terms *Doctor* and *Medicus* in a much broader sense[638]. We also examined how the spheres of translational research are included in this paradigm, and how from a specific radical reductionistic sphere, as opposed to a vitalistic one, as base for the modern scientific method in medicine in the Western world, we suggested further steps aimed at a better understanding of (once again) disorders, patients, and interactions patient-provider. In fact, as we postulated, and *also* observed through our empirical research, lack of proper communication and more general misunderstandings contribute to problems that affect the whole spectrum of patient's care, for instance the tendency patients have to decline elective surgeries and diseases screenings, which could ultimately lead to risks from false positives and unnecessary interventions. To address these problems, we included a debate on premises, conceptual standpoint and therapeutic and social action within palliative care and advance care planning. Through this discussion we also analyzed issues connected to the conceptual evolution, starting from the XIX century on, of a scientific method whose epistemological analysis is rational, realist and methodologically skeptical, and whose philosophical viewpoint and ontological nature is materialist and systemic. Advance care includes a discussion on a sphere of possible non-action, which is not necessarily inaction, due to the practical, and again, realist (even pragmatic) impossibility of therapeutic outreach beyond certain, definitely not well understood within this scientific paradigm, *punto di non ritorno*. This problematic discussion is by no means completed in this volume, albeit we did include non ordinary states of consciousness and near death experiences as an important part of both our philosophical study and surveys within empirical research.

In medical decision making the concept of intuition is, as we have seen, connected with neurological models such as short-, mid-, and long-term memory. The imprecision of human intuitive powers, when these can be linked with memory-related phenomena such as *source misattribution* and *confabulation* and non-linear time, are part of our analysis, in the sense that there are translational views involving an ethical sensibility to issues which (still) ap-

---

[637]   Thus, it is not merely a form of Translational Science.
[638]   Including "hero", in a Vichian sense.

pear to be unsolvable, at least under the modern lenses of Western scientific method. Once more, *intueor* carries a reference to the action of literally "enter with the sight" this form of (patient, provider, and beyond) perceptual knowledge, even in a holotropic sense. The non-empirical/experimental forms of knowledge of the pure form of intuition of Kantian *memory* are therefore very important to "*increase the focus* of our *perceptual understanding.*"

Thus, a correct interpretation of a disorder needs to address a correct interpretation of the patient. This is possible through philosophical work targeting the learning perspective of behaviorism, the biological perspective, the cognitive perspective of cognitivism, situated cognition and cognitive science, the socio-cultural perspective, the analysis on elaboration and contrastive method, and the hypothesis-based reasoning method. We also made sure to indicate how this philosophical basis impacts humanistic and positive psychology. In particular, we discussed how the psychological tradition of existentialism and phenomenology underlies the humanistic approach. We have seen how humanistic psychology often provides further references to the theological debate, as well as to the hermeneutic analysis of psychological science. The form of understanding defined in hermeneutics is prereflective as well as parareflective, and provides important strategies focused on what is the right way to achieve a goal, not in the epistemological sense of universal, unchanged, unchangeable, stable (and still, often with reference to homeostatic effects) truth (or truths), but in the sense of Aristotelian phronesis. In fact, we are not talking about the mere ability to decide how to achieve a particular goal but also the ability to reflect and decide what should be the *end* on the base of experience. Therefore, the focus (which is also an important target of this study) is on what is good and what is bad, what is desirable for man and society. It is therefore represented by a series of actions, which are conducted according to a specific criterion.

These criteria are the core of the connection between our philosophical investigation and the empirical research. In fact, the questions presented in the surveys were structured in a way which allowed the patients to take into account different issues related to perception, therapeutic progress, and progress in general (once again opening up perspectives on the linearity and the conceptual, even ethical weight of time), among others. In particular, the focus was on *patient* perception in diagnostics and therapy. The patient was at the center, which is also the *central* viewpoint of *central*(ized) medicine. This appeared to be especially important in discussing concepts such as therapeutic effectiveness, patient satisfaction and general happiness (levels). As we have discussed in Chapter four, this type[639] of morality is not necessarily related to the way, the method, the doctrine of how we may make ourselves happy, but how we may make ourselves *worthy* of happiness. This is fundamental in addressing problems of (lack of) self-esteem, depression, and sense of meaning and purpose; especially in a psychiatric unit, which is the medical-social environment of choice in our study. Patients were asked to identify a series of questions addressing this separation of selves, which is also a separation of self, in psychological terms. It is the relation with a higher self, which is higher in different stages and different senses. In Nietzschean terms this is connected to man's attempt to separate himself from a "higher self", often channeled into religion or scientific rationalism of the Enlightenment, as further discussed by Feuerbach. Moreover, this new contemplation of self is therapy in itself, in the sense that the origins of empirical methodologies (which were after all used in the questionnaires we administered to our patients) in philosophy are combinations of classical philosophy with the experimental rigor of social sciences. This is actually not diminishing, but increasing the weight of philosophical discipline, both in conceptual and ethical terms, since this rigor can also be (just, only, merely) perceived as such. In other words, philosophy uses this rigor to make the process *rigorous*, and also makes sure that it does not turn into *rigidity*, which could possibly affect the singularities of perceptions (of the single patient) and thereby also affect the results of the research. The cognitive perspective on critical thinking is used in modern psychological science and practice, especially in the form of the previously discussed Socratic Method, undoubtedly a philosophical form of inquiry. Common examples are Cognitive Behavioral Therapy and Dialectic Behavioral Therapy, therapeutically very effective, as research has shown multiple times. Thus, modern scientific *field* research *also* indicates how philosophy plays a major role in medicine. This truth was after all suggested throughout history, not only history of philosophy, but history in general. This is evident when we *contemplate* the absence of a clear separation between science, religion and philosophy up until around the V century, in the cultural and scientific centers of the ancient world. As we have seen, the separation between the external part of medicine (the physical) from the internal part of medicine (the psychical, but also spiritual, in the sense of sacred science) has been beneficial in developing the core values, and methods of modern science, to be intended both in post-Galilean as well as post-

---

[639]   Again, in a theoretical comparison between Aristotle and Kant.

Cartesian sense. However, in complex medical fields such as psychiatry, this separation represents (also in the sense of "creates") a problem. In fact, we asked whether the individual (in our case the patient) is really indivisible or there are several parts of the self which are contributing to the image that one has of self, or that others have of him. We certainly define ourselves as (human) beings by comparing each other, and by sharing knowledge, ultimately by communicating in one form or the other. Modern science has often attempted to get rid of the complexity and the mystery of human life. Although there are several very good reasons for this endeavour, the ultimate result has unfortunately been "alienating ourselves from ourselves" and also making a better (if not full, complete) understanding *of* ourselves even more difficult. In fact, some ultra-materialistic and biologico-reductionist approaches in modern science made the mistake (through mere assumptions) of reducing our "essence" in (or only as a result of or production by) our brains, even beyond the most conservative views in embodied cognition (which is again very interesting and not completely reductionist, since it is technically not em*brained* cognition). This process is beyond reducing essence to existence (some would argue that is indeed the opposite), it is an attempt to locate the *Geist* in an organ, possibly a single one.[640] In other terms, we think that the equation mind=brain has to be reevaluated. The same applies to reason, a faculty far larger than mere objective thought. To continue in our parallel, and to stress the importance of going beyond these categories and the way *certain philosophies and sciences* have often depicted the relationship between body and spirit, self, soul, essence and existence, we quoted the Vichian expression *"coscienza non è conoscenza."*[641] Furthermore, the choice of psychiatry and psychology has been especially important in our analysis because in these medical and scientific subfields, the connection with a higher (or lower) sphere was very much evidenced by our interaction with the patients, and by the way patient relate to themselves, to each other, to the environment (providers included) and to the metaphysical, transcendental, and spiritual sphere. In the Heideggerian "process of becoming" we observed the coming-to-oneself of the existential future, more of a dimension rather than a sequence of single not-yet-present moments. Discussing factors such as belief in God and in the afterlife opened up new dimension

---

[640]   In this context, we should also remember how in Traditional Chinese Medicine and other CAM disciplines, the definition of a specific organ goes often beyond what the physical organ appears to be, in physical and *geographical-directional* terms within our bodies.

[641]   Especially in regard to epistemological consideration of causal relationship.

to our speculations, since *Sein-zum-Tode* is a true way of being, a towardness rather than an orientation, a revelation of the process of Dasein as a threefold condition of Being.

In our study, all the data collected showed a very clear picture of patients' perspectives on perception, life's meaning and purpose, spiritual/religious beliefs and therapy. Of note, 72.63% of the total number of patients who responded to the Focus Group Questionnaire also responded to the Health Perception Survey. The highest score on the first question regarding factors affecting patient's health was found in the patient's personal ability to get better ("You", with 89% of the patients indicating either "I absolutely agree" or "I mostly agree"), was closely followed by "Therapist" (86%), and "Medications" (85%) in this sense slightly differentiating between the therapeutic effectiveness of the provider and pharmacological interventions. The lowest score was found in "destiny" (53%) and "randomness" (60%), thus suggesting a strong emphasis on the scientific-clinical aspects of the treatment. Regarding question number 2 on patients' view on life's purpose or meaning, the highest score was "Whether or not there is a purpose or meaning in life depends upon whether one gives it meaning or not" (82%), followed by "life depends upon one's beliefs" (80%), and "there is a meaning or purpose in life, and it can be discovered or known" (64%). The lowest scores were 34% for "there is a meaning or purpose in life, but it cannot be discovered or known," and "life's meaning depends entirely upon external factors (such as environment, relationships, social structures)" and "life is randomness," with 44% of patients agreeing on these possibilities as answers for the question "How would you define life's meaning or purpose." The third part of the Health Perception Survey, focused on patients' specific beliefs reported the highest score (between 8 – "strongly agree" and 7 – "mostly agree") in "Belief in your ability to get better" (79% of patients), followed by "Belief in God" (60%) and "Life after Death" (58%). For the lowest score (between 1 – "absolutely disagree" and 2 – "mostly disagree") we found, respectively, 6%, 21%, and 18%. The data also suggests strong correlations:

a) Between patient's perception of the causes of his/her health conditions and perceived positive/negative health outcomes, and

b) Between patient's perception of life's meaning and purpose and his/her ability to get better.

Further details are presented in the Appendix at the end of this volume, and certainly more data is needed to infer a generalizability of the information gathered through our surveys and questionnaires. However, by combining the theoretical-philosophical debate on medical philosophy, especially through considerations of psychological and psychiatric nature, with empirical data collected directly from the patients, we can achieve a more balanced approach which will allow us to frame new questions and open up new conversations in a more appropriate and efficient (in a therapeutic sense) way. Moreover, this approach has been proven successful through a series of scientific studies conducted with a special focus on these concepts, which are debated and understood under appropriate philosophical lenses. A good example is represented by the evidence of a strong correlation between the effects of practices such as mindfulness, and mindful awareness and perception (of all the aforementioned categories) on mental health issues, including depression and mood disorders. Important considerations on a neurobiological level also arise from the realization of the importance of such practices, for instance in the modifications in density of grey matter in the amygdala.

Generally speaking, the image we obtained from the examination of these data is that patients value every aspect of the multilayered dimension making up their own perception and their interaction with the clinical/medical environment, as well as the scientific-therapeutic and the religious-spiritual perspective. Furthermore, the majority of patients seems to indicate that the combination of their personal ability to get better, the medical strength of the therapies provided and the more spiritual/metaphysical spheres of life's meaning and purpose, including a spiritual dimension represents very important values in their effort to get better. Moreover, since the vast majority of data was comprised between the highest scores on our scale (values 7–8), with much lower scores on the opposite side of the spectrum (values 1–2 on our scale) –thus leaving very few outliers indicating uncertainties in answering the questions one way or the other (values between 3 and 6, "somewhat" or "slightly" agree/disagree)– the patients seemed to indicate a relatively strong belief in the answers they chose. Therefore, the data collected up to this point seem to confirm our predictions on the importance of such elements in our efforts to better understand patients and provide a better care, which takes into account those very spheres of investigation, interaction, and a possible therapeutic action. To be sure, we were not interested, at this stage, to find a direct causal link between the aforementioned concepts and the effectiveness of therapy. Our focus was on the way patients see themselves and/within the environment in diagnostics and therapy.

In the first survey of our empirical analysis, the Focus Group, we also found very interesting data. After 6 months, two important figures captured our attention. First, a great number of comments were explicitly addressing patient-provider communication (251). Second, out of the total of patients who decided to attend the focus group, 72.63 % answered the questions in the survey. Two figures which directly target the issues of patient-provider relationship. Interestingly, the biggest difference between negative and positive responses were found in the comments on Activity Therapists, which had the biggest amount of positive comments *and* the smallest amount of negative comments among all the professionals within the Multidisciplinary Treatment Team (ATs, MDs, RNs, and SWs) as well as by comparing ATs with every other category in the survey. More in detail, Activity Therapists achieved 1 point more than the total of the second best positive comments, found in Registered Nurses, and 17 points less than the total of the most negative comments, interestingly also found in RNs. Furthermore, the positive comments achieved by Activity Therapists were 74.97% of the total comments, versus the 5.92% negative comments. Certainly, the results might have been affected by the fact that both the Health Perception Survey and the Focus Group Questionnaires were administered by ATs. In order to reduce the possible bias, we decided to implement our research with two devices.

First, we decided that surveys and questionnaires be administered by ATs except for the Principal Investigator, who had never been present during the writing process, the introduction and the collecting of the completed questionnaires and surveys. Second, we provided every patient with a separate document on which they could write comments on ATs, a document which was directly collected by the nurse manager and not by ATs. Although completely avoiding bias in this kind of research is impossible, we were still able to make few inferences on the analysis of the numbers obtained from patients' responses. In fact, the data seem to suggest that a special emphasis in patient's attention and preference was found in those categories which directly work in strong connection (communicative, personal, and psychotherapeutic) with the patients, e.g. Activity Therapists, Psychiatrists, Mental Health Technicians, Licensed Nurse Assistants, and Social Workers. As we previously observed, Registered Nurses also obtained an important number of positive responses, albeit together with a great number (the greatest among staff on both units) of negative comments. The latter consideration is perhaps another confirmation of the importance of patient-provider communication, which not only underlies every clinical intervention (at least in a psychiatric unit) but turns out to be fundamental in therapeutic effectiveness. In other words, the results of our research suggest that, in order to guarantee an improvement in our care, we need to understand and work on all those aforementioned layers which constitute a patient *as* human being. Communication and (philosophical and medical) understanding are the keys. On a more individual, case-by-case level, many comments appear to follow the same perspective, in the sense that they seem to confirm the importance of concepts such as perception, sense of meaning, spirituality and communication-relation in diagnostics and therapy. We hereby report few examples and refer to the *Appendix: Empirical Research* for a comprehensive list of patients' comments:

"They listened to me and didn't judge I felt comfortable enough to be honest."

(November 2014, Physician/Attending, Things done well, Shepardson 3 Unit)

"I was scared and everyone did their best to make me comfortable my first weeks here."

(November 2014, Admission Process, Things done well, Shepardson 3 Unit)

"Do Not Like patronization or Testing Like Zoo Animals. I AM HUMAN I AM A MAN..."

(November 2014, Nursing, Concerns, Shepardson 6 Unit)

"Love thy neighbor as thyself."

(November 2014, Admission Process, Concerns, Shepardson 6 Unit)

"I believe doctors should take more time to listen to their patients before making decisions or suggestions. If they don't have the time or feel rushed the doctors should minimize their patient lists so they do have time to listen to their patients. And make life changing suggestions. In my opinion it's part of their fiduciary responsibility as a health professional."

(December 2014, Physician/Attending, Recommendations, Shepardson 6 Unit)

"Dr. [...]: good bedside manner, helpful suggestions and mental-emotional suggestions."

(January 2015, Residents, Things done well, Shepardson 3 Unit)

"I feel that I should have a say if I'm not ready to leave or not. My feelings should count; no one knows how I feel better that myself."

(February 2015, Physician/Attending, Concerns, Shepardson 3 Unit)

"Hated him some days which meant he was doing his job."

(February 2015, Physician/Attending, Things done well, Shepardson 3 Unit)

To be sure, we used statistical data to obtain a general picture of the situation, but (as we often discussed throughout this study) we refrain from adding to every aspect of our data a principle of generalizability. Among the main reasons we find the very complexity of the issue, and the difficulties, in statistical and epidemiological terms, to convert such data into a well-formed, hard-structured image. Furthermore, every time we have found outliers in our data, a series of important philosophical/theoretical consideration arose. This was not only to provide justification for a skewed curve, or a diagram which did not reflect a perfectly regular shape (certainly not symmetry). The wonderful experience with this data was and is the realization of the beauty of the individual, which is a full, whole and complete (yet not perfect, in the sense that it is ever morphing) combination of subject and object. It is a person, a human being, a man who is dealing with (the sense of) himself/herself, and with an incredible amount of environments, from the temporal, to the historical and experiential, the relational and social, all the way to the spiritual, and possibly even religious, with a Levinasian "Other" somewhere in the middle of the path. As we have seen, this Other becomes several people/persons in different contexts, sometimes even the patient himself/herself. Medical Philosophy focuses on this relation, a relationship between the patient and the environment (provider, therapy, clinical setting, but also cultural, religious/spiritual, and social), as well as with himself/herself.

Throughout this study, we investigated several philosophical positions, in order to find a solid ground upon which to build the best possible perspective on medical diagnosis and therapy keeping in mind the above mentioned human complexity. The data suggests that a metaphysical, transcendental, and even spiritual perspective is absolutely needed to address those very issues that underlie patient's view of themselves and of their environment, especially when dealing with illness or disease, and especially when these medical issues are related to psychological and psychiatric interventions. To be sure, this does not mean that our duty as medical/mental health care providers is one of preaching, sermonizing and/or attempting to convert patients to this or that philosophical, spiritual or religious perspective. However, our theoretical analysis and the empirical data spurs an honest look at reality as we see it, perceive it, understand it by addressing questions and interact directly with our patients, e.g. making sure that those existential questions, questions of meaning and purpose are not forgotten in our therapeutic efforts. As example, some philosophers believe that disease is generally speaking a concept linked to time, in the sense that it is a moment (-um) of human choice or decision. In other words, when human beings feel that they do not meet the needs of everyday life, health problems arise, and illnesses are created. In fact, health is a phenomenon, an epiphany, a manifestation of (human) existence, structured on a philosophical level of social, ethical, and moral responsibility, toward nature, mankind and values. We agree with this point of view in the sense that we proposed and investigated (both through philosophical analysis as well as empirical research) a deeper connection between levels of (human) existence: from an external, phenomenological ground, to an experiential (thus time- and environment- connected, especially in the sense of *Erlebnis*) ground, to an essential—both personal as well as social—ground. Since health and disease are also philosophical (more specifically phenomenological) concepts, we suggest they be analyzed under the theoretical lenses of (Medical) Philosophy.

Furthermore, "health" means understanding and (self) knowledge of identity and role in life as opposed to "disease", or loss of (part of) identity. The investigation is between these spheres of human action/interaction and the (effectiveness/non-effectiveness on) the healing process. Medical Philosophy is central in suggesting the combination of evidence-based medicine and a patient-centered (or at least patient-informed) practice, both supported by a strong theoretical (philosophical-scientific) basis, in order to produce positive outcomes in clinical-therapeutic settings, in particular diagnosis, prognosis, and treatment. Moreover, since Medicine is a science, a technical skill and an art, we need to understand that there are several pathways to the (several) truths behind the healing process: the scientific, the mechanical-finalistic, the philosophical-theoretical, the artistic-interpretative, etc., including different models of Reasoning in Medicine: Induction, Deduction, and Abduction.[642] This perspective has a practical application in scientific research, namely the integration of qualitative and quantitative methods, as we first proposed, and then applied in our study. In fact, this modus operandi is not a brand-new strategy in science, since it dates back to the Aristotelian definition of knowledge as *theoria* and as *praxis*. Furthermore, this strategy has been proven very successful as evidenced by the great and ever increasing amount of studies in psychological research which employ qualitative and quantitative approaches,

---

[642]   See Pahal, J.S., and Li, H.Z. 2006. *The dynamics of resident-patient communication: Data from Canada*. Communication & Medicine 3(2) (2006), pp. 161–170.

which include important philosophical methods and theories.[643] Since at the center of our research there were questions of perception, meaning, and purpose, we believed that the best investigative strategy to answer them is by *interacting with* –instead of just *acting upon*– the subjects of our investigation. The ultimate purpose, once again, is not only successful (therapeutic, behavioral) scientific predictions, but also the (ethical, social, philosophical, moral) inclination/orientation toward goals (such as deeper understanding, empathy, sympathy and tolerance) which go far beyond the common use and appreciation of medicine. Since, similarly to the placebo effect, completely avoiding bias[644] is impossible, we not only raise awareness on the possible bias of both investigator and investigated subject, but also on the possible positive use of this bias with the aforementioned ethical goal in mind... and brain... and heart.

---

[643] "In addition to experimentation, researchers might freely engage in case studies, introspection, ethnography, field observation, and phenomenology. However, with the advent of behaviorism and its linkage to logical positivism, the aims of psychological inquiry began to narrow. [...] The hermeneutic, the constructionist, and the praxis orientation [offer] alternatives to the traditional emphasis on the empirical grounding of generalized theory. [...] Although the aims of traditional research are to establish value-neutral knowledge, these particular conceptions of inquiry open more direct paths to value expression." Gergen, K.J., Josselson, R., Freeman, M. 2015. *The promises of Qualitative Inquiry*. American Psychologist, Vol. 70, No. 1, 1–60. Washington, DC: American Psychological Association, p. 3

[644] Especially in the above mentioned context of inclination/orientation.

Afterword

David Tomasi is privileged to be both a practicing psychotherapist and a scholar with doctoral degree in philosophy. What a better position could one hope for in order to write on medical philosophy? In regard to medicine, this book draws mainly on psychology and psychiatry but it touches upon a much broader range of clinical experience and medical research. The philosophical approach mastered by the author lies within the continental philosophy tradition. Philosophy, as it has emerged and developed on the European Continent and then influenced various thinkers all over the world, is a fertile ground for pondering health, malady, and medicine as a human fate and human endeavor.

The principle goal of this book are philosophical reflections on actual and potential patients: the healing process as well as prevention, diagnostics, and prognostics. There is no surprise that patient centered medicine occupies a special place in this study although a substantial part of this work is dedicated to evidence based medicine. Viewing medicine in the perspective of patients, David Tomasi succeeds to comprehend patients as integral human beings and not just as a particular case of a disease. Realizing a patient's uniqueness, and not considering him/her simply as an individual variation of a biomedical set of rules and social patterns, is an essential prerequisite for successful clinical practice. Addressing patients as humans engaged in looking for and constituting the sense of their life, while structuring their actions teleologically within the life world, is believed to impact immensely the process and outcomes of any treatment. Each patient is not just a living body and rational mind capable of judging about their health condition or perhaps of interacting with the attending physician; being a human, the patient is a source of undisclosed possibilities and unpredictable strength or disappointment.

Following Gadamer, the author regards health as an expression of dynamic equilibrium within specific human existence, as a phenomenon embodying the responsibility to fellow humans and nature. Furthermore, various value systems are embodied in the notion of health. That is why viewing disease and health in the light of philosophical categories is hoped to contribute to get a better comprehension of these phenomena. Hermeneutics, understood as answering right questions within a certain tradition, is also instrumental in taking care of chronic patients or turning malady into healthy equilibrium. The diagnosis, therapy, and the prognosis never rely on mere fact based knowledge, but are accomplished through explanation and interpretation, which make them more adequate to reality; and reality always surpasses empirical data. Hermeneutical interpretation begins with a vague notion of the final outcome or final end that is believed to be reached. In the light of such a vague premise, the current stage is grasped and new steps in reflecting on the further developments and the telos are taken. Going in this kind of circles, hermeneutical cognition proceeds gradually coming closer to a more adequate opinion about what the person in a predicament suffers from.

Nomothetical sciences infer deductively (in a non-contradictory manner and necessarily) particular items from general laws. Clinical medicine, however, is an ideographic science or at least many researchers and practicing clinicians regard it as such. Ideographic sciences, unlike nomothetical, are occupied with the task of explaining particular events that cannot be deduced by general principles. Typical questions for an idiographic science would be linked with the reasons why a given historical event has occurred, what made a certain language disappear, why a patient has recovered much faster and with fewer complications than expected.

To answer the above questions ideographic sciences cannot depend only on the formal logic identity principle. They have no other option but to stick to the concrete identity, in which inevitably an element of difference is present. It is like the identity of different states and manifestations of one and the same thing often called dialectical. No doubt, there is an identity of one and the same person, who has passed through the stage of a five-month old baby, and has now reached his fiftieth birthday.

This is especially true for the clinical diagnosis, which cannot be limited to an entity that manifests itself always in the same way. Its manifestations are linked to the difference which inevitably accompanies the concrete, and not the abstract (uniformity like), identity. In this case, the concrete identity consists in the differences in the manifestation of one and the same disease in different patients. Clinical individuality, however, is not absolute and does not herald extreme nominalism. Concrete identity is compatible with moderate conceptualism. Applied to diagnostics, the conceptualist approach to concrete identity would mean to establish a typology of individual patients and in accordance to this typology to foresee the specific manifestation of a disease. Helping in dealing with these issues, medical philosophy is not simply a translational science (although it can serve this purpose, as David Tomasi rightly points out) but can take part in constituting the sense of life of the patient in the course of his sickness, treatment, and convalescence.

* * *

The idea of establishing a series in Medical Philosophy was launched by Christian Schön, the ibidem-Verlag Manager. His suggestion reached me in Sofia in early December 2015 at the eve of David Tomasi's Ph.D. dissertation defense. After the outstanding defense, we discussed this proposal with Friedrich Luft and decided it was really worth to pursue it. We agreed Mr. Tomasi's dissertation to open the series, while Dr. Luft and I were to become the series general editors. It is our great hope that *Medical Philosophy: A Philosophical Analysis of Patient Self-Perception in Diagnostics and Therapy* will turn out as an appealing reading not only for medical professionals and philosophers but for various experts in related fields as well as for a much broader audience interested in the philosophical foundations of medicine. We have no doubts that this book will serve as a key milestone in David Tomasi's forthcoming productive and exciting career as a scholar, lecturer, and psychotherapist.

The *Studies in Medical Philosophy* (SMP) book series aims at putting philosophy and medicine in the perspective of interdependence: the series provides opportunity both to views which discuss how medicine can benefit from philosophy and to those showing how philosophy is able to be enriched by medicine. The possible need of philosophy in medicine will be searched in terms of elucidation and stimulation of certain aspects of medical research and clinical practice by philosophical heritage such as ethics, epistemology, logic, ontology, social philosophy, and philosophical anthropology. On the other hand, medicine is considered to be a valuable and unique resource of individual cases and statistical tendencies for reflection and further conclusions in philosophical fields. It will be a source of special reward for us if *Studies in Medical Philosophy* contribute to establishing closer ties between philosophy and medicine for the sake of actual and potential patients and for the better understanding what constitutes a human being.

Alexander L. Gungov

Appendix
Empirical Research at the University of Vermont Medical Center

1. Introduction

This study has been conducted at the University of Vermont Medical center in Burlington, Vermont, USA and supplemented the Research for the volume "Medical Philosophy. Philosophical Analysis of Patient Self-Perception in Diagnostics and Therapy". The statistical data have been analyzed using the statistical software Stata©13.

2. Objective

The following research focused on psycho-social determinants of health perception from the perspective of patient self-analysis underlying aspects of diagnostics and therapy directly linked to the patient's personal experience, for Quality Improvement Purposes. In particular, the study analyzed the importance of factors such as environment, personal belief and perspective on life, as a way to relate the patient's viewpoint within the specific structure of therapeutic groups led by the University of Vermont Medical Center (UVMMC, former Fletcher Allen Health Care) Inpatient Psychiatry Activities Therapists on the units Shepardson 3 and 6. Of note, following this research the position and title of Activities Therapist (AT) has been changed into "Group Therapist".

3. Methods

The research is comprised of two parts: Part 1 has been represented by the Focus Group Questionnaire (FGQ), as previously approved by UVMMC Quality Council Meeting and administered verbally (through printed handouts) on both units by UVMMC Activities therapists. Part 2, the Health Perception Survey, has been presented as printed attachment to the FGQ and followed the same structure, rules and requirements of the FGQ. The data collected have been part of a retrospective cohort study in the case of the FGQ and have been implemented by the HPS, an empirical research questionnaire conducted over a period of six months, as approved by the Institutional Review Boards (IRBs). Patients have been able to choose to participate in the therapeutic focus group and not allow their responses to be used for research. Furthermore, patients have been able to decide to only answer the questions in the FGQ and not take part in the HPS. In the case of patients changing their mind after the focus group interview has been completed and wishing to withdraw from the study, the information collected has been used as part of the research study because the information was recorded with no identifiers, and with no link to patients' name.

4. Protocol

No personal, clinical and medical information regarding the single patient has been collected and presented as part of this research. All the information has been collected without any identifiers and used only for statistical purposes, and it has not been connected or linkable to clinical/medical records of single patients and/or groups / categories / diagnosis. A request for Alteration of Authorization—HIPAA has been submitted to the University of Vermont Research Protections Office / Committee on Human Research, together with the Common Protocol Cover Form, the Human Subjects Research Protocol and the Request for UVM Net ID for Required Training. The research has been quantitative and qualitative in nature and entirely anonymous, and involved no more than minimal risk to the subjects (breach of confidentiality/protected health information).

5. Approvals

This study has been approved by:

- The University of Vermont Medical Center, Inpatient Psychiatry Unit Quality Committee
- The University of Vermont College of Medicine, Research and Education Committee
- The University of Vermont Integrity and Compliance Department
- The University of Vermont Research Protocol Committee
- The University of Vermont Institutional Review Board, Committee on Human Research in the Medical Sciences

6. Structure

At the beginning of each Focus Group, the Activities Therapist (AT) read the informed consent information and procedure to the patients. Every patient has been free to decline to take part in the focus group and attached survey. 15 minutes before the beginning of each group, the AT asked the patient to decide whether he/she wanted to take part in the group. The total time allowed to complete both Focus Group and Health Perception Survey, from beginning to end, has been 60 minutes. The PI discussed the structure and procedure with each Activities Therapist (AT) and handed out a written description of the informed content process. Each week one AT has been present for the initial and subsequent informed consent discussions with the subject.

Each Activities Therapist (AT) documented on paper the number of patients participating in the group and the number of patients absent or patients who declined to take part in the group. Each patient has been documented using initials only, not the full name. Each Activities Therapist (AT) actively monitored the activity and the safety of patients and environment. The AT also documented on paper the adverse event and patient(s) involved using initials only, not the full name. In the case of extreme, dangerous or potentially harmful events, the AT also notified staff on the unit and Nurse Manager, both verbally as well as through SOAP notes on UVMMC Prism system and through incident reports on UVMMC S.A.F.E. reports. Each Activities Therapist (AT) provided constant information and updates on safety at the beginning of each group, after discussing details and structure with the Nurse Manager, the Unit staff and the other ATs. Each Activities Therapist (AT) assured confidentiality both verbally as well as in writing through discussion of privacy/informed consent with every patient at the beginning of each group. ATs held constant (weekly) meetings to review and examine the progress of the groups. The hardcopy data has been archived in the locked Activities Therapist Office on the Unit Patrick 4, separated from both Inpatient Psychiatry Units Shepardson 3 and Shepardson 6.

7. Subject Selection

The research has been purely quantitative in structure and addressed quality improvement of patients' care. The focus of the research has been the therapeutic work on FAHC Inpatient Psychiatry Unit. Subjects have been recruited on Shepardson 3 and Shepardson 6 after clinical evaluation by the Unit Multidisciplinary Treatment Team (MDs, ATs, RNs, and SWs) in order to monitor patient's safety, capacity, and clinical/medical ability to join in the focus group and complete the survey.

The study and questionnaire administrators (UVMMC Inpatient Psychiatry ATs), in cooperation with the Medical Unit Staff (RNs and MDs) constantly monitored the therapeutic, clinical and medical presentation and availability of each patient before, throughout and after each group, in order to guarantee complete safeness of procedure and interactions within the group and to prevent physical and psychological harmful situations and minimize risks.

A total of 198 subjects enrolled within a six months period at UVMMC Inpatient Psychiatry Unit. Every patient on both Units Shepardson 3 and Shepardson 6 has been eligible to take part in the study, unless declared medically and/or clinically unfit by the clinical and medical staff on both Units Shepardson 3 and Shepardson 6 (Activities Therapists—ATs, Nurses—RNs, Physicians—MDs). The study has been open to the entire Inpatient Psychiatry patient population on the Unit, regardless of their age, race, creed, color, sex, national origin, religion, sexual orientation, gender identity, marital status, and socioeconomic status. All the details of the research regarding inclusion and exclusion criteria, consent, structure, administration, purpose, withdrawal procedures, references, objectives, risks and benefits, data safety and monitoring, design and statistical consideration have been discussed with the Inpatient Psychiatry Interim Nurse Manager, Sponsor, Staff and the Quality Council.

8. Administration

Prior to signing the informed consent form the subject:

- Read the consent form
- Discussed the protocol participation with researcher including:

    - Purpose of the study
    - Risks/benefits
    - inclusion and exclusion criteria
    - consent
    - structure
    - administration
    - data safety and monitoring
    - design and statistical consideration
    - Withdrawal rights and procedure

- Asked questions; and
- Consulted with other clinicians / physicians.

9. Personnel involved in the Study

- PI: David Tomasi, AT
- Contact Person: Katharine Monje, RN, BSN
- Faculty Sponsor: William Tobey Horn, MD
- Enman, Lindsay, AT
- Rapaport, Ann, AT
- Melo, Kevin, AT
- Derivan, John, AT
- Tudor, Adoria, AT
- Shupp-Star, Joshua, AT
- Gates, Sheri, AT

10. Presenting the Data

a) General Considerations

The Health Perception Survey (HPS) was conducted over a 6-month period, from December 2014 to May 2015. For the Focus Group Questionnaire (FGQ) we started monitoring the data starting a month earlier (November 2014), to verify possible impact and influence of group attendance and participation. From November 2014 to December 2014 we observed a decrease in patient response by 52.94% on Shepardson 3, and by 44.44% on Shepardson 6. Patient attendance dropped by 42.85% on Shepardson 3, while it stayed the same on Shepardson 6. However, the trend disappeared statistically in January. By February the curve changed and we observed an actual increase of attendance. On Shepardson 3 attendance increased by 18.18% and on Shepardson 6 by 35.71%, with $p < 0.001$.

The FGQ was structured by indicating the following categories: Medication teaching, Pain management, MDs, Residents, RNs, SWs, ATs, Admission process, Food, Housekeeping, MHT/LNA/Secretaries, Environment, and religious/spiritual. Responses for each of the categories were divided into "Concerns", "Recommendations", and "Things done well". A further analysis was dedicated to the medical professionals working on the units:

- Multisciplinary Treatment Team: MDs (Physicians/Attendings) and Residents (Psychiatrists in Training), ATs (Activities Therapists), RNs (Registered Nurses), and SWs (Social Workers);
- MHTs (Mental Health Technicians), LNAs (Licensed Nurse Assistants), and Unit Secretaries.

Patients were asked to rate the medical professionals by answering the following question:

1) [Category] treated you with courtesy & respect?
2) [Category] listened carefully to you?
3) [Category] explained in a way you could understand?

Using the following scale:

Always Most of the time Sometimes Rarely Never

In the HPS survey, patients were asked to answer the survey and rate their responses following the scale:

1) = Absolutely Disagree
2) = Mostly Disagree
3) = Somewhat Disagree
4) = Slightly Disagree (can't say)
5) = Slightly Agree (can't say)
6) = Somewhat Agree
7) = Mostly Agree
8) = Absolutely Agree

In order to provide a more accurate quantitative and qualitative analysis of the percentages, we indicate with TP (Total Positive) all the ratings comprising the upper values 5,6,7,8 and added the RP (Relative Positive) comprising the two top values (7,8), followed by RN (Relative Negative) with the two lowest values (1,2). At the end of the 6-months period, 72.63 % of the total number of patients who attended the FGQ responded to the Survey. Between November 2014 and February 2015, 48.71 % of the total number of patients who responded to the FGQ also responded to the HPS. At the end of the 6-months period, the figure increased to 68.49 %.

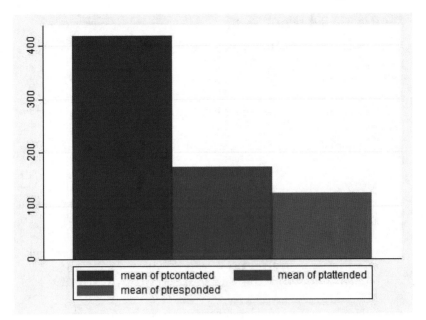

Figure 3. –   Graph Bar percentages for FGQ of the total number of patients who were contacted, patients who attended the 1-hour meeting, and patients who responded to the questions.

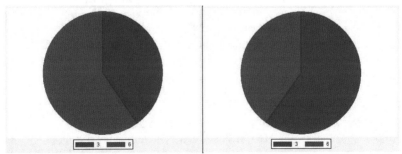

Figure 4 –   **(left) and 4bis (right)**. Pie charts percentages of the total numbers of patients who responded to the questionnaire, divided by floors Shepardson 3 (3) and Shepardson 6 (6): On the left, first 3 months data and on the right the complete 6-month period, indicating the fluctuation of response between floors.

Variables with relative percentages:

- destiny = [...] your health depends on: destiny → TP: 53%; RP: 30%; RL: 23%.
- medications = [...] your health depends on: medications → TP: 85%; RP: 60%; RL: 8%.
- therapy = [...] your health depends on: therapy → TP: 77%; RP: 51%; RL: 7%.
- therapistandp = [...] your health depends on: therapist and physician → TP: 86%; RP: 64%; RL: 4%.
- random = [...] your health depends on: randomness → TP: 60%; RP: 26%; RL: 19%.
- extfactors = [...] your health depends on: external factors → TP: 80%; RP: 43%;
- RL: 6%.
- you = [...] your health depends on: yourself → TP: 89%; RP: 74%; RL: 5%.
- brainchemistry = [...] your health depends on: brain chemistry → TP: 77%; RP: 57%; RL: 6%.
- genpred = [...] your health depends on: genetic predisposition → TP: 78%; RP: 50%;
- RL: 9%.
- meaningknown = there is a meaning or purpose in life, and it can be discovered or known → TP: 64%; RP: 49%; RL: 11%.
- meaningunkown = there is a meaning or purpose in life, but it cannot be discovered or known → TP: 34%; RP: 13%; RL: 36%.
- randomness = life is randomness → TP: 44%; RP: 22%; RL: 27%.
- beliefs = life depends upon one's beliefs → TP: 80%; RP: 56%; RL: 6%.
- togive = whether or not there is a purpose or meaning in life depends upon whether one
- gives it meaning or not → TP: 82%; RP: 57%; RL: 7%.
- meaningextfact = life's meaning depends entirely upon external factors (such as environment, relationships, social structures) → TP: 54%; RP: 23% ; RL: 31%.
- lifeafterdeath = how much do you believe in life after death? → TP: 58%; RP: 48%;
- RL: 18%.
- believeingod = how much you believe in God? → TP: 60%; RP: 49%; RL: 21%.

- yourability = how much do you believe in your ability to get better? →
  TP: 79%;
- RP: 59%; RL: 6%.

b) Views on Life's Meaning and Purpose

In the following pie charts, we present the data relative to the three parts of the HPS:

- Part A) Factors that affect your health—How much do you think your health depends on
- Part B) Your view on life's purpose or meaning—How would you define life's meaning or purpose
- Part C) Your specific beliefs

The highest score in Part A) was observed in the patient's personal ability to get better ("You", with 89% and was closely followed by "Therapist" (86%), and "Medications" (85%) in this sense slightly differentiating between the therapeutic effectiveness of the provider and pharmacological interventions. The lowest score was found in "Destiny" (53%) and "Randomness" (60%), thus suggesting a strong emphasis on the scientific-clinical aspects of the treatment. In Part B), the highest score was "Whether or not there is a purpose or meaning in life depends upon whether one gives it meaning or not" (82%), followed by "Life depends upon one's beliefs" (80%), and "There is a meaning or purpose in life, and it can be discovered or known" (64%). The lowest scores were 34% for "There is a meaning or purpose in life, but it cannot be discovered or known", and "Life is randomness", with 44% of patients agreeing on these possibilities as answers for the question "How would you define life's meaning or purpose". Part C) yielded the highest score in "Belief in your ability to get better" (79% of patients), followed by "Belief in God" (60%) and "Life after Death" (58%). For the lowest score (between 1 – "absolutely disagree" and 2 – "mostly disagree") we found, respectively, 6%, 21%, and 18%, with $p < 0.001$.

Part A) Factors that affect your health—How much do you think your health depends on:

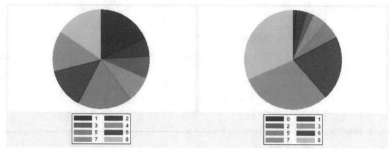

Figure 5. –   (left) – Destiny
Figure 6. –   (right)– Medications

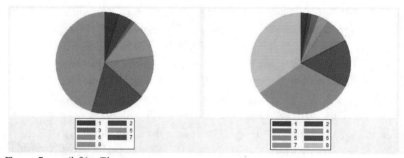

Figure 7. –   (left) – Therapy
Figure 8. –   (right) – Therapist and Physician

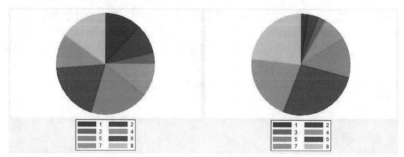

Figure 9. –   (left) – Random
Figure 10. –   (right) – External Factors

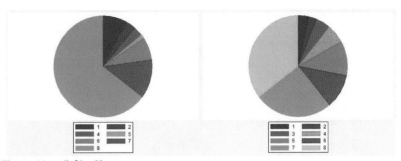

Figure 11. – (left) – You
Figure 12. – (right) – Brain Chemistry

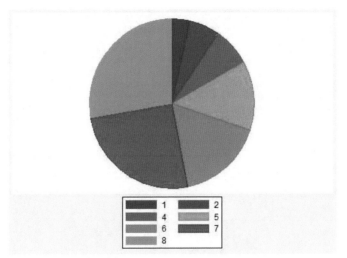

Figure 13. – Genetic Predisposition

From these first images, we got the clear impression that the combination of therapeutic effort, pharmacological intervention and personal role play the most important part in the path to health and well-being, in patients' perception. "You" as main factor affecting patients' health appeared clear and evident. Before we continue in our description of part B and C, let us take a closer look at the 95% confidence interval of Means and Standard Deviation for each of the categories listed in our Survey for the 38-patients subsample in the first three months of the research:

Variable	Obs	Mean	Std. Err.	[95% Conf.	Interval]
destiny	34	4.941176	.415693	4.095443	5.78691
medications	36	5.888889	.3939579	5.089112	6.688666
therapy	36	6.333333	.3518658	5.619008	7.047659
therapista~p	36	6.305556	.33998	5.615359	6.995752
random	35	4.971429	.4047734	4.14883	5.794027
extfactors	37	5.783784	.3336376	5.107135	6.460432
you	36	6.777778	.3653898	6.035997	7.519558
brainchemi~y	34	5.735294	.3712215	4.980038	6.49055
genpred	35	5.485714	.3875617	4.698094	6.273334
meaningknown	33	6.454545	.3643459	5.712397	7.196694
meaningunk~n	31	3.129032	.4489939	2.212064	4.046
randomness	32	4.03125	.4611617	3.090705	4.971795
beliefs	33	6.151515	.35919	5.419869	6.883161
togive	33	6.363636	.3764321	5.596869	7.130403
meaningext~t	34	4.470588	.4724784	3.509324	5.431853
lifeafterd~h	31	6.451613	.4444126	5.544001	7.359225
believeingod	31	6.129032	.4513824	5.207186	7.050878
yourability	32	6.53125	.3756295	5.765149	7.297351

Table 3. –   95% confidence interval for the mean in the subsample of 38 patients in the HPS.

As we can observe, the highest value for mean is found in "You" (6.77), followed by "Your ability to get better" (6.53), and "Life after death" (6.45). To help with the interpretation of the values, please note that the categories reported in the graphs are coded in the following way:

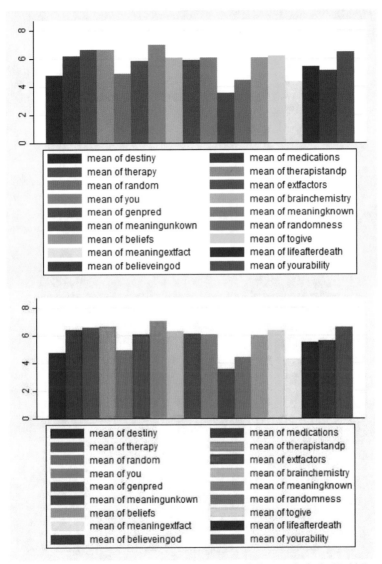

Figure 14 (top) and 14 bis (bottom). – Comparative means of all categories in the Health Perception Survey. Above the results after three months, below the data at the end of the 6-month period.

Part B) Your view on life's purpose or meaning—How would you define life's meaning or purpose

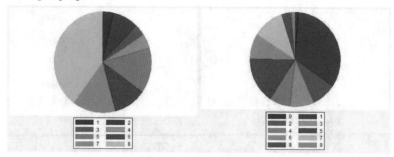

Figure 15. – (left) – there is a meaning or purpose in life, *and* it *can* be discovered or known
Figure 16. – (right) – there is a meaning or purpose in life, *but* it *cannot* be discovered or known

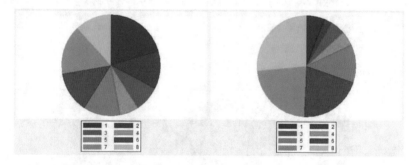

Figure 17. – (left) – life is randomness
Figure 18. – (right) – life depends upon one's beliefs

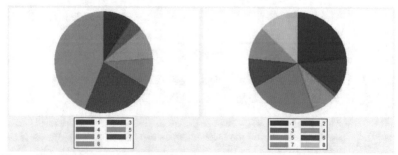

Figure 19. – (left) – Whether or not there is a purpose or meaning in life depends upon whether one gives it meaning or not
Figure 20. – (right) – life's meaning depends entirely upon external factors (such as environment, relationships, social structures)

Part C) Your specific beliefs

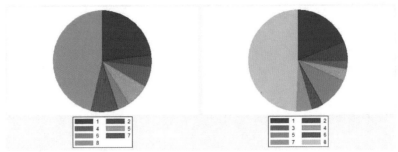

Figure 21. – (left) – How much do you believe in life after death?
Figure 22. – (right) – How much you believe in God?

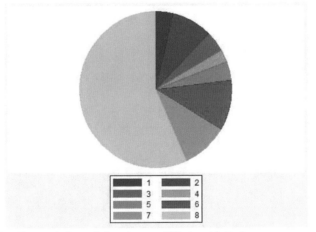

Figure 23. – How much do you believe in your ability to get better?

As we have observed, all three aspects "(Personal) Ability to get better", "Belief in God", and "Life after death" are absolutely relevant in patient perception. We therefore investigated the possible connection between variables. Again, the results were very interesting, indicating:

- a strong correlation between a strong belief in life after death and a strong belief in (personal) ability to get better, and
- a strong correlation between a strong belief in God and a strong belief in (personal) ability to get better.

Following, two scatter plot graphs representing this correlation in our sample:

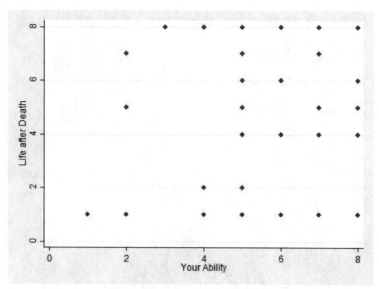

Table 4. –   Scatter plot subsample of the correlation between "life after death" and "your ability to get better".

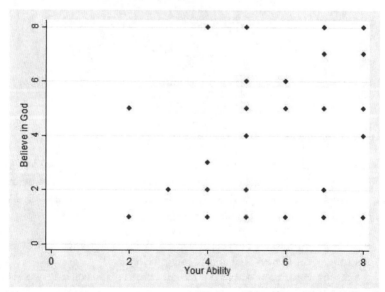

Table 5. –   Scatter plot subsample of the correlation between "life after death" and "your ability to get better".

c) Patient Perception in Diagnostics and Therapy

As we previously mentioned, 72.63 % of the total number of patients who attended the FGQ responded to the Survey. Between November 2014 and February 2015, 48.71 % of the total number of patients who responded to the FGQ also responded to the HPS. At the end of the 6-months period, the figure increased to 68.49 %. Furthermore, a great number of comments (251) were explicitly addressing patient-provider communication. These figures directly target the issues of patient-provider relationship. The biggest difference between negative and positive responses was found in the comments on Activity Therapists, which had the biggest amount of positive comments (100) *and* the smallest amount of negative comments (8) among all professionals within the Multidisciplinary Treatment Team (ATs, MDs, RNs, and SWs) as well as by comparing ATs with every other category in the survey. More in detail, Activity Therapists achieved 5 points more than the total of the second best positive comments, found in Registered Nurses, and 27 points less than the total of the most negative comments, interestingly also found in RNs. Furthermore, the positive comments achieved by Activity Therapists were 74.97 % of the ATs' total comments, versus the 5.92 % of negative comments.

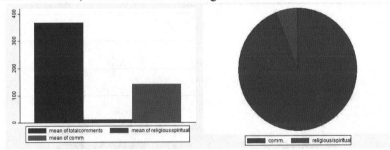

Figure 24. – (left) – Bar Chart Means of total number of comments (totalcomments) in the Focus Group Survey compared to the total amount of comments directly focused on patient-provider communication (comm.) and with a religious or spiritual content (religiousspiritual).

Figure 25. – (right) – Pie Chart Means of total number of *general* comments directly focused on patient-provider communication (comm.) and comments with a religious or spiritual content (religiousspiritual).

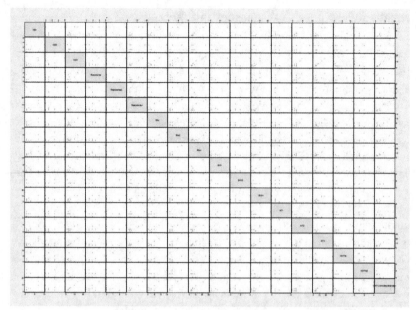

Table 6. –   First 3 months – Scatter plot analysis of all categories in the Health Perception survey with relative values.

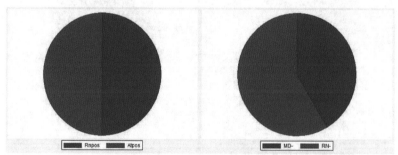

Figure 26. – (left) – Comparison between the total number of the first most positive comments received by a provider (AT pos, Activities Therapists) and the total number of the second most positive comments received by a provider (RNpos, Registered Nurses).

Figure 27. – (right) – Comparison between the total number of the first most negative comments received by a provider (RN-, Registered Nurses) and the total number of the second most negative comments received by a provider (MD-, Physician).

Certainly the results might have been affected by the fact that both the Health Perception Survey and the Focus Group Questionnaires were administered by ATs. In order to reduce the possible bias, we decided to implement our research with two devices. First, we decided that surveys and questionnaires be administered by ATs except for the Principal Investigator, who had never been present during the writing process, the introduction and the collecting of the completed questionnaires and surveys. Second, we provided every patient with a separate document on which they could write comments on ATs, a document which was directly collected by the nurse manager and not by ATs. Although completely avoiding bias in this kind of research is impossible, we were still able to make few inferences on the analysis of the numbers obtained from patients' responses.

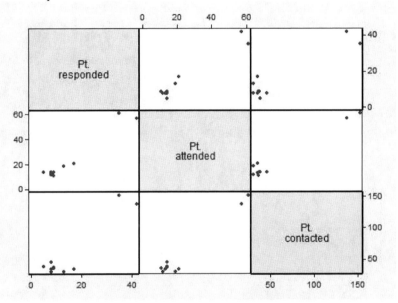

Table 7. –   First 38 patients – Scatterplot analysis of the total number of patients who were contacted, patients who attended the 1-hour meeting, and patients who responded to the questions.

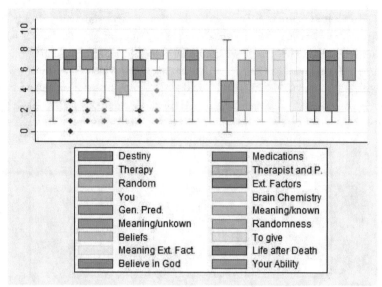

Figure 28. – Box plot analysis of all categories in the Health Perception survey with relative values.

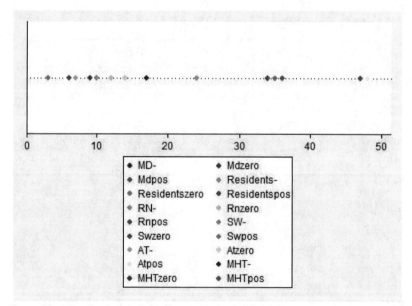

Figure 29. – Dot Graph analysis of all categories in the Health Perception survey with relative values.

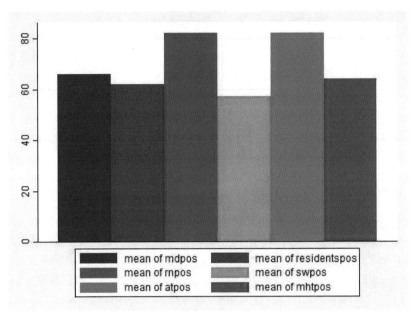

Figure 30. – Comparison of the *most positive* comments received by providers, divided by categories: MDpos (Physicians), RNpos (Registered Nurses), ATpos (Activities Therapists), Residentpos (Residents), SWpos (Social Workers), and MHTPos (Mental Health Technicians + Licensed Nurse Assistants + Unit Secretaries).

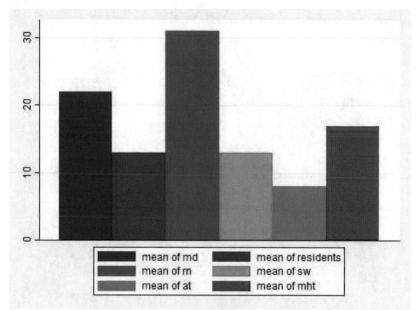

Figure 31. – Comparison of the *most negative* comments received by providers, divided by
categories: MDpos (Physicians), RNpos (Registered Nurses), ATpos (Activities
Therapists), Residentpos (Residents), SWpos (Social Workers), and MHTPos
(Mental Health Technicians + Licensed Nurse Assistants + Unit Secretaries).

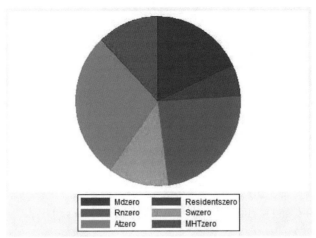

Figure 32. – Pie Chart comparison of the *general/average* comments and recommendations received by providers, divided by categories: MDpos (Physicians), RNpos (Registered Nurses), ATpos (Activities Therapists), Residentpos (Residents), SWpos (Social Workers), and MHTPos (Mental Health Technicians + Licensed Nurse Assistants + Unit Secretaries).

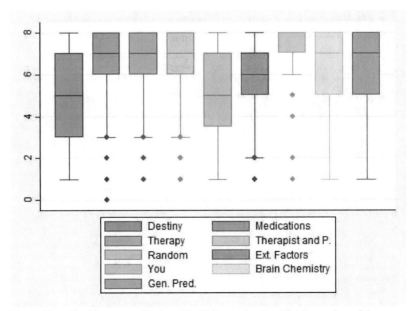

Figure 33. – Final Summary of Patients' Health Perception: Box Plot Comparison of the answers provided by patients in regard to the question "Your health depends on".

Brief Summary of the data collected:

- Total number of patients taking part in the research: 198
- Total number of admissions Shepardson 3: 131.
- Total number of patients Shepardson 3: 119.
- Patient with multiple admissions on Shepardson 3: 12
- Total number of admissions Shepardson 6: 93.
- Total number of patients Shepardson 6: 79.
- Patient with multiple admissions on Shepardson 6: 14
- Total number of patients attending the HPS and FGQ: 198.
- Total number of patients answering the HPS: 100.
- Total number of patients answering the FGQ: 146.
- MDs – positive comments: 81; suggestions: 20; negative comments: 23.
- Residents – positive comments: 71; suggestions: 11; negative comments: 16.
- RNs – positive comments: 95; suggestions: 28; negative comments: 35.
- ATs – positive comments: 100; suggestions: 27; negative comments: 8.
- SWs – positive comments: 62; suggestions: 13; negative comments: 23.
- MHTs – positive comments: 75; suggestions: 13; negative comments: 19.
- Total comments focused on patient-provider communication in the FGQ: 251.
- Total comments with spiritual/religious content in the FGQ: 13.
- Highest scores for "How much do you think your health depends on": "You" 89%; "Therapist" (86%); "Medications" (85%).
- Highest scores for "How would you define life's meaning or purpose": "Whether or not there is a purpose or meaning in life depends upon whether one gives it meaning or not" 82%; "life depends upon one's beliefs" 80%; "there is a meaning or purpose in life, and it can be discovered or known" 64%.

11. Survey & Questionnaires, Original Format

STUDY:

Medical Philosophy.

Philosophical Analysis of Patient Self-Perception in Diagnostics and Therapy.

Part 1: Patient Satisfaction Focus Group Survey

Floor:_____ Date:_____ Name (AT):_____

Areas of concern and need for improvement in the Quality of Care, Recommendations and Things Done Well. *Thank you for completing the survey. Your input makes a difference!*

1)   Medication Teaching: Concerns:

    Recommendations:

    Things done well:

2)   Pain Management: Concerns:

    Recommendations:

    Things done well:

3)   Attending Physicians: Concerns:

    Recommendations:

    Things done well:

4)   Residents (Psychiatrists in training): Concerns:

    Recommendations:

    Things done well:

5)   Nursing: Concerns:

Recommendations:

Things done well:

6)   Social Workers: Concerns:

Recommendations:

Things done well:

7)   Activities Therapy: Concerns:

Recommendations:

Things done well:

8)   The Admission Process: Concerns:

Recommendations:

Things done well:

9)   Food Service: Concerns:

Recommendations:

Things done well:

10)   Housekeeping: Concerns:

Recommendations:

Things done well:

11)   Techs/ LNAs/ Secretaries: Concerns:

Recommendations:

Things done well:

12)   Environment: <u>Concerns:</u>

       Recommendations:

       Things done well:

<u>Circle Best Response</u>

<u>Nurses</u>

1)   Nurses treated you with courtesy & respect?

       Always Most of the time Sometimes Rarely Never

2)   Nurses listened carefully to you?

       Always Most of the time Sometimes Rarely Never

3)   Nurses explained in a way you could understand?

       Always Most of the time Sometimes Rarely Never

<u>Physicians/Attendings</u>

1)   Physicians treated you with courtesy & respect?

       Always Most of the time Sometimes Rarely Never

2)   Physicians listened carefully to you?

       Always Most of the time Sometimes Rarely Never

3)   Physicians explained in a way you could understand?

       Always Most of the time Sometimes Rarely Never

Residents (Psychiatrists in Training)

1)   Residents treated you with courtesy & respect?

  Always Most of the time Sometimes Rarely Never

2)   Residents listened carefully to you?

  Always Most of the time Sometimes Rarely Never

3)   Residents explained in a way you could understand?

  Always Most of the time Sometimes Rarely Never

Social Workers

1)   Social Workers treated you with courtesy & respect?

  Always Most of the time Sometimes Rarely Never

2)   Social Workers listened carefully to you?

  Always Most of the time Sometimes Rarely Never

3)   Social Workers explained in a way you could understand?

  Always Most of the time Sometimes Rarely Never

Activity Therapists

1)   Activity Therapists treated you with courtesy & respect?

  Always Most of the time Sometimes Rarely Never

2)   Activity Therapists listened carefully to you?

  Always Most of the time Sometimes Rarely Never

3)   Activity Therapists explained in a way you could understand?

  Always Most of the time Sometimes Rarely Never

Mental Health Techs/Unit Secretary

1)   Mental Health Techs/Unit Secretary treated you with courtesy & respect?

   Always Most of the time Sometimes Rarely Never

2)   Mental Health Techs/Unit Secretary listened carefully to you?

   Always Most of the time Sometimes Rarely Never

3)   Mental Health Techs/Unit Secretary explained in a way you could understand?

   Always Most of the time Sometimes Rarely Never

Part 2: Health Perception Survey

Please score each item on the following scale:

   1)   = Absolutely Disagree
   2)   = Mostly Disagree
   3)   = Somewhat Disagree
   4)   = Slightly Disagree (can't say)
   5)   = Slightly Agree (can't say)
   6)   = Somewhat Agree
   7)   = Mostly Agree
   8)   = Absolutely Agree

Factors that affect your health

How much do you think your health depends on:

destiny	
medications	
therapy	
therapist and psychiatrist	
randomness	
external factors	
you	

brain chemistry	
genetic predisposition	

A) Your view on life's purpose or meaning

How would you define life's meaning or purpose:

there is a meaning or purpose in life, and it can be discovered or known	
there is a meaning or purpose in life, but it cannot be discovered or known	
life is randomness	
life depends upon one's beliefs	
Whether or not there is a purpose or meaning in life depends upon whether one gives it meaning or not	
life's meaning depends entirely upon external factors (such as environment, relationships, social structures)	

B) Your specific beliefs

How much do you believe in life after death?	
How much you believe in God?	
How much do you believe in your ability to get better?	

Comments

_____

_____

_____

_____

_____

_____

_____

_____

_____

_____

_____

_____

_____

12. Selection of Comments

Part 1: Patient Satisfaction Focus Group Survey

"Everyone listened to my concerns and discontinued the medication immediately."

(November 2014, Medication Teaching, Things done well, Shepardson 3 Unit)

"Read the history so they can know more about the patients."

(November 2014, Physician/Attending, Recommendations, Shepardson 3 Unit)

"Dr. [...] does a good job making sure I understand everything he says."

(November 2014, Physician/Attending, Things done well, Shepardson 3 Unit)

"Time taken to talk with patients."

(November 2014, Physician/Attending, Things done well, Shepardson 3 Unit)

"They listened to me and didn't judge I felt comfortable enough to be honest."

(November 2014, Physician/Attending, Things done well, Shepardson 3 Unit)

"Discuss meds & alternatives before making a decision."

(November 2014, Residents, Recommendations, Shepardson 3 Unit)

"Very helpful about concerns and questions about treatment."

(November 2014, Residents, Things done well, Shepardson 3 Unit)

"I loved all the nurses but one. And that was only because she has a brisk personality."

(November 2014, Nurses, Things done well, Shepardson 3 Unit)

"They never forced me to participate in group. They waited until I was ready and then made me feel welcome. The activities are fun and keep me focused on things other than my unhealthy thoughts/anxieties."

(November 2014, Activities Therapy, Things done well, Shepardson 3 Unit)

"Although the admission process was lengthy, treated with caring and respect."

(November 2014, Admission Process, Things done well, Shepardson 3 Unit)

"I was scared and everyone did their best to make me comfortable my first weeks here."

(November 2014, Admission Process, Things done well, Shepardson 3 Unit)

"[...] is my favorite. He interacts & has a good personality."

(November 2014, Techs/LNAs/Secretaries, Things done well, Shepardson 3 Unit)

"It's a calmer atmosphere than I expected."

(November 2014, Environment, Things done well, Shepardson 3 Unit)

"Describe how meds work, if asked."

(November 2014, Medication Training, Things done well, Shepardson 6 Unit)

"What if punching yourself in the head causes your head to stop thinking so much? That's what monks do and they are very peaceful and they meditate a lot." NOTE: The patient was asked what he meant with this response, and he stated that he has been hitting himself in the head to stop his thoughts. Pt was offered alternative suggestions.

(November 2014, Pain Management, Things done well, Shepardson 6 Unit)

"They always ask how my pain is—good."

(November 2014, Pain Management, Things done well, Shepardson 6 Unit)

"Listen to your patients. If they say they don't want to talk about something, don't talk about it!"

(November 2014, Physician/Attending, Recommendations, Shepardson 6 Unit)

"Sincerity"

(November 2014, Physician/Attending, Things done well, Shepardson 6 Unit)

"Listened to what I wanted—good."

(November 2014, Physician/Attending, Things done well, Shepardson 6 Unit)

"Need love and Bible study."

(November 2014, Residents, Concerns, Shepardson 6 Unit)

"Get them to talk about their feelings."

(November 2014, Residents, Recommendations, Shepardson 6 Unit)

"Nice, kind patient peaceable friendly caring sympathetic soothing."

(November 2014, Residents, Things done well, Shepardson 6 Unit)

"Do Not Like patronization or Testing Like Zoo Animals. I AM HUMAN I AM A MAN..."

(November 2014, Nursing, Concerns, Shepardson 6 Unit)

"Most of them always wanted to help and listen."

(November 2014, Nursing, Things done well, Shepardson 6 Unit)

"Sincere, nice, caring, sympathetic, awesome."

(November 2014, Nursing, Things done well, Shepardson 6 Unit)

"Friendly kind patient helpful sweet caring."

(November 2014, Activities Therapy, Things done well, Shepardson 6 Unit)

"I would have preferred if they told me beforehand that I wouldn't be able to leave."

(November 2014, Admission Process, Concerns, Shepardson 6 Unit)

"Love thy neighbor as thyself."

(November 2014, Admission Process, Concerns, Shepardson 6 Unit)

"They listen and make accommodations according to our needs and desires."

(November 2014, Food, Things done well, Shepardson 6 Unit)

"Need to talk to patients more."

(November 2014, Techs/LNAs/Secretaries, Recommendations, Shepardson 6 Unit)

"Too many code calls too loud too many security used. Security shouldn't be on psych unit."

(November 2014, Environment, Concerns, Shepardson 6 Unit)

"All groups interesting, informative, and facilitate therapeutic dialogue between patients."

(December 2014, Activities Therapy, Things done well, Shepardson 3 Unit)

"Best care/concern for the most part comes from these people."

(December 2014, Activities Therapy, Things done well, Shepardson 3 Unit)

"Kept it brief and recognized my distress thus expedited the process."

(December 2014, Admission Process, Things done well, Shepardson 3 Unit)

"Sometimes some communication glitches since so many of them."

(December 2014, Techs/LNAs/Secretaries, Concerns, Shepardson 3 Unit)

"Everyone is different and has needs to be addressed. Proceed with caution."

(December 2014, Medication Teaching, Recommendations, Shepardson 6 Unit)

"I believe doctors should take more time to listen to their patients before making decisions or suggestions. If they don't have the time or feel rushed the doctors should minimize their patient lists so they do have time to listen to their patients. And make life changing suggestions. In my opinion it's part of their fiduciary responsibility as a health professional."

(December 2014, Physician/Attending, Recommendations, Shepardson 6 Unit)

"They only had a short time available. It takes at least 20 minutes to arrive at a proper diagnosis."

(December 2014, Resident, Concerns, Shepardson 6 Unit)

"All—demeanor—calmness—calming. Thank you, it's relaxing to converse with such people that are confident!"

(December 2014, Social Workers, Things done well, Shepardson 6 Unit)

"The techs and mental health staff here on the floor are fantastic. The patience and overall kindness I've witnessed is stellar. They are probably the least paid and have to be on the front lines. They don't get to hide behind bullet-proof glass and choose whether or not to deal with a patient. They [...] have no choice, they are stuck most of the time. I've seen them carry out their duties like true professionals. They all deserve to get a pay raise and much credit and thanks from all doctors and nurses."

(December 2014, Techs/LNAs/Secretaries, Things done well, Shepardson 6 Unit)

"Meds just shoved at you. No info given unless you refuse to take the med until you have med up on it." NOTE: In a post-session discussion, the patient was offered a consult with management, but declined.

(January 2015, Medication Teaching, Concerns, Shepardson 3 Unit)

"Explaining how medications should help my symptoms; explaining side effects."

(January 2015, Medication Teaching, Things done well, Shepardson 3 Unit)

"Don't spend enough time."

(January 2015, Physician/Attending, Concerns, Shepardson 3 Unit)

"Incorporating counseling/therapy with meds management (I wasn't expecting that)."

(January 2015, Physician/Attending, Things done well, Shepardson 3 Unit)

"Dr. [...]: good bedside manner, helpful suggestions and mental-emotional suggestions."

(January 2015, Residents, Things done well, Shepardson 3 Unit)

"She seemed to go out of her way to help me and others. She seemed to care deeply."

(January 2015, Social Workers, Things done well, Shepardson 3 Unit)

"Overall the groups I attended (which were many) were very good. Some therapists gave me individual attention outside the groups, which I appreciated."

(January 2015, Activities Therapy, Things done well, Shepardson 3 Unit)

"Everyone is professional and helpful, polite and friendly. Also non-judgmental."

(January 2015, Techs/LNAs/Secretaries, Things done well, Shepardson 3 Unit)

"Avoid all violence. Love because Christ first loved us."

(January 2015, Environment, Recommendations, Shepardson 6 Unit)

"Believe the patient about truly hurting and the certain meds are not working need something stronger no matter what their background is."

(February 2015, Pain Management, Recommendations, Shepardson 3 Unit)

"I wasn't ready to leave last time, I don't want to have Dr. [...] again. When doctor says you are ready to go apparently you should be fine. They don't listen, they do what they want to do."

(February 2015, Physician/Attending, Concerns, Shepardson 3 Unit)

"I feel that I should have a say if I'm not ready to leave or not. My feelings should count; no one knows how I feel better that myself."

(February 2015, Physician/Attending, Concerns, Shepardson 3 Unit)

"Hated him some days which meant he was doing his job."

(February 2015, Physician/Attending, Things done well, Shepardson 3 Unit)

"Very easy to talk to and knowledgeable. They give me hope."

(February 2015, Residents, Things done well, Shepardson 3 Unit)

"How much medication is too much medication? How does it affect me?"

(February 2015, Medication Training, Concerns, Shepardson 6 Unit)

"Too many young physicians, which often leads to group think."

(February 2015, Physician/Attending, Recommendations, Shepardson 6 Unit)

"Less time here and more time with [...] and his studies. The bedrock is family, friends, religion."

(February 2015, Activities Therapy, Things done well, Shepardson 6 Unit)

"Went smooth... very good transition felt cared for in a human & importantly humane way... good sense of humor which is the best medicine."

(February 2015, Admission Process, Things done well, Shepardson 6 Unit)

"Could keep their eyes open a little more. So much going on that is being missed. This is true of all staff. Many things went on that shouldn't have, which put a lot of stress on my taking care of myself."

(March 2015, Techs/LNAs/Secretaries, Recommendations, Shepardson 3 Unit)

"Dr. [...] was very caring and helpful to me. She heard from me that I was pursuing faith healing locally and was supportive of that as being a part of what I needed for treatment—as well as medication. I really appreciated her."

(April 2015, Physician/Attending, Things done well, Shepardson 6 Unit)

"I appreciate very much that this group honored by religious values, and this was very important need that I had. I was very open to many—that I was a Christian, and this group honored that, and some let me share a little bit with them, and some had questions for me—and that all worked out quite well—and this was a very important need that I had."

(April 2015, Activities Therapy, Things done well, Shepardson 6 Unit)

"Explanation of neurochemistry of meds."

(May 2015, Medication Training, Things done well, Shepardson 3 Unit)

"Clear lines of communication between patient and staff."

(May 2015, Pain Management, Things done well, Shepardson 3 Unit)

"It was evident that the people are highly skilled. However I found it difficult to grasp everything that was taught."

(May 2015, Activities Therapy, Things done well, Shepardson 3 Unit)

"Im a animal that belongs outside. Stop caging me in your hypnotizing medication schemes. I have no money, & refuse to be part of/support your figments of your imagination. In other words, there is no such things as a mentally ill person;--just a person. If anyone were to be pushed/pulled around enough, they would react in a crazy way. We're just animals. Im not sick. I need freedom. We need freedom."

(May 2015, Environment, Recommendations, Shepardson 6 Unit)

Part 2: Health Perception Survey

"The extra steps everyone has taken to help me be who I really am is heartfelt and appreciated greatly."

(January 2015, Shepardson 3 Unit)

"My well-being is much better at home with family and my stuff."

(January 2015, Shepardson 6 Unit)

"I thank you for soliciting my opinions. Because my medicines are given to me with no explanation as to their use or even their function, I appreciate this opportunity to speak on paper. At this time, I end hoping that if you need me to clarify these opinions, I will answer."

(January 2015, Shepardson 6 Unit)

"Improving health relies on people around for support and structure on lifestyle, happy friends, family."

(February 2015, Shepardson 6 Unit)

"Knowing people care makes all things better."

(February 2015, Shepardson 6 Unit)

"I had a life changing experience and this place made me into a better man."

(February 2015, Shepardson 6 Unit)

"I think the groups do help with the recovery."

(March 2015, Shepardson 3 Unit)

"I was a wreck when I came in here, honestly. Coming here and meeting so many new friends and people I would say really helped me out and get me through some hard times. I would say the 2 biggest factors that got me through this place would be Love and Faith. Without those 2 things, I would already be dead. I thank God every day for the second chance he gave and how much he smiles on my family, immediate and distant. I can't wait to get back into the real world and start helping people and saving lives, like I was put on this planet to do."

(April 2015, Shepardson 6 Unit)

"Yes, [answering: "How much do you believe in your ability to get better?"] improved in health, until I reach other stage of life when I'm on my way to death."

(May 2015, Shepardson 6 Unit)

13. Conclusions

At the end of this research, the image we obtained from the examination of these data is that patients value every aspect of the multilayered dimension making up their own perception and their interaction with the clinical/medical environment, as well as the scientific-therapeutic and the religious-spiritual perspective. Furthermore, the majority of patients seem to indicate that the combination of their personal ability to get better, the medical strength of the therapies provided and the mores spiritual/metaphysical spheres of life's meaning and purpose, including a spiritual dimension represents very important values in their effort to get better. In this regard, the data also suggests strong correlations between patient's perception of the causes of his/her health conditions and perceived positive/negative health outcomes, and between patient's perception of life's meaning and purpose and his/her ability to get better.

Moreover, since the vast majority of data was comprised between the highest scores on our scale (values 7–8), with much lower scores on the opposite side of the spectrum (values 1–2 on our scale) –thus leaving, *especially in negative answers* very few outliers indicating uncertainties in answering the questions (values 3 and 4, "somewhat" or "slightly" disagree)– the patients seemed to indicate a relatively strong belief in the answers they chose. More in detail, since the highest scores were found in those elements particularly connected to the patient's ability to get better, in cooperation (which is interaction) with his/her provider and to give meaning to his/her own life, also on the base of one's beliefs, we should definitely pay more attention to: a) what really matters to the patients, and b) to what really seems beneficial, in terms of therapeutic effectiveness, in patient's opinion and perception. Therefore, the data collected up to this point seem to confirm our predictions on the importance of such elements in our efforts to better understand patients and provide a better care, which takes into account those very spheres of investigation, interaction, and a possible therapeutic action. To be sure, we were not interested, at this stage, to find a direct causal link between the aforementioned concepts and the effectiveness of therapy. Our focus was on the way patients see themselves and/within the environment in diagnostics and therapy, therefore by investigating the relationship between patients and providers. The study suggests that a special emphasis in patient's attention and preference was found in those categories which directly work in strong connection (communicative, personal, and psychotherapeutic) with the patients, e.g. Activity Therapists, Psychiatrists, Mental Health Technicians, Licensed Nurse Assistants, and Social Workers. As we previously observed, Registered Nurses also obtained an important number of positive responses, albeit together with a great number (the greatest among staff on both units) of negative comments. The latter consideration is perhaps another confirmation of the importance of patient-provider communication, which not only underlies every clinical intervention (at least in a psychiatric unit) but turns out to be fundamental in therapeutic effectiveness. In other words, the results of our research suggest that, in order to guarantee an improvement in our care, we need to understand and work on all those aforementioned layers which constitute a patient *as* human being. Communication and (philosophical and medical) understanding are the keys. On a more individual, case-by-case level, many comments appear to follow the same perspective, in the sense that they seem to confirm the importance of concepts such as perception, sense of meaning, spirituality and communication-relation in diagnostics and therapy.

References and Further Readings

1. Bibliography

AA.VV. 1913. *Medical Philosophy*. The Lancet, Volume 181, No. 4662, p50, 4 January, Amsterdam, NL: Elsevier.

Abbagnano, N. and Fornero, G. 1986. *Filosofi e filosofie nella storia* (Philosophers and Philosophies in history), Torino: Paravia, II ed. 1992; for the analysis on the body-mind related issues, see in particular Vol. I, Chapters 2–6 and Vol. II, part 2; for a further debate on the contemporary logical debate on the relationship conscious - unconscious, please see Vol. 3, Chapter 5.

Abbot, N.C.; Harkness, E.F.; Stevinson, C.; Marshall, F.P.; Conn, D.A.; Ernst, E. 2001. *Spiritual healing as a therapy for chronic pain: a randomized, clinical trial*. Pain 91 (1–2): 79–89

Achinstein, P. 1983. *The nature of explanation*. Oxford: Oxford University Press.

Achtenberg J. 1996. *What is medicine*. Alternative therapy. 2(3): 58–61. For further information: http://www.alternatives_therapiescom/pdfarticle/9605-achterberg

Andersen, H. 2001. The history of reductionism versus holism approaches to scientific research. *Endeavor* 25: 153–156.

Antiseri, D., and Cagli, V. 2008. *Dialogo sulla diagnosi. Un filosofo e un medico a confronto*. Roma, I: Armando

Antiseri, D., and Timio, M. 2000. *La medicina basata sulle evidenze*. Milano, I: Edizioni Memoria.

Antiseri, D., and Vattimo, G. 2008. *Ragione filosofica e fede religiosa nell'era postmoderna*. Soveria Mannelli, I: Rubbettino Editore.

Aristotle. 1966. *Metaphysics*. H.G. Apostle, trans. Bloomington: Indiana University Press.

Baglivi, G. 1723. *Practice of physick*, 2nd edition. London: Midwinter.

Barnett, J.E., and Shale, A.J. 2013. *Alternative techniques. Today's psychologists are increasingly integrating complementary and alternative medicine techniques into their work with clients. Here's an overview of the most popular treatments, the research on their efficacy and the ethical concerns they raise*. Monitor on Psychology. Washington, DC: American Psychological Association, Vol 44, No. 4

Bartlett, E. 1844. *Essay on the philosophy of medical science*. Philadelphia: Lea & Blanchard.

Bassman, L. 1998. *The Whole Mind: The Definitive Guide to Complementary Treatment for Mind, Mood, and Emotion*. Novato, CA: New World Library

Beauchamp, T., and Childress, J.F. (2001) *Principles of biomedical ethics*, 5th edition. Oxford:Oxford University Press.

Beauregard, M., O'Leary, D. 2008. *The Spiritual Brain. A Neuroscientist's Case for the Existence of the Soul*. New York, NY: HarperCollins.

Behnke, S.H. 2014. *Always a cultural perspective. The Society of Indian Psychologists comments on the APA Ethics Code*. In Ethically Speaking, Monitor on Psychology, Vol. 45, N. 10

Bersoff, D.N. 1996. *Ethical Conflicts in Psychology*. Washington, DC: American Psychological Association.

Bettini, M. (Editor) 1991. *La maschera, il doppio e il ritratto. Strategie dell'identità* (The mask, the double and the portrait: strategies of Identity), Rome-Bari: Editori Laterza

Bialosky J.E., George S.Z., Horn M.E., at al. 2014. *Spinal manipulative therapy-specific changes in pain sensitivity in individuals with low back pain* (NCT01168999). The Journal of Pain; 15(2): 136–148.

Black, D.A.K. 1968. *The logic of medicine*. Edinburgh: Oliver & Boyd.

Blois, M. S. 1990. Medicine and the nature of vertical reasoning. New England Journal of Medicine, 318, 847–851.

Bobrow, D. G. (Ed.). 1985. *Qualitative reasoning about physical systems*. Cambridge, MA: MIT Press.

Bock, G.R., and Goode, J.A., eds. 1998. *The limits of reductionism in biology*. London: John Wiley.

Boncinelli, E. 2011. *La vita della nostra mente* (Our mind's life), Rome: Editori Laterza.

Bonelli, R., Dew, R.E., Koenig, H.G.; Rosmarin, D.H.; and Vasegh, S. 2012. *Religious and Spiritual Factors in Depression: Review and Integration of the Research*. Depression Research and Treatment.

Boorse, C. 1975. On the distinction between disease and illness. *Philosophy and Public Affairs* 5: 49–68.

Boorse, C. 1987. Concepts of health. In *Health care ethics: an introduction*, D. VanDeVeer and T.

Brianese, G. (Editor) 1998. *"Congetture e confutazioni" di Popper e il dibattito epistemologico post-popperiano* (Popper's Conjectures and Refutations and the post-Popper epistemological debate). I ed. – XIII, Turin: Paravia.

Boshuizen, H.P.A., and Schmidt, H. G. 1992. *On the role of biomedical knowledge in clinical reasoning by experts, intermediates, and novices.* In: Cognitive Science, 16(2), 153–184.

Buchler, J. 1955. Nature and judgment. New York, NY: Columbia University Press.

Bunge, M. 1989. Treatise on Basic Philosophy, Vol. 8: Ethics: The Good and the Right. Dordrecht & Boston: Reidel

Bunge, M. 2013. *Medical Philosophy. Conceptual Issues in Medicine*, Singapore: World Scientific Publishing

Breggin, P.R. 1991. *Toxic Psychiatry: Why Therapy, Empathy, and Love Must Replace the Drugs, Electroshock, and Biochemical Theories of the "new Psychiatry"*, New York, NY: St. Martin's Press

Britton W.B., Lepp N.E., Niles H.F., et al. 2014. *A randomized controlled pilot trial of classroom-based mindfulness meditation compared to an active control condition in sixth-grade children.* Journal of School Psychology. 2014; 52(3): 263–278;

Brody, H. 1992. *The healer's power.* New Haven, CT: Yale University Press.

Brooks, L. R., Norman, G. R., & Allen, S. W. 1991. *Role of specific similarity in a medical diagnostic task.* Journal of Experimental psychology: General, 120(3), 278–287.

Brown, L., and Jellison, J. 2011. *Auditory Perception of Emotion in Sung and Instrumental Music in Children with Autism Spectrum Disorders.* AMTA Published Journals Posters Research Catalog. Silver Spring, MD: American Music Therapy Association

Brown, W.S., Murphy N., and Maloney H. N. (eds.). 1998. *Whatever Happened of the Soul? Scientific and Theological Portraits of Human Nature.* Minneapolis: Fortress Press

Byron, P.B. (Ed.) 2011. *The Science of Emotion*, Boston, MA: Harvard Medicine

Cacciari, M. 2000. *L'ubiquità del centro* (The ubiquity of the Centre), in: Tema Celeste, n. 79–80, Milan: Gabrius, p. 94.

Caplan, A.L. 1986 Exemplary reasoning? A comment on theory structure in biomedicine. *Journal of Medicine and Philosophy* 11: 93–105.

Caplan, A.L. 1992. Does the philosophy of medicine exist? *Theoretical Medicine* 13: 67–77.

Carpenter, S. 2012. *That gut feeling. With a sophisticated neural network transmitting messages from trillions of bacteria, the brain in your gut exerts a powerful influence over the one in your head, new research suggests.* Monitor on Psychology, Vol 43, No. 8, Washington, DC: American Psychological Association, pp. 50–55

Carlat, D. 2010. *Unhinged: The Trouble with Psychiatry. A Doctor's Revelations about a Profession in Crisis*. New York, NY: Simon & Schuster

Carlson, N.R. 1994 (5th Ed.). *Physiology of Behavior*. Needham Heights, MA: Allyn and Bacon/Paramount Publishing,

Carter, K.C. 2003. *The rise of causal concepts of disease: case histories*. Burlington, VT: Ashgate.

Cassell, E.J. 2004. *The nature of suffering and the goals of medicine*, 2nd edition. New York: Oxford University Press.

Castel, A., Salvat, M., Sala, J., and Rull, M. 2009. *Cognitive-behavioural group treatment with hypnosis: A randomized pilot trial in fibromyalgia*. Contemporary Hypnosis, 26, 48–59

Cavalli-Sforza, L. L. and M. Feldman. 1981. *Cultural Transmission and Evolution: A Quantitative Approach*. Princeton, New Jersey: Princeton University Press.

Cefalù W.T., Floyd Z.E., Stephens J.M., et al. 2014. *Botanicals and translational medicine: a paradigm shift in research approach. Nutrition*. NIH PubMed. 2014; 30(7–8S): S1–S68

Chabris, C., and Simons, D. *The Invisible Gorilla*. New York, NY: Crown Publishing Group

Chandrasekaran, B., Smith, J. W., and Sticklen, J. 1989. *Deep models and their relation to diagnosis. Artificial Intelligence in Medicine*, 1, 29–40.

Chapman, G. B., and Elstein, A. S. 2000. *Cognitive processes and biases in medical decision making*. In G. B. Chapman & A. Frank (Eds.), Decision making in health care: Theory, psychology, and applications, pp. 183–210.

Cherkin D.C., Sherman K.J., Kahn J., et al. 2011. *A comparison of the effects of 2 types of massage and usual care on chronic low-back pain: a randomized, controlled trial*. Annals of Internal Medicine; 155(1): 1–9.

Christopher, J.C., Wendt, Marecek, J., D.C., Goodman, D.M. 2014. *Critical Cultural Awareness. Contributions to a Globalizing Psychology*. In *American Psychologist*. Vol. 69, Num. 7: 645–655 Washington, DC: APA, American Psychological Association.

Churchland, P. S. 2002. *Brain-Wise: Studies in Neurophilosophy*, Cambridge, MA: MIT Press.

Churchland, P. S. 2013. *Touching a nerve. The self as brain*, W.W. Norton & Company, New York, NY.

Clay, R.A. 2014. *Random Sample. James E. Maddux, PhD*. In: Monitor on Psychology, Vol. 45, N. 11, Washington, DC.: American Psychological Association

Clouser, K.D., and Gert, B. 1990. A critique of principlism. *Journal of Medicine and Philosophy* 15: 219–236.

Coiera, E. 2000. *When conversation is better than computation*. Journal of the American Medical Informatics Association, 7(3), 277–286.

Collingwood, R.G. 1940. *An essay on metaphysics*. Oxford: Clarendon Press.

Collins, F.S. 2006. *The Language of God. A Scientist presents Evidence for Belief*. New York, NY: Free Press Simon & Schuster.

Conboy L.A., Macklin E., Kelley J., et al. 2010. *Which patients improve: characteristics increasing sensitivity to a supportive patient-practitioner relationship*. Social Science & Medicine; 70(3): 479–484.

Cotton S., Roberts Y.H., Tsevat J., et al. 2010. *Mind-body complementary alternative medicine use and quality of life in adolescents with inflammatory bowel disease*. Inflammatory Bowel Disease; 16(3): 501–506.

Cook, C. 2004. *Addiction and spirituality*. Addiction, 99, 539–551.

Crichton, P. 2004. *When philosophy meets psychiatry*. The Lancet, Volume 363, No. 9410, p. 741, 28 February, Amsterdam, NL: Elsevier.

Coulter, A. 1999. Paternalism or partnership? *British Medical Journal* 319: 719–720.

Crespin D.J., Griffin K.H., Johnson J.R., Miller C., Finch M.D., Rivard R.L., Anseth S., Dusek J.A. 2015. *Acupuncture Provides Short-Term Pain Relief for Patients in a Total Joint Replacement Program*. Pain Med

Crumbaugh, J. C., & Maholick, L. T. 1964. *An experimental study in existentialism: The psychometric approach to Frankl's concept of noogenic neurosis*. Journal of Clinical Psychology, 20, 200–207.

Culver, C.M., and Gert, B. 1982. *Philosophy in medicine: conceptual and ethical issues in medicine and psychiatry*. New York: Oxford University Press.

Cutter, P. 1979. *Problem solving in clinical medicine*. Baltimore: Williams & Wilkins.

Daschle, T. 2008. *Critical: what we can do about the health-care crisis*. New York: Thomas Dunne Books.

Davis, R.B. 1995. *The principlism debate: a critical overview*. In: *Journal of Medicine and Philosophy* 20: 85–105.

Davis-Floyd, R., and St. John, G. 1998. *From doctor to healer: the transformative journey*. New Brunswick, NJ: Rutgers University Press.

Dawkins, R. 1989. *The Selfish Gene* (2 ed.), Oxford, UK: Oxford University Press.

DeAngelis, T. 2013. *Therapy gone wild. More psychologist are using the wilderness as a backdrop and therapeutic too in their work*. Monitor in Psychology, Vol. 44, No. 8. Washington, DC: American Psychological Association, pp. 48–52.

Desbordes G., Negi L.T., Pace T.W.W., et al. 2012. *Effects of mindful-attention and compassion meditation training on amygdala response to emotional stimuli in an ordinary, non-meditative state*. Frontiers in Human Neuroscience.

Dickinson H., Campbell F., Beyer F., et al. 2008. *Relaxation therapies for the management of primary hypertension in adults: a Cochrane review*. Journal of Human Hypertension; 22(12): 809–820.

Diener, E., Emmons, R. A., Larsen, R. J., Griffin, S. 1985. *The satisfaction with life scale*. Journal of Personality Assessment, 49, 71-75.

Diener, E. 2000. *Subjective well-being: The science of happiness and a proposal for a national index*. American Psychology, 55(1), 34–43.

Diener, E, and Oishi, S. 2003. *Personality, culture and subjective wellbeing: Emotional and cognitive evaluations of life*. Annual Review of Psychology 54: 403–425.

Dilthey, W. 1883. *Einleitung in die Geisteswissenschaften. Versuch einer Grundlegung für das Studium der Gesellschaft und der Geschichte*. Bd. 1, Leipzig, D: Duncker & Humblot.

Dimitrova, M. 2011. *In Levinas' Trace*. Newcastle upon Tyne, UK: Cambridge Scholars Publishing.

Dossey, L., Chopra, D., and Roy, R. 2010. *The Mythology Of Science-Based Medicine*. Huffpost Healthy Living. New York, NY: The Huffington Post

Dretske, F. 1971. *Conclusive Reasons* in *Australasian Journal of Philosophy* v. 49, London: Routledge, pp. 1–22.

Doubilet, P., &McNeil, B.1985. *Clinical decision making*. Medical Care, 23, 648–662.

Dowie, J., & Elstein, A. S. (Eds.). 1988. *Professional judgment: A reader in clinical decision making*. Cambridge, MA: Cambridge University Press.

Dummett, M.A.E. 1991. *The logical basis of metaphysics*. Cambridge: Harvard University Press.

Duncan, L.E., Pollastri, A.R., Smoller, J.W. 2014. *Mind the Gap. Why Many Geneticists and Psychological Scientists Have Discrepant Views About Gene–Environment Interaction (GxE) Research*. In *American Psychologist*. Vol. 69, Num. 3: 218–324 Washington, DC: APA, American Psychological Association.

Dusek, J. 2015. *Effectiveness of Integrative Therapies on Pain and Anxiety in Hospitalized Oncology Patients and Cardiovascular, Joint Replacement Patients*. A Series in Integrative Medicine. Jointly sponsored by Vanderbilt University School of Medicine Department of Medicine, Division of General Internal Medicine and Public Health and the Consortium of Academic Health Centers for Integrative Medicine (CAHCIM).

Earhart, G.M. 2009. *Dance as therapy for individuals with Parkinson disease*. European journal of physical and rehabilitation medicine 45 (2): 231–8

Eliade, M. 1984. *Immagini e Simboli* (Images and Symbols), I ed. Milan: Jaca Book.

Eliade, M. 1985. *Miti Sogni e Misteri* (Myths, Dreams and Mysteries), I ed. Milan: Rusconi Editore.

Ellis, A. 1994. *Reason and Emotion in Psychotherapy: Comprehensive Method of Treating Human Disturbances*. New York, NY: Citadel Press

Elsassar, W.M. 1998. *Reflections on a theory of organisms: holism in biology*. Baltimore: Johns Hopkins University Press.

Elstein, A. S., Kleinmuntz, B., Rabinowitz, M., McAuley, R., Murakami, J., Heckerling, P. S., et al. 1993. *Diagnostic reasoning of high- and low-domain-knowledge clinicians: a reanalysis*. Medical Decision Making, 13(1), 21–29.

Elstein, A. S., Shulman, L. S., & Sprafka, S. A. 1978. *Medical problem solving: An analysis of clinical reasoning*. Cambridge, MA: Harvard University Press.

Emanuel, E.J., and Emanuel, L.L. 1992 Four models of the physician-patient relationship. *Journal of American Medical Association* 267: 2221–2226.

Endres H.G., Zenz, M., Schaub, C., Molsberger, A., Haake, M., Streitberger, K., Skipka, G., Maier, C., 2005. *German Acupuncture Trials (GERAC) address problems of methodology associated with acupuncture studies*. Schmerz. Jun; 19(3): 201–4, 206, 208–10

Engel, G.L. 1977. The need for a new medical model: a challenge for biomedicine. *Science* 196: 129–136.

Engelhardt, Jr., H.T., ed., 2000. *Philosophy of medicine: framing the field*. Dordrecht: Kluwer.

Engelhardt, Jr., H.T., and Erde, E.L. 1980. Philosophy of medicine. In *A guide to culture of science, technology, and medicine*, P.T. Durbin, ed. New York: Free Press, pp. 364–461.

Engelhardt, Jr., H.T., and Wildes, K.W. Philosophy of medicine. 2004. In *Encyclopedia of bioethics*, 3rd edition, S.G. Post, ed. New York: Macmillan, pp. 1738–1742.

Engeström, Y., and Middleton, D. (Eds.) 1996. *Cognition and communication at work*. New York, NY: Cambridge University Press

Emanuel E.J., and Emanuel, L.L. 1992. *Four Models of the Physician-Patient Relationship*. JAMA. 1992; 267(16): 2221–2226

Ernst, E. 2004. *Anthroposophical medicine: A systematic review of randomised clinical trials*. Wien, A: Wiener klinische Wochenschrift 116 (4): 128–30

Evans, A.S. 1993. *Causation and disease: a chronological journey*. New York: Plenum.

Evans, M., Louhiala, P. and Puustinen, P., eds. 2004. *Philosophy for medicine: applications in a clinical context*. Oxon, UK: Radcliffe Medical Press.

Evidence-Based Medicine Working Group. 1992. *Evidence-based medicine: a new approach to teaching the practice of medicine*. In: *Journal of American Medical Association* 268: 2420–2425.

Feinstein, A.R. .1967. *Clinical judgment*. Huntington, NY: Krieger.

Feltovich, P. J., Johnson, P. E., Moller, J. H., & Swanson, D. B. 1984. *LCS: The role and development of medical knowledge in diagnostic expertise*. In W. J. Clancey & E. H. Shortliffe (Eds.), *Readings in medical artificial intelligence: the first decade* (pp. 275–319). Reading, Mass: Addison-Wesley.

Ferré, F., Kockelmans, J.J., Smith, J.E. 1982. *The Challenge of Religion. Contemporary Readings in Philosophy of Religion*. New York, NY: The Seabury Press.

Fleming, M.H. 1991. *Clinical Reasoning in Medicine Compared With Clinical Reasoning in Occupational Therapy*. American Journal of Occupational Therapy, November 1991, Vol. 45, 988–996.

Flyvbjerg, B. 1993. *Aristotle, Foucault and Progressive Phronesis: Outline of an Applied Ethics for Sustainable Development*; in: Winkler, Earl R., and Coombs Jerold R., *Applied Ethics*, Cambridge : Blackwell Publishers.

Fogassi et al. 2005. *Parietal Lobe: From Action Organization to Intention Understanding*, In: Science, Washington, D.C: American Association for the Advancement of Science.

Foglia, L. 2005. *Rappresentazioni Mentali. Modelli teorici a confronto*. Arkete, I (2), 17–42

Foglia, L. and Grush, R. 2010. *Neural reuse: A fundamental organizational principle of the brain*. Behavioral and Brain Sciences, Vol, 33, pp. 245–313

Foglia, L. and Grush, R. 2011. *The Limitations of a Purely Enactive (Non-Representational) Account of Imagery*. Journal of Consciousness Studies, 18, No. 5–6

Foglia, L. and Wilson, R.A. 2013. *Embodied Cognition*, Focus Article. Volume 4, Issue 3, pp. 319–325.

Fox, C. 2006. *A brain-based philosophy of life*. The Lancet, Volume 5, No. 3, p212, March, Amsterdam, NL: Elsevier.

Foucault, M. 1966. *The Order of Things: An Archaeology of the Human Sciences* (Les Mots et les choses: Une archéologie des sciences humaines), New York: Pantheon Books

Frankl, V. E. (1984). *Man's search for meaning* (3rd ed.). New York, NY: Washington Square Press. (Original work published 1946).

Fuchs, T., Birbaumer, N., Lutzenberger, W., Gruzelier, J., & Kaiser, J. 2003. *Neurofeedback treatment for attention-deficit/hyperactivity disorder in children: A comparison with methylphenidate*. Applied Psychophysiology and Biofeedback, 28, 1–12.

Fulford, K.W.M. 1989. *Moral theory and medical practice*. Cambridge: Cambridge University Press.

Fulford, K.W.M. 1991. The potential of medicine as a resource for philosophy. *Theoretical Medicine*. Dordrecht, NL: Kluwer Academic Publishers, 12: 81–85.

Gadamer. H.-G. 1960. *Wahrheit und Methode. Grundzüge einer philosophischen Hermeneutik*. Tübingen, D: Mohr Siebeck [Unveränd. Nachdr. d. 3. erw. Aufl. Tübingen 1975]

Gadamer, H.-G. 1993.*Über die Verborgenheit der Gesundheit*, Frankfurt a. M., D: Suhrkamp.

Gaizo M. Del. 1909. *L'opera scientifica di Giovanni Alfonso Borelli e la scuola di Roma nel secolo XVII*, Rome: Memorie della Pontificia Accademia Romana dei Nuovi Licei.

Galimberti, U. 1983. *Il corpo* (The body), XII ed. Universale Economica Saggi 2003. Milan: Feltrinelli

Gardiner, P. 2003. A virtue ethics approach to moral dilemmas in medicine. *Journal of Medical Ethics* 29: 297–302

Gawande, A. 2002. *Complications: A Surgeon's Notes on an Imperfect Science*. New York, NY: Metropolitan Books.

Gawande, A. 2007. *Better: A Surgeon's Notes on Performance*, New York, NY: Picador.

Gawande, A. 2014. *Being Mortal: Medicine and What Matters in the End*. London, UK: Macmillan

Gert, B., Culver, C.M., and Clouser, K.D. 1997. *Bioethics: a return to fundamentals*. Oxford, Oxford University Press.

Gergen, K.J., Josselson, R., Freeman, M. 2015. *The promises of Qualitative Inquiry*. American Psychologist, Vol. 70, No. 1, 1–60. Washington, DC: American Psychological Association, pp. 1–9

Gettier, E. 1963. *Is Justified True Belief Knowledge?*, in Martinich P. and Sosa D. (editors) 2001, *Analytic Philosophy*, Oxford: Blackwell Publishers.

Giardina, S., and Spagnolo, A.G. 2014. *I medici e il camice bianco. Note storico-culturali e implicazioni per la formazione dello studente di medicina*. Medicina e Morale 2014/2, Rome, I: Università Cattolica del Sacro Cuore.

Giddens, A. 1984. *The Constitution of Society. Outline of a Theory of Structuration*. Oakland, CA: The University of California Press

Gillies, D.A. 2005. Hempelian and Kuhnian approaches in the philosophy of medicine: the Semmelweis case. *Studies in History and Philosophy of Science Part C: Studies in History and Philosophy of Biological and Biomedical Science* 36: 159–181.

Gillon, R. 1986. *Philosophical medical ethics*. New York: John Wiley and Sons.

Giovetti, P. 2000 (Editor). *L'uomo e il mistero* (Man and Mystery). I ed, Vol. 8. Rome: Edizioni Mediterranee.

Gomora, X. 2003. *Ansichten eines Wilden über die zivilisierten Menschen* (Perspectives of a wild man on a civilized society), Klagenfurt: NOI-Verlag.

Gorski, T.N. 2002. The Eisenberg Data: Flawed and Deceptive. Quackwatch, article posted on March 16, available on http://www.quackwatch.org/11Ind/eisenberg.html

Greenhalgh T, Hurwitz B. 1999. *Narrative based medicine: why study narrative?* US National Library of Medicine, National Institutes of Health, PubMed BMJ. Jan 2, 1999; 318(7175): 48–50.

Goldacre, B. 2007. Benefits and risks of homoeopathy. The Lancet, Amsterdam, NL: Elsevier Volume 370, No. 9600, p. 1672–1673

Goldman, G.M. 1990. The tacit dimension of clinical judgment. *Yale Journal of Biology and Medicine* 63: 47–61.

Goldman, A. 1967. *A Causal Theory of Knowing* in *The Journal of Philosophy* v. 64 New York, NY: Columbia University Press

Goldman, L., and Ausiello, D.. 2004. *Cecil Textbook of Medicine, Philadelphia*, PA: Saunders, p. 45

Golub, E.S. 1997. *The limits of medicine: how science shapes our hope for the cure*. Chicago: University of Chicago Press.

Goodyear-Smith, F., and Buetow, S. 2001. Power issues in the doctor-patient relationship. *Health Care Analysis* 9: 449–462.

Gorowitz, S., & McIntyre, A. 1978. *Toward a theory of medical fallibility*. Journal of Medicine and Philosophy, 1, 51–71.

Griffin, D.R. (Ed.) 1998. *Reenchantment of Science: Postmodern Proposals*, New York, NY: State University of New York Press

Groopman, J. 2007. *How doctors think*. New York: Houghton Mifflin.

Guénon, R. 1962. *Simboli della Scienza sacra* (Symbols of the Sacred Science), VII ed. 2005, Milan: Adelphi, Original: *Symboles fondamentaux de la Science sacrée*, 1962 Paris: Gallimard.

Gungov, A.L. 2012. *Logic in Medicine: Approaches to Patient Safety*. Sofia, BG: Avangard.

Gungov, A.L. 2013. *Diagnostics in a Logical Perspective*, in Gungov, A.L., Kaneva V., and Kasabov, O. (eds). 2003. *Normativity: Contemporary Challenges*, Sofia, BG: St. Kliment Ohridski University Press.

Guyatt G., Rennie D., Meade M.O., and Cook D.J., 2014. *Users' Guides to the Medical Literature: A Manual for Evidence-Based Clinical Practice*, 2nd Edition: JAMA & Archives Journals, American Medical Association, New York: McGraw-Hill.

Haas M., Spegman A., Peterson D., et al. 2010. *Dose response and efficacy of spinal manipulation for chronic cervicogenic headache: a pilot randomized controlled trial*. Spine Journal; 10(2): 117–128.

Halpern, J. 2001. *From detached concern to empathy: humanizing medical practice*. New York: Oxford University Press.

Hameroff, S.R. 2006. *The entwined mysteries of anesthesia and consciousness*. Anesthesiology 105 (2): 400–412. doi: 10.1097/00000542-200608000-00024. PMID 16871075.

Hammrick, H.J., & Garfunkel, J.M. 1991. *Editor's Column-Clinical decisions: How much analysis and how much judgment?* Journal of Pediatrics, 118, 67

Hampton, J.R. 2002. Evidence-based medicine, opinion-based medicine, and real-world medicine. *Perspectives in Biology and Medicine* 45: 549–568.

Hardin E.E., Robitschek, C., Flores, L.Y., Navarro, R.L., Ashton, M.W. 2014. *The Cultural Lens Approach to Evaluating Cultural Validity of Psychological Theory*. In *American Psychologist*. Vol. 69, Num. 7: 656–668 Washington, DC: APA, American Psychological Association

Harman, G.H. 1965. The inference to the best explanation. *Philosophical Review* 74: 88–95.

Haug, M.R., and Lavin, B. 1983. *Consumerism in medicine: challenging physician authority*. Beverly Hills, CA: Sage Publications.

Häyry, H. 1991. *The limits of medical paternalism*. London: Routledge.

Hegel, G.W.F. *Phänomenologie des Geistes*, Suhrkamp Verlag Frankfurt am Main, I. Auflage (edition), 1986.

Heintzelman, S.J., and King, L.A. 2014. *Life is Pretty Meaningful*. In *American Psychologist*. Vol. 69, Num. 6561–6574. Washington, DC: APA, American Psychological Association

Herman P.M., Szczurko O., Cooley K., et al. 2008. *Cost-effectiveness of naturopathic care for chronic low back pain*. Alternative Therapies in Health and Medicine; 14(2): 32–39.

Heyting, A. 1956. *Intuitionism. An introduction.* Amsterdam: North-Holland Publishing

Hempel, C.G. 1965. *Aspects of scientific explanation and other essays in the philosophy of science.* New York: Free Press.

Hempel, C.G., and Oppenheim, P. 1948. Studies in the logical of explanation. *Philosophy of science* 15: 135–175.

Hill, A.B. 1965. The environment and disease: association or causation? *Proceedings of the Royal Society of Medicine* 58: 295–300.

Hiroshi, H. 1998. *On Vis medicatrix naturae and Hippocratic Idea of Physis.* In: Memoirs of School of Health Sciences, Faculty of Medicine, Kanazawa University 22: 45–54

Hollifield, M., Sinclair-Lian, N., Warner, T.D., and Hammerschlag, R. 2007. *Acupuncture for Posttraumatic Stress Disorder: A Randomized Controlled Pilot Trial.* The Journal of Nervous and Mental Disease.

Hofmann, E. 2003. *Progressive Muskelentspannung, ein Trainingsprogramm.* 2. Aufl. Göttingen, D: Hogrefe.

Holyoak, K., Morrison, R.G. 2012. *The Oxford Handbook of Thinking and Reasoning.* Oxford Library of Psychology. Oxford, UK: Oxford University Press

Howick, J.H. 2011. The philosophy of evidence-based medicine. Hoboken, NJ: Wiley-Blackwell.

Hölzel B.K., Carmody J., Vangel M., et al. 2011. *Mindfulness practice leads to increases in regional brain gray matter density.* Psychiatry Research: Neuroimaging; 191(1): 36–43.

Hudziak JJ, Albaugh MD, et al. 2014. *Cortical thickness maturation and duration of music training: Health-promoting activities shape brain development.* JAACAP. 2014; 11: 1153–1161.

Illari, P.M., Russo, F., and Williamson, J., eds. 2011. *Causality in the sciences.* New York: Oxford University Press.

Illich, I. 1976. *Limits to Medicine; Medical Nemesis: The Expropriation of Health.* London, UK: Marion Boyars Publishers.

Illingworth, P.M.L. 1988. The friendship model of physician/patient relationship and patient autonomy. *Bioethics* 2: 22–36.

Jackson, M. 2005. *Existential Anthropology—Events, Exigencies, and Effects (Methodology and History in Anthropology)*, California: Berghahn Books.

James, D.N. 1989. *The friendship model: a reply to Illingworth. Bioethics* 3: 142–146.

Jansen, K.L.R. 1998. *The Ketamine Model of the Near Death Experience: A Central Role for the NMDA Receptor.* Journal Article, London, UK: The Maudsley Hospital, Denmark Hill.

Jedel S., Hoffman A., Merriman P., et al. 2014. *A randomized controlled trial of mindfulness-based stress reduction to prevent flare-up in patients with inactive ulcerative colitis.* Digestion. NIH PubMed; 89: 142–155

Jensen, M. P., Ehde, D. M., Gertz, K. J., Stoelb, B. L., Dillworth, T. M., Hirsh, A. T., .Kraft, G. H. 2011. *Effects of self-hypnosis training and cognitive restructuring on daily pain intensity and catastrophizing in individuals with multiple sclerosis and chronic pain.* International Journal of Clinical and Experimental Hypnosis, 59, 45–63.

Johansson, I., and Lynøe, N. 2008. *Medicine and philosophy: a twenty-first century introduction.* Frankfurt: Ontos Verlag.

Jonsen, A.R. 2000. *A short history of medical ethics.* New York: Oxford University Press.

Jonsen, A., Siegler, M., and Winslade, W. 2002. *Clinical ethics: a practical approach to ethical decisions in clinical medicine.* New York, NY: McGraw-Hill.

Joseph, G. M., & Patel, V. L. 1990. *Domain knowledge and hypothesis generation in diagnostic reasoning.* Medical Decision Making, 10(1), 31–46.

Jung, C.G. 1963 (1990 ed.), *Mysterium Coniunctionis. Untersuchungen über die Trennung und Zusammensetzung der seelischen Gegensätze in der Alchemie*, Olten und Freiburg im Breisgau: Walter-Verlag

Kaku, M. 2011. *Physics of the Future: How Science will Shape Human Destiny and our Daily Lives by the Year 2100.* New York, NY: Doubleday

Kaku, M. 2014. *The Future of the Mind: The Scientific Quest to Understand, Enhance, and Empower the Mind.* New York, NY: Doubleday

Kaptchuk, T.J. 2000. *The web that has no weaver: understanding Chinese medicine.* Chicago, IL: Contemporary Books.

Kassirer, J.P. 1989. *Diagnostic reasoning.* Annals of Internal Medicine, 110(11), 893–900.

Kadane, J.B. 2005. Bayesian methods for health-related decision making. *Statistics in Medicine* 24: 563–567.

Kaliman P., Álvarez-López M.J., Cosín-Tomás M., et al. 2014. *Rapid changes in histone deacetylases and inflammatory gene expression in expert meditators.* Psychoneuroendocrinology; 40: 96–107

Kearney, R. and Rainwater M. 1996. The Continental Philosophy Reader, London & New York: Routledge.

Katz, J. 2002. *The silent world of doctor and patient.* Baltimore: Johns Hopkins University Press.

Kay, J. and Kay, R.L. 2003. *Ethnocultural Issues in psychotherapy*, in: Psychiatry: Therapeutics, Chapter 1: Individual Psychoanalytic Psychotherapy, II edition, Chichester, West Sussex, England: John Wiley & Sons

Kessler, R.C., Berglund, P., Demler, O., Jin, R., Merikangas, K.R., and Walters, E.E. 2005. *Lifetime prevalence and age-of-onset distributions of DSM-IV disorders in the National Comorbidity Survey Replication*. Archives of General Psychiatry, 62(6), 593–602.

Keysers, C. 2010. *Mirror Neurons*. Current Biology 19 (21): R971–973. doi: 10.1016

Kiecolt-Glaser, J.K., Graham J.E., Malarkey W.B., et al. 2008. *Olfactory influences on mood and autonomic, endocrine, and immune function. Psychoneuroendocrinology*; 33(3): 328–339.

Kiecolt-Glaser, J.K., Christian L., Preston H., et al. 2010. *Stress, inflammation, and yoga practice*. Psychosomatic Medicine; 72(2): 113–121.

Kienle, S.G., Kiene H. und Albonico H.-U. 2006. *Anthroposophische Medizin in der klinischen Forschung. Wirksamkeit, Nutzen, Wirtschaftlichkeit, Sicherheit*. Stuttgart, D: Schattauer

Kihlstrom J.F. 2002. *Mesmer, the Franklin Commission, and hypnosis: a counterfactual essay*. The International Journal of Clinical and Experimental Hypnosis 50 (4): 407–19

King, L.S. 1978. *The philosophy of medicine*. Cambridge: Harvard University Press.

Kleinman, A. 1988. *The illness narratives: suffering, healing and the human condition*. New York: Basic Books.

Klinger, B. 2015. *Non-Pharmacological Interventions to Chronic Pain. An evidence-based review of the use of integrative approaches including mind-body therapies and acupuncture to the management of chronic pain conditions*. University of Vermont College of Medicine / Laura Mann Integrative Healthcare Lecture Series, Burlington, VT.

Knight, J.A. 1982. The minister as healer, the healer as minister. *Journal of Religion and Health* 21: 100–114.

Knobe, J. and Nichols, S. 2008. *Experimental philosophy*. Oxford, UK: Oxford University Press.

Knobe, J. and Prinz, J. 2008. *Intuitions about Consciousness: Experimental Studies*. In: Phenomenology and Cognitive Science. University of North Carolina, Chapel Hill

Koyré A. 1966. *La rivoluzione astronomica. Copernico, Keplero, Borelli*, Milan: Feltrinelli.

Kong J., Kaptchuk T.J., Polich G., et al. 2009. *Expectancy and treatment interactions: a dissociation between acupuncture analgesia and expectancy evoked placebo analgesia*. NeuroImage; 45(3): 940–949.

Konner, M. 1993. *Medicine at the crossroads: the crisis in health care*. New York: Pantheon Books.

Kovács, J. 1998. The concept of health and disease. *Medicine, Health Care and Philosophy* 1: 31–39.

Kulkarni, A.V. 2005. The challenges of evidence-based medicine: a philosophical perspective. *Medicine, Health Care and Philosophy* 8: 255–260.

Kuipers, B., & Kassirer, J. P. 1984. *Causal reasoning in medicine: Analysis of a protocol*. Cognitive Science, 8(4), 363–385.

Kunstler, R., Greenblatt, F., & Moreno, N. 2004. *Aromatherapy and hand massage: Therapeutic recreation interventions for pain management*. Therapeutic Recreation Journal, 38, 133–147.

Lad, V.D. 2002. *Textbook of Ayurveda: fundamental principles of Ayurveda*, volume 1. Albuquerque, NM: Ayurvedic Press.

Lang, E.V., Berbaum, K.S., Faintuch, S. et al. 2006. *Adjunctive self-hypnotic relaxation for outpatient medical procedures: A prospective randomized trial with women undergoing large core breast biopsy*. Pain. PubMed.

Larson, J.S. 1991. *The measurement of health: concepts and indicators*. New York: Greenwood Press.

Le Fanu, J. 2002. *The rise and fall of modern medicine*. New York: Carroll & Graf.

Leder, D. 1990. *Clinical interpretation: The hermeneutics of medicine*. In: Theoretical Medicine March 1990, Volume 11, Issue 1, Dordrecht, the Netherlands: Kluwer Academic Publishers

Ledley, R. S., & Lusted, L. B. 1959. *Reasoning foundations of medical diagnosis*. In: Science, 130, 9–21.

Lee, M.S., Pittler, M.H., Ernst, E. 2008. *Effects of Reiki in clinical practice: a systematic review of randomized clinical trials*. International Journal of Clinical Practice 62 (6): 947–54

Lee, M.S., Oh, B., Ernst E. 2011. *Qigong for healthcare: an overview of systematic reviews*. JRSM Short Rep 2(2): 7.

Leontyev, A.N., Luria, A.R., and Smirnov, A. (Eds.) 1966. *Psychological Research in the USSR*. Moscow: Progress Publishers.

Leurent, B., Nazareth, I., Bellón-Saameño, j., Geerlings, M.I., Maaroos, H., Saldivia, S., Švab, I., Torres-González, F., Xavier, M., and Kin, M. 2013. *Spiritual and religious beliefs as risk factors for the onset of major depression: an international cohort study*. Psychological Medicine. London, UK: Cambridge University Press.

Levi, B.H. 1996. Four approaches to doing ethics. *Journal of Medicine and Philosophy* 21: 7–39.

Levinas, E. 1961. *Totality and Infinity. An Essay on Exteriority.* Pittsburg, PA: Duquesne University Press, 3rd ed. 1969.

Levinas, E. 1947. *Time and The Other.* Pittsburg, PA: Duquesne University Press, English Translation by Richard A, Cohen, 1987.

Leung, L. 2012. *Neurophysiological basis of acupuncture-induced analgesia–an updated review.* Journal of acupuncture and meridian studies, 5 (6), 261–270

Liberati, A. Vineis, P. 2004. Introduction to the symposium: what evidence based medicine is and what it is not. *Journal of Medical Ethics* 30: 120–121.

Licciardone J.C., Buchanan S., Hensel K.L., et al. 2010. *Osteopathic manipulative treatment of back pain and related symptoms during pregnancy: a randomized controlled trial.* American Journal of Obstetrics and Gynecology. 2010; 202(1): 43.e1–43.e8.

Lipton, P. 2004. *Inference to the best explanation*, 2nd edition. New York: Routledge.

Little, A.C., Jones, B.C., DeBruine, L.M. 2014. *Primacy in the Effects of Face Exposure: Perception Is Influenced More by Faces That Are Seen First.* Archives of Scientific Psychology, Washington, DC: APA, American Psychological Association, pp. 43–47

Little, M. 1995. *Humane medicine* Cambridge: Cambridge University Press.

Loewy, E.H. 2002. Bioethics: past, present, and an open future. *Cambridge Quarterly of Healthcare Ethics* 11: 388–397.

Loftus, S.F. 2006. *Language in clinical reasoning: using and learning the language of collective clinical decision making.* Sydney, AUS: Faculty of Health Sciences, School of Physiotherapy, University of Sydney.

Looijen, R.C. 2000. *Holism and reductionism in biology and ecology: the mutual dependence of higher and lower level research programmes.* Dordrecht: Kluwer.

Lowen, A. 1975. *Bioenergetics.* New York, NY: Coward, McCarin & Geoghen.

Lutz A., Brefczynski-Lewis J., Johnstone T., et al. 2008. *Regulation of the neural circuitry of emotion by compassion meditation: effects of meditative expertise.* PLoS ONE. 2008; 3(3):e1897

Maier, B., and Shibles, W.A. 2010. *The philosophy and practice of medicine and bioethics: a naturalistic-humanistic approach.* New York: Springer.

Malcolm, N. 1996. *Bosnia: a short history.* New York, NY: New York University Press.

Marchianò, G. 1991 (editor). *La religione della terra* (The religion of the Earth). Como, IT: Red Edizioni

Marcum, J.A. 2005. *Metaphysical presuppositions and scientific practices: reductionism and organicism in cancer research*. In: International Studies in the Philosophy of Science 19: 31–45.

Marcum, J.A. 2008. *An introductory philosophy of medicine: humanizing modern medicine*. New York: Springer.

Marcum, J.A., and Verschuuren, G.M.N. 1986. Hemostatic regulation and Whitehead's philosophy of organism. *Acta Biotheoretica* 35: 123–133.

Maslow, A.H. 1943. *A Theory of Human Motivation*. Originally published in *Psychological Review*, 1943, Vol. 50 #4, Washington, DC: APA, pp. 370–396

Matthews, J.N.S. 2000. *An introduction to randomized controlled clinical trials*. London: Arnold.

May, W.F. 2000. *The physician's covenant: images of the healer in medical ethics*, 2nd edition. Louisville: Westminster John Knox Press.

McDaniel, S.H., and deGruy III, F.V. 2014. *An Introduction to Primary Care and Psychology*. American Psychologist, Vol. 69, No. 4, 325–331. Washington, DC: American Psychological Association, p. 327

McKenzie, E. et al. 1998. *Healing Reiki*. Hamlyn Health & Well Being: Hamlyn

Meehl, P.E. 1954. *Clinical versus statistical prediction: a theoretical analysis and a review of the literature*. Minneapolis: University of Minnesota Press.

Miller, A. 2014. *Friends wanted. New research by psychologists uncovers the health risks of loneliness and the benefits of strong social connections*. Monitor on Psychology, Vol 45, No. 1 Washington, DC: American Psychological Association, pp. 54–58

Montgomery G.H., Bovbjerg D.H., Schnur J.B., David D., Goldfarb A., et al. 2007. *A Randomized Clinical Trial of a Brief Hypnosis Intervention to Control Side Effects in Breast Surgery Patients*. J National Cancer Institute; 99: 1304–1312

Montgomery, K. 2006. *How doctors think: clinical judgment and the practice of medicine*. New York, NY: Oxford University Press.

Moody, R. 1975. *Life After Life: the investigation of a phenomenon – survival of bodily death*, San Francisco, CA: Harper San Francisco

Morabia, A. 1996. P.C.A. Louis and the birth of clinical epidemiology. *Journal of Clinical Epidemiology* 49: 1327–1333.

Murphy, E.A. 1997. *The logic of medicine*, 2nd edition. Baltimore: The Johns Hopkins University Press.

Murphy N., and Brown, W.S. 2007. *Did My Neurons Make Me Do It? : Philosophical and Neurobiological Perspectives on Moral Responsibility and Free Will*. Oxford, U.K.: Oxford University Press.

Napolitano J.G., Lankin D.C., Graf T.N., et al. 2013. *HiFSA fingerprinting applied to isomers with near-identical NMR spectra: the silybin/isosilybin case*. Journal of Organic Chemistry; 78(7): 2827–2839

Naylor, T.H., Willimon, W.H., Naylor, M.R. 1994. *The Search for Meaning*. Nashville, TN: Abigdon Press

Nesse, R.M. 2001. *On the difficulty of defining disease: a Darwinian perspective*. Medicine, Health Care and Philosophy 4: 37–46.

Nestoriuc, Y., Martin, A., Rief, W., & Andrasik, F. 2008. *Biofeedback treatment for headache disorders: A comprehensive efficacy review*. Applied Psychophysiology and Biofeedback, 33, 125–140.

Nguyen H.T., Grzywacz J.G., Lang W., et al. 2010. *Effects of complementary therapy on health in a national U.S. sample of older adults*. Journal of Alternative and Complementary Medicine; 16(7): 701–706.

Nicolelis, M.A.L. 2011. *Beyond Boundaries: The New Neuroscience of Connecting Brains with Machines — and How It Will Change Our Lives*. New York, NY: Times Books.

Nidich S.I., Rainforth M.V., Haaga D.A.F., et al. 2009. *A randomized controlled trial on effects of the Transcendental Meditation program on blood pressure, psychological distress, and coping in young adults*. American Journal of Hypertension. 2009; 22(12): 1326–1331

Nordenfelt, L. 1995. *On the nature of health: an action-theory approach*, 2nd edition. Dordrecht: Kluwer.

Norman, G. R., & Brooks, L. R. 1997. *The non-analytical basis of clinical reasoning*. Advances in Health Sciences Education, 2(2), 173–184.

Norman, G.R., Brooks, L.R., Colle, C.L. and Hatala, R.M. 2010. *The Benefit of Diagnostic Hypotheses in Clinical Reasoning: Experimental Study of an Instructional Intervention for Forward and Backward Reasoning*. In: Cognition and Instruction, 17(4), 433–488, Hamilton, Ontario, CA: Lawrence Erlbaum Associates

Novotney, A. 2013. *Music as medicine. Researchers are exploring how music therapy can improve health outcomes among a variety of patient populations, including premature infants and people with depression and Parkinson's disease*. Monitor on Psychology, Vol. 44, N.10, Washington, DC: American Psychological Association, pp. 46–49.

Nozick, R. 1981. *Philosophical Explanations*. Boston: Harvard University Press

Overby, P. 2005. The moral education of doctors. *New Atlantis* 10: 17–26.

Pagnini, A. (Ed.). 2010. *Filosofia della medicina. Epistemologia, ontologia, etica, diritto*. Roma, I: Carocci.

Pahal, J.S., and Li, H.Z. 2006. *The dynamics of resident-patient communication: Data from Canada.* In: Communication & Medicine, 3(2), pp. 161–170. New York, NY: Mouton de Gruyter.

Papakostas, Y.G., and Daras, M.D. 2001. *Placebos, placebo effects, and the response to the healing situation: the evolution of a concept.* Epilepsia 42: 1614–1625.

Parker, M. 2002. Whither our art? Clinical wisdom and evidence-based medicine. *Medicine, Health Care and Philosophy* 5: 273–280.

Patel, V. L., & Arocha, J. F. 2001. *The nature of constraints on collaborative decision making in health care settings.* In E. Salas & G. Klein (Eds.), *Linking expertise and naturalistic decision making.* pp. 383–405. Mahwah, NJ: Lawrence Erlbaum Associates.

Patel, V.L., Arocha, J.F., Zhang, J. 2004. *Thinking and reasoning in medicine.* In: Holyoak, K. 2004: *Cambridge Handbook of Thinking and Reasoning.* Cambridge, UK: Cambridge University Press.

Patel, V. L., Evans, D. A., & Kaufman, D. R. 1989. *Cognitive framework for doctor-patient communication.* In D. A. Evans & V. L. Patel (Eds.), *Cognitive science in medicine: Biomedical modeling,* pp. 257–312. Cambridge, MA, US: MIT Press.

Patel, V. L., & Kaufman, D. R. 1994. *Diagnostic reasoning and expertise.* Psychology of Learning and Motivation, 31, 137–252.

Patel, V. L., & Kaufman, D. R. 1995. *Clinical reasoning and biomedical knowledge: Implications for teaching.* In J. Higgs & M. Jones (Eds.), *Clinical reasoning in the health professions,* pp. 117–128. Oxford: Butterworth Heinemenn.

Patel, V.L., Arocha, J., Zhang, J. 2010. *Medical Reasoning and Thinking.* In K. Holyoak and Morrison (Eds.), Oxford Handbook of Thinking & Reasoning. New York, NY: Oxford University Press.

Pellegrino, E.D., and Thomasma, D.C. 1981. *A philosophical basis of medical practice: toward a philosophy and ethic of the healing professions.* New York: Oxford University Press.

Penrose, R. 1989. *Shadows of the Mind: A Search for the Missing Science of Consciousness.* Oxford, UK: Oxford University Press.

Phillips, C.V., and Goodman K.J. 2004. *The missed lessons of Sir Austin Bradford Hill.* Epidemiologic Perspectives and Innovations 1 (3): 3. doi: 10.1186/1742-5573-1-3

Pinker, S. 2004. *The evolutionary psychology of religion.* Presented at the annual meeting of the Freedom from Religion Foundation, Madison, Wisconsin, October 29, 2004, on receipt of "The Emperor's New Clothes Award."

Pinker, S. 2007. *The mystery of consciousness.* New York, NY: Time Magazine

Pinker, S. 2010. *Ethics and the Ethical Brain*. In: Reuter-Lorenz, P.A., Baynes, K., Mangun, G.R., and Phelps, A.E. 2010. The Cognitive Neuroscience of Mind. A Tribute to Michael S. Gazzaniga. Boston, MA: Massachusetts Institute of Technology

Pole, S. 2006. *Ayurvedic medicine: the principles of traditional practice*. Philadelphia, PA: Elsevier.

Plantinga A.C. and Dennet, D. 2010. *Science and Religion*. Oxford: Oxford University Press

Post, S.G. 1994. Beyond adversity: physician and patient as friends? *Journal of Medical Humanities* 15: 23–29.

Prietula, M. 1981. *Expertise and error in diagnostic reasoning*. In: Cognitive Science, 5, 235–283.

Project of the ABIM Foundation, ACP-ASIM Foundation, and European Federation of Internal Medicine 2002. Medical professionalism in the new millennium: a physician charter. *Annals of Internal Medicine* 136: 243–246.

Power, D'Arcy 1897. *William Harvey: Masters of Medicine*, London: T. Fisher Dunwin

Quante, M., and Vieth, A. 2002. Defending principlism well understood. *The Journal of Medicine and Philosophy* 27: 621–649.

Raiffa, H. 1970. *Decision analysis*. Reading, MA: Addison-Wesley.

Ramoni, M. F., Stefanelli, M., Magnani, L., & Barosi, G. 1992. *An epistemological framework for medical knowledge based system*. IEEE Transactions on Systems, Man, and Cybernetics, 22, 1361–1375.

Rank, O. 1925. *Der Doppelgänger – Eine psychoanalytische Studie* (The Double: a psychoanalytic study), Wien: Turia+Kant, Wien 1993. Reprint der 1925 Wiener Ausgabe, Internat. Psychoanalytischer Verlag, The Estate of Otto Rank, Becket, Mass., USA

Rao R.P.N., Stocco A., Bryan M., Sarma D., Youngquist T.M., et al. 2014. *A Direct Brain-to-Brain Interface in Humans*. PLoS ONE 9(11): e111332. doi: 10.1371/journal.pone.0111332

Reason, J. T. 1990. *Human error*. Cambridge, UK: Cambridge University Press.

Reeder, L.G. 1972. The patient-client as a consumer: some observations on the changing professional-client relationship. *Journal of Health and Social Behavior* 13: 406–412.

Reich, W. 1927. *Die Funktion des Orgasmus*. Revidierte Fassung 1982: Genitalität in der Theorie und Therapie der Neurose/Frühe Schriften II, Köln, D: Kiepenheuer & Witsch

Reiser, S.J. 1978. *Medicine and the reign of technology*. Cambridge: Cambridge University Press.

Relman, A.S. 2007. *A second opinion: rescuing America's healthcare*. New York: Perseus Books.

Reznek, L. 1987. *The nature of disease*. London: Routledge & Kegan Paul.

Rho, K., Han, S., Kim, K., & Lee, M. S. 2006. *Effects of aromatherapy massage on anxiety and self-esteem in Korean elderly women: A pilot study*. International Journal of Neuroscience, 116, 1447–1455.

Ritenbaugh C., Hammerschlag R., Dworkin S.F., et al. 2012. *Comparative effectiveness of traditional Chinese medicine and psychosocial care in the treatment of temporomandibular disorders-associated chronic facial pain*. Journal of Pain; 13(11): 1075–1089.

Rizzi, D.A., and Pedersen, S.A. 1992. Causality in medicine: towards a theory and terminology. *Theoretical Medicine* 13: 233–254.

Rizzolatti, G., and Craighero, L. 2004. *The mirror-neuron system*. Annual Review of Neuroscience 27: 169–192.

Rizzolatti G., and Sinigaglia C. 2006. *So quel che fai. Il cervello che agisce e i neuroni specchio*. Milan, I: Raffaello Cortina Editore.

Rizzolatti G., Sinigaglia C. 2010. *The functional role of the parieto-frontal mirror circuit: interpretations and misinterpretations*. Nature reviews neuroscience, 11(4) 264–274.

Robiner, W.N, Dixon, K.E., Miner, J.L., and Hong, B.A. *Psychologists in Medical Schools and Academic Medical Centers. Over 100 Years of Growth, Influence, and Partnership*. In: *American Psychologist*. Vol. 69, Num. 3: 217–315 Washington, DC: APA, American Psychological Association.

Robinson, P. and Ellis N.C. (Eds.) 2008. *Handbook of Cognitive Linguistics and Second Language Acquisition*. London, UK: Routledge.

Rosenblueth, A. 1970, *Mind and Brain: A Philosophy of Science*. Cambridge, MA: MIT Press.

Rosenblueth, A. and Wiener, N. 1945. *The role of models in science*. Philos. Sci. 1945; 12: 316–321.

Roter, D. 2000. The enduring and evolving nature of the patient-physician relationship. *Patient Education and Counseling* 39: 5–15.

Rothman, K.J. 1976. Causes. *Journal of Epidemiology* 104: 587–592.

Russell, B. 1912. *The problems of Philosophy*. Barnes & Noble edition, New York, NY: Barnes & Noble

Ryff, C.D., and Singer, B. 1998. Human health: new directions for the next millennium. *Psychological Inquiry* 9: 69–85.

Sackett, D.L., Richardson, W.S., Rosenberg, W., and Haynes, R.B. 1998. *Evidence-based medicine: how to practice and teach EBM*. London: Churchill Livingstone.

Safranski, R. 1999. *Martin Heidegger – Between Good and Evil*. Cambridge, MA: Harvard University Press.

Salmon, W. 1984. *Scientific explanation and the causal structure of the world*. Princeton: Princeton University Press.

Saper R.B., Phillips R.S., Sehgal A., et al. 2008. *Lead, mercury, and arsenic in U.S. and Indian-manufactured Ayurvedic medicines sold via the Internet*. Journal of the American Medical Association; 300(8): 915–923

Satel, S., Lilienfeld, S.O. 2013. *Brainwashed. The seductive appeal of Mindless Neuroscience*. New York, NY: Basic Books

Saunders J. 2000. *The practice of clinical medicine as an art and as a science*. Medical Humanities. 26: 18–22

Schaef, A.W. 1992. *Beyond Therapy, Beyond Science*. New York, NY: HarperCollins

Schaffner, K.F., and Engelhardt, Jr., H.T. 1998. Medicine, philosophy of. In *Routledge Encyclopedia of Philosophy*, E. Craig, ed. London: Routledge, pp. 264–269.

Schönemann, D. 1999. *Der Spiritismus*. In: *Spiritismus. Sind paranormale Phänomene unumstößliche Beweise für ein Fortleben nach dem Tode?*. NOI International, Jahrgang 34, N. 128. Klagenfurt, A: NOI-Verlag, pp. 9–28

Schönemann, D. 2002. *Warum verstehen wir uns gegenseitig so oft nicht?*, NOI International 139/140, I. Aufl. Klagenfurt, A: NOI-Verlag.

Schwartz, W.B., Gorry, G.A., Kassirer, J.P., and Essig, A. 1973. Decision analysis and clinical judgment. *American Journal of Medicine* 55: 459–472.

Scotton, B.W., Chinen, A.B., and Battista, J.R. 1996. *Textbook of Transpersonal Psychiatry and Psychology*. New York, NY: Basic Books.

Seifert, J. 2004. *The philosophical diseases of medicine and their cures: philosophy and ethics of medicine, vol. 1: foundations*. New York: Springer.

Senn, S. 2007. *Statistical issues in drug development*, 2nd edition. Hoboken, NJ: John Wiley & Sons.

Simon, J.R. 2010. Advertisement for the ontology of medicine. *Theoretical Medicine and Bioethics* 31: 333–346.

Slagter, H.A., Lutz, A., Greischar, L.L., Francis, A.D., Nieuwenhuis, D., Davis, J.M., and Davidson, R.J. 2007. *Mental training affects distribution of limited brain resources*. PLOS Biology

Smart, J.J.C. 1963. *Philosophy and scientific realism*. London: Routledge & Kegan Paul.

Smuts, J. 1926. *Holism and evolution*. New York: Macmillan.

Slayton, S.C., D'Archer, J., and Kaplan, F. 2010. *Outcome Studies on the Efficacy of Art Therapy: A Review of Findings*. Art Therapy: Journal of the American Art Therapy Association, 27(3) pp. 108–111

Solomon, M.J., and McLeod, R.S. 1998. Surgery and the randomized controlled trial: past, present and future. *Medical Journal of Australia* 169: 380–383.

Spagnolo, A.G. 1997. *Bioetica nella ricerca e nella prassi medica*. Torino: Edizioni Camilliane

Spagnolo, A.G. 2008. *Quality of life and Ethical decisions in medical practice*. Journal of Medicine and The Person, vol.6, number 3: 118–122

Spagnolo, A.G. 2014. *La valutazione della ricerca in bioetica*. Medicina e Morale 2014/3: 355–365. Rome, I: Università Cattolica del Sacro Cuore.

Spodick, D.H. 1982. The controlled clinical trial: medicine's most powerful tool. *The Humanist* 42: 12–21, 48.

Stefanelli, M., & Ramoni, M. F. 1992. *Epistemological constraints on medical knowledge-based systems*. In D. A. Evans & V. L. Patel (Eds.), *Advanced models of cognition for medical training and practice* Vol. 97, pp. 3–20. Heidelberg, D: Springer-Verlag.

Steger, M. F., Frazier, P., Oishi, S., & Kaler, M. 2006. *The Meaning in Life Questionnaire: Assessing the presence of and search for meaning in life*. Journal of Counseling Psychology, 53, 80–93

Steiner, R. 1912.*Von Jesus zu Christus* (From Jesus to Christ). I. Aufl. Berlin. 1980 Dornach, CH: Rudolf Steiner Verlag.

Steiner, R. 2001 (Ed.) *Das esoterische Christentum und die geistige Führung der Menscheit* (Exoteric Christianity and the spiritual guidance of humanity). IV Taschenbuchausgabe aus der 4. Gesamtausgabe 1995. Dornach, CH: Rudolf Steiner Nachlaßverwaltung,

Steinhart, E.C. 2014. *Your Digital Afterlives: Computational Theories of Life after Death (Palgrave Frontiers in Philosophy of Religion)*. New York, NY: Palgrave McMillan

Steinpach, R. 2006 (Aufl.; Schönemann, D., Red.). *Wieso wir nach dem Tode leben und welchen Sinn das Leben hat*. In: *Der Tod, ein Übergang; das Jenseits, eine andere Realität*. NOI International, Jahrgang 41, N. 154. Klagenfurt, A: NOI-Verlag, pp. 8–43

Stempsey, W.E. 2004. The philosophy of medicine: development of a discipline. *Medicine, Health Care and Philosophy* 7: 243–251.

Stevenson, C.L. 1944. *Ethics and Language*, New Haven, CT: Yale University Press.

Stevenson, I. 1974 (2nd Ed.) *Twenty Cases Suggestive of Reincarnation*. Charlottesville, VA: University Press of Virginia.

Straus, S.E., and McAlister, F.A. 2000. *Evidence-based medicine: a commentary on common criticisms*. in *Canadian Medical Association Journal* 163: 837–840.

Summer, W.G. 1963. *Social Darwinism: Selected Essays*, ed. Stow Persons— Englewood Cliff, New Jersey: Prentice-Hall.

Svenaeus, F. 2000. *The hermeneutics of medicine and the phenomenology of health: steps towards a philosophy of medical practice*. Dordrecht: Kluwer.

Tallis, R.C. 2006. *Doctors in society: medical professionalism in a changing world*. in *Clinical Medicine* 6: 7–12.

Tasman, A., Kay, J., Lieberman, J.A. 2003. *Psychiatry. Second Edition. Therapeutics*. Chichester, West Sussex, UK: John Wiley & Sons.

Tauber, A.I. 2005. *Patient autonomy and the ethics of responsibility*. Cambridge: MIT Press.

Teyber, E. 2000. *Interpersonal Process in Psychotherapy. A relational approach*. (4th Ed).Belmont, CA: Wadsworth/Thomson Learning.

Thagard, P. 1999. *How scientists explain disease*. Princeton: Princeton University Press.

Tillich, P.J. 1983. *Gesammelte Werke*, 14 Bände + 6 Ergänzungs- und Nachlassbände, 1958–1983, Hg. Renate Albrecht, Stuttgart, D: Evangelisches Verlagswerk, (new edition by Verlag Walter de Gruyter, Berlin)

Tjeltveit, A.C., and Gottlieb, M.C. 2012. *Avoiding ethical missteps. By drawing on the science of prevention, psychologists can develop skills, relationships and personal qualities to bolster ethical resilience and minimize risks related to unethical behavior*. Monitor on Psychology, Vol 43, No. 4. Washington, DC: American Psychological Association, Vol 44, No. 4, pp. 68–74.

Todorov, I., Kornell, N., Larsson Sundqvist, M., Jönsson, F.U. 2014. *Phrasing Questions in Terms of Current (Not Future) Knowledge Increases Preferences for Cue-Only Judgments of Learning*. Archives of Scientific Psychology, Washington, DC: APA, American Psychological Association, pp. 7–13

Tonelli, M.R. 1998. *The philosophical limits of evidence-based medicine*. In *Academic Medicine* 73: 1234–1240.

Toombs, S.K. 1993. *The meaning of illness: a phenomenological account of the different perspectives of physician and patient*. Dordrecht: Kluwer.

Tracey, J.G., Wampold, B.E., Lichtenberg, J.W., Goodyear, R.K. 2014. *Expertise in Psychotherapy. An Elusive Goal?* In: *American Psychologist*. Vol. 69, Num. 3: 217–315. Washington, DC: APA, American Psychological Association, pp. 225–226

Trosseau A. *Lectures on clinical medicine*, The New Sydenham Society, 1869 Submitted by AL Wyman: Filler. Medicine: art or science. 1869 May; 2(320): 1322

Tucker N.H. 1999. *Presidential message Art vs Science*. Jacksonville Medicine. Dec., 50(12)

Unschuld, P.U. 2010. *Medicine in China: a history of ideas*, 2nd edition. Berkeley, CA: University of California Press.

Van Dalen, D. 2012. *L.E.J. Brouwer – Topologist, Intuitionist, Philosopher: How Mathematics Is Rooted in Life*. London: Springer

Van der Steen, W.J., and Thung, P.J. 1988. *Faces of medicine: a philosophical study*. Dordrecht: Kluwer.

van Gijn, J. 2005. From randomized trials to rational practice. *Cardiovascular Diseases* 19: 69–76.

Vassallo, N. 2002, *Epistemologia*, in D'Agostini F. and Vassallo N. (editors) 2002. *Storia della filosofia analitica*, Torino: Einaudi.

Vattimo, G., and Zabala, S. 2011. *Hermeneutic Communism: From Heidegger to Marx*, New York, NY: Columbia University Press.

Veatch, R.M. 1991. *The patient-physician relations: the patient as partner, part 2*. Bloomington, IN: Indiana University Press.

Velanovich, V. 1994. *Does philosophy of medicine exist?* A commentary on Caplan. *Theoretical Medicine* 15: 88–91.

Verene, D.P. 1997. *Philosophy and the Return to Self-Knowledge*. New Haven, CT: Yale University Press.

Vickers A.J., Cronin A.M., Maschino A.C., Lewith G., MacPherson H., Foster N.E., Sherman K.J., Witt C.M., Linde K., & Acupuncture Trialists' Collaboration 2012. *Acupuncture for chronic pain: individual patient data meta-analysis*. Archives of internal medicine, 172 (19), 1444–1453

Vickers A.J., and Linde, K. 2014. *Acupuncture for chronic pain*. JAMA: the journal of the American Medical Association, 311 (9), 955–956

Villar, F. 1996. *Gli Indoeuropei e le origini dell'Europa* (The Indoeuropeans and the origins of Europe), Bologna: Società editrice Il Mulino, 1997—Original Edition: *Los Indoeuropeos y los orígenes de Europa. Lenguaje e historia*, Madrid: Gredos, Madrid.

Vis, J., & Boynton, H. 2008. *Spirituality and transcendent meaning making: Possibilities for enhancing posttraumatic growth.* Journal of Religion & Spirituality in Social Work, 27, 69–86

Volk, S. 2011. *Fringe-ology: How I tried to Explain Away the Unexplainable—And Couldn't*, New York, NY: HarperCollins.

Vygotsky, L.S. 1962. *Thought and Language.* Cambridge, MA: MIT Press.

Vygotsky, L.S. 1978. *Mind in Society.* Cambridge, MA: Harvard.

Wade, C., Tavris, C., and Garry, M. 2014. *Invitation to Psychology.* 6th Edition. New York, NY: Person

Waterman, A.S. 2013. *The Humanistic Psychology-Positive Psychology Divide. Contrasts in Philosophical Foundations.* In *American Psychologist.* Vol. 68, Num. 3: 123–196 Washington, DC: APA

Weatherall, D. 1996. *Science and the quiet art: the role of medical research in health care.* New York: Norton.

Weindling, P.J. 2004. *Nazi Medicine and the Nuremberg Trials. From Medical War Crimes to Informed Consent.* Houndmills, Basingstoke, Hampshire, UK: Palgrave Macmillan.

Westen, D., and Weinberger, J. 2005. In praise of clinical judgment: Meehl's forgotten legacy. *Journal of Clinical Psychology* 61: 1257–1276.

Whitaker, R. 2001. *Mad In America: Bad Science, Bad Medicine, and The Enduring Mistreatment of the Mentally Ill*, New York, NY: Perseus Publishing

Whitaker, R. 2010. *Anatomy of an Epidemic: Magic Bullets, Psychiatric Drugs, and the Astonishing Rise of Mental Illness in America*, New York, NY: Crown

Whitbeck, C. 1981. *A theory of health.* In *Concepts of health and disease: interdisciplinary perspectives*, A.L. Caplan, H.T. Engelhardt, Jr., and J.J. McCartney, eds. London: Addison- Wesley, pp. 611–626.

Wildes, K.W. 2001. The crisis of medicine: philosophy and the social construction of medicine. *Kennedy Institute of Ethics Journal* 11: 71–86.

Wilson, C. 1971. *Das Okkulte*, (Original: The Occult) Lizenzausgabe für Parkland Verlag, Köln/Deutschland, 2004 Neu Isenburg: Melzer Verlag.

Wilson, R.A. and Foglia, L. 2011. *Embodied Cognition.* Stanford Encyclopedia of Philosophy. Palo Alto, CA: Stanford University Press.

Witt C.M., Berling N.E.J., Rinpoche N.T., Cuomo M.; Willich S.N. 2009. *Evaluation of medicinal plants as part of Tibetan medicine prospective observational study in Sikkim and Nepal.* Journal of Alternative & Complementary Medicine, 2009-01-0115:1, 59(7)

Wittgenstein, L. 1958. *Preliminary Studies for the "Philosophical Investigations", Generally known as The Blue and Brown Books*. Hoboken, NJ: Blackwell Publishers

Woodward, J. 2003. *Making things happen: a theory of causal explanation*. Oxford: Oxford University Press.

Wortman, J., Donnellan, M.B., and Lucas, R.E. 2014. *Can Physical Warmth (or Coldness) Predict Trait Loneliness? A Replication of Bargh and Shalev (2012)*. Archives of Scientific Psychology, Washington, DC: APA, American Psychological Association, pp. 13–19

Wrathall, M. 2006. *How to Read Heidegger*, New York, NY: W. W. Norton, p. 100

Wulff, H.R., Pedesen, S.A., and Rosenberg, R. 1990. *Philosophy of medicine: an introduction*, 2nd edition. Oxford: Blackwell.

Yeh G.Y., McCarthy E.P., Wayne P.M., et al.. 2011. *Tai chi exercise in patients with chronic heart failure: a randomized controlled trial.. Archives of Internal Medicine*; 171(8): 750–757; Wang C., Schmid C.H., Rones R., et al. 2010. *A randomized trial of tai chi for fibromyalgia*. New England Journal of Medicine; 363(8): 743–754..

Zaner, R.M. 1981. *The context of self: a phenomenological inquiry using medicine as a clue*. Athens, OH: Ohio University Press.

Zhang, J., Patel, V.L., Johnson, T.R., and Shortliffe, E.H. 2004. *A cognitive taxonomy of medical errors*. Journal of Biomedical Informatics 37 (2004) 193–204

Zürrer, R. 1989. *Reinkarnation. Die umfassende Wissenschaft der Seelenwanderung* (Reincarnation: the omni-comprehensive science of the migration of the body), IV. Aufl. 2000. Neuhausen, CH: Govinda-Verlag

Žižek, S., and Gunjević, B. 2012. *God in Pain: Inversions of Apocalypse*. New York, NY: Seven Stories Press

2. Quoted Works

Abbot, N.C.; Harkness, E.F.; Stevinson, C.; Marshall, F.P.; Conn, D.A.; Ernst, E. 2001. *Spiritual healing as a therapy for chronic pain: a randomized, clinical trial*. Pain 91 (1–2): 79–89

Andersen, H. 2001. The history of reductionism versus us holism approaches to scientific research. *Endeavor* 25: 153–156.

Aristotle. 1966. *Metaphysics*. H.G. Apostle, trans. Bloomington: Indiana University Press.

Barnett, J.E., and Shale, A.J. 2013. *Alternative techniques. Today's psychologists are increasingly integrating complementary and alternative medicine techniques into their work with clients. Here's an overview of the most popular treatments, the research on their efficacy and the ethical concerns they raise.* Monitor on Psychology. Washington, DC: American Psychological Association, Vol 44, No. 4

Bassman, L. 1998. *The Whole Mind: The Definitive Guide to Complementary Treatment for Mind, Mood, and Emotion.* Novato, CA: New World Library.

Beauregard, M., O'Leary, D. 2008. *The Spiritual Brain. A Neuroscientist's Case for the Existence of the Soul.* New York, NY: HarperCollins.

Behnke, S.H. 2014. *Always a cultural perspective. The Society of Indian Psychologists comments on the APA Ethics Code.* In Ethically Speaking, Monitor on Psychology, Vol. 45, N. 10

Bersoff, D.N. 1996. *Ethical Conflicts in Psychology.* Washington, DC: American Psychological Association.

Bialosky J.E., George S.Z., Horn M.E., at al. 2014. *Spinal manipulative therapy-specific changes in pain sensitivity in individuals with low back pain* (NCT01168999). The Journal of Pain; 15(2): 136–148.

Blois, M.S. 1990. Medicine and the nature of vertical reasoning. New England Journal of Medicine, 318, 847–851.

Bonelli, R., Dew, R.E., Koenig, H.G.; Rosmarin, D.H.; and Vasegh, S. 2012. *Religious and Spiritual Factors in Depression: Review and Integration of the Research.* Depression Research and Treatment.

Boshuizen, H.P.A., and Schmidt, H.G. 1992. *On the role of biomedical knowledge in clinical reasoning by experts, intermediates, and novices.* In: Cognitive Science, 16(2), 153–184.

Buchler, J. 1955. Nature and judgment. New York, NY: Columbia University Press.

Bunge, M. 2013. *Medical Philosophy. Conceptual Issues in Medicine*, Singapore: World Scientific Publishing

Breggin, P.R. 1991. *Toxic Psychiatry: Why Therapy, Empathy, and Love Must Replace the Drugs, Electroshock, and Biochemical Theories of the "new Psychiatry"*, New York, NY: St. Martin's Press

Britton W.B., Lepp N.E., Niles H.F., et al. 2014. *A randomized controlled pilot trial of classroom-based mindfulness meditation compared to an active control condition in sixth-grade children.* Journal of School Psychology. 2014; 52(3): 263–278;

Brooks, L. R., Norman, G. R., & Allen, S. W. 1991. *Role of specific similarity in a medical diagnostic task.* Journal of Experimental psychology: General, 120(3), 278–287.

Brown, L., and Jellison, J. 2011. *Auditory Perception of Emotion in Sung and Instrumental Music in Children with Autism Spectrum Disorders*. AMTA Published Journals Posters Research Catalog. Silver Spring, MD: American Music Therapy Association

Brown, W.S., Murphy N., and Maloney H. N. (eds.). 1998. *Whatever Happened of the Soul? Scientific and Theological Portraits of Human Nature*. Minneapolis: Fortress Press

Byron, P.B. (Ed.) 2011. *The Science of Emotion*, Boston, MA: Harvard Medicine

Caplan, A.L. 1992. Does the philosophy of medicine exist? *Theoretical Medicine* 13: 67–77.

Carpenter, S. 2012. *That gut feeling. With a sophisticated neural network transmitting messages from trillions of bacteria, the brain in your gut exerts a powerful influence over the one in your head, new research suggests*. Monitor on Psychology, Vol 43, No. 8, Washington, DC: American Psychological Association, pp. 50–55

Carter, K.C. 2003. *The rise of causal concepts of disease: case histories*. Burlington, VT: Ashgate.

Castel, A., Salvat, M., Sala, J., and Rull, M. 2009. *Cognitive-behavioural group treatment with hypnosis: A randomized pilot trial in fibromyalgia*. Contemporary Hypnosis, 26, 48–59

Cefalù W.T., Floyd Z.E., Stephens J.M., et al. 2014. *Botanicals and translational medicine: a paradigm shift in research approach. Nutrition*. NIH PubMed. 2014; 30(7–8S): S1–S68

Chabris, C., and Simons, D. *The Invisible Gorilla*. New York, NY: Crown Publishing Group

Chandrasekaran, B., Smith, J. W., and Sticklen, J. 1989. *Deep models and their relation to diagnosis. Artificial Intelligence in Medicine*, 1, 29–40.

Chapman, G. B., and Elstein, A. S. 2000. *Cognitive processes and biases in medical decision making*. In G. B. Chapman & A. Frank (Eds.), Decision making in health care: Theory, psychology, and applications, pp. 183–210.

Cherkin D.C., Sherman K.J., Kahn J., et al. 2011. *A comparison of the effects of 2 types of massage and usual care on chronic low-back pain: a randomized, controlled trial*. Annals of Internal Medicine; 155(1): 1–9.

Christopher, J.C., Wendt, Marecek, J., D.C., Goodman, D.M. 2014. *Critical Cultural Awareness. Contributions to a Globalizing Psychology*. In *American Psychologist*. Vol. 69, Num. 7: 645–655 Washington, DC: APA, American Psychological Association.

Churchland, P. S. 2013. *Touching a nerve. The self as brain*, W.W. Norton & Company, New York, NY, p. 11

Clay, R.A. 2014. *Random Sample. James E. Maddux, PhD*. In: Monitor on Psychology, Vol. 45, N. 11, Washington, DC.: American Psychological Association

Collins, F.S. 2006. *The Language of God. A Scientist presents Evidence for Belief*. New York, NY: Free Press Simon & Schuster.

Cotton S., Roberts Y.H., Tsevat J., et al. 2010. *Mind-body complementary alternative medicine use and quality of life in adolescents with inflammatory bowel disease*. Inflammatory Bowel Disease; 16(3): 501–506.

Cook, C. 2004. *Addiction and spirituality*. Addiction, 99, 539–551.

Crespin D.J., Griffin K.H., Johnson J.R., Miller C., Finch M.D., Rivard R.L., Anseth S., Dusek J.A. 2015. *Acupuncture Provides Short-Term Pain Relief for Patients in a Total Joint Replacement Program*. Pain Med

Crumbaugh, J. C., & Maholick, L. T. 1964. *An experimental study in existentialism: The psychometric approach to Frankl's concept of noogenic neurosis*. Journal of Clinical Psychology, 20, 200–207.

Culver, C.M., and Gert, B. 1982. *Philosophy in medicine: conceptual and ethical issues in medicine and psychiatry*. New York: Oxford University Press.

Cutter, P. 1979. *Problem solving in clinical medicine*. Baltimore: Williams & Wilkins.

Daschle, T. 2008. *Critical: what we can do about the health-care crisis*. New York: Thomas Dunne Books.

Davis-Floyd, R., and St. John, G. 1998. *From doctor to healer: the transformative journey*. New Brunswick, NJ: Rutgers University Press.

Dawkins, R. 1989. *The Selfish Gene* (2 ed.), Oxford, UK: Oxford University Press.

DeAngelis, T. 2013. *Therapy gone wild. More psychologist are using the wilderness as a backdrop and therapeutic too in their work*. Monitor in Psychology, Vol. 44, No. 8. Washington, DC: American Psychological Association, pp. 48–52.

Desbordes G., Negi L.T., Pace T.W.W., et al. 2012. *Effects of mindful-attention and compassion meditation training on amygdala response to emotional stimuli in an ordinary, non-meditative state*. Frontiers in Human Neuroscience.

Dickinson H., Campbell F., Beyer F., et al. 2008. *Relaxation therapies for the management of primary hypertension in adults: a Cochrane review*. Journal of Human Hypertension; 22(12): 809–820.

Diener, E., Emmons, R. A., Larsen, R. J., Griffin, S. 1985. *The satisfaction with life scale*. Journal of Personality Assessment, 49, 71–75.

Diener, E. 2000. *Subjective well-being: The science of happiness and a proposal for a national index*. American Psychology, 55(1), 34–43.

Diener, E., and Oishi, S. 2003. *Personality, culture and subjective wellbeing: Emotional and cognitive evaluations of life*. Annual Review of Psychology 54: 403–425.

Dossey, L., Chopra, D., and Roy, R. 2010. *The Mythology Of Science-Based Medicine*. Huffpost Healthy Living. New York, NY: The Huffington Post

Dummett, M.A.E. 1991. *The logical basis of metaphysics*. Cambridge: Harvard University Press.

Duncan, L.E., Pollastri, A.R., Smoller, J.W. 2014. *Mind the Gap. Why Many Geneticists and Psychological Scientists Have Discrepant Views About Gene–Environment Interaction (GxE) Research*. In *American Psychologist*. Vol. 69, Num. 3: 218–324 Washington, DC: APA, American Psychological Association.

Dusek, J. 2015. *Effectiveness of Integrative Therapies on Pain and Anxiety in Hospitalized Oncology Patients and Cardiovascular, Joint Replacement Patients*. A Series in Integrative Medicine. Jointly sponsored by Vanderbilt University School of Medicine Department of Medicine, Division of General Internal Medicine and Public Health and the Consortium of Academic Health Centers for Integrative Medicine (CAHCIM).

Earhart, G.M. 2009. *Dance as therapy for individuals with Parkinson disease*. European journal of physical and rehabilitation medicine 45 (2): 231–238

Emanuel, E.J., and Emanuel, L.L. 1992 Four models of the physician-patient relationship. *Journal of American Medical Association* 267: 2221–2226.

Endres H.G., Zenz, M., Schaub, C., Molsberger, A., Haake, M., Streitberger, K., Skipka, G., Maier, C., 2005. *German Acupuncture Trials (GERAC) address problems of methodology associated with acupuncture studies*. Schmerz. Jun; 19(3): 201–204, 206, 208–210

Engelhardt, Jr., H.T., ed., 2000. *Philosophy of medicine: framing the field*. Dordrecht: Kluwer.

Emanuel E.J., and Emanuel, L.L. 1992. *Four Models of the Physician-Patient Relationship*. JAMA. 1992; 267(16): 2221–2226

Ernst, E. 2004. *Anthroposophical medicine: A systematic review of randomised clinical trials*. Wien, A: Wiener klinische Wochenschrift 116 (4): 128–30

Evans, M., Louhiala, P. and Puustinen, P., eds. 2004. *Philosophy for medicine: applications in a clinical context*. Oxon, UK: Radcliffe Medical Press.

Ferré, F., Kockelmans, J.J., Smith, J.E. 1982. *The Challenge of Religion. Contemporary Readings in Philosophy of Religion*. New York, NY: The Seabury Press.

Fleming, M.H. 1991. *Clinical Reasoning in Medicine Compared With Clinical Reasoning in Occupational Therapy*. American Journal of Occupational Therapy, November 1991, Vol. 45, 988–996.

Flyvbjerg, B. 1993. *Aristotle, Foucault and Progressive Phronesis: Outline of an Applied Ethics for Sustainable Development*; in: Winkler, Earl R., and Coombs Jerold R., *Applied Ethics*, Cambridge : Blackwell Publishers.

Foglia, L. 2005. *Rappresentazioni Mentali. Modelli teorici a confronto*. Arkete, I (2), 17–42

Foglia, L. and Grush, R. 2010. *Neural reuse: A fundamental organizational principle of the brain*. Behavioral and Brain Sciences, Vol, 33, pp. 245–313

Foglia, L. and Grush, R. 2011. *The Limitations of a Purely Enactive (Non-Representational) Account of Imagery*. Journal of Consciousness Studies, 18, No. 5–6

Fox, C. 2006. *A brain-based philosophy of life*. The Lancet, Volume 5, No. 3, p. 212, March, Amsterdam, NL: Elsevier.

Foucault, M. 1966. *The Order of Things: An Archaeology of the Human Sciences* (Les Mots et les choses: Une archéologie des sciences humaines), New York: Pantheon Books

Frankl, V. E. (1984). *Man's search for meaning* (3rd ed.). New York, NY: Washington Square Press. (Original work published 1946).

Fuchs, T., Birbaumer, N., Lutzenberger, W., Gruzelier, J., & Kaiser, J. 2003. Neurofeedback treatment for attention-deficit/hyperactivity disorder in children: A comparison with methylphenidate. *Applied Psychophysiology and Biofeedback*, 28: 1–12.

Fulford, K.W.M. 1991. The potential of medicine as a resource for philosophy. *Theoretical Medicine*. Dordrecht, NL: Kluwer Academic Publishers, 12: 81–85.

Gadamer. H.-G. 1960. *Wahrheit und Methode. Grundzüge einer philosophischen Hermeneutik*. Tübingen, D: Mohr Siebeck [Unveränd. Nachdr. d. 3. erw. Aufl. Tübingen 1975]

Gadamer, H.-G. 1993. *Über die Verborgenheit der Gesundheit*, Frankfurt a. M., D: Suhrkamp.

Gawande, A. 2002. *Complications: A Surgeon's Notes on an Imperfect Science*. New York, NY: Metropolitan Books.

Gawande, A. 2014. *Being Mortal: Medicine and What Matters in the End*. London, UK: Macmillan

Gergen, K.J., Josselson, R., Freeman, M. 2015. *The promises of Qualitative Inquiry*. American Psychologist, Vol. 70, No. 1, 1–60. Washington, DC: American Psychological Association, pp. 1–9

Giardina, S., and Spagnolo, A.G. 2014. *I medici e il camice bianco. Note storico-culturali e implicazioni per la formazione dello studente di medicina*. Medicina e Morale 2014/2, Rome, I: Università Cattolica del Sacro Cuore

Gillon, R. 1986. *Philosophical medical ethics*. New York: John Wiley and Sons.

Gorski, T.N. 2002. The Eisenberg Data: Flawed and Deceptive. Quackwatch, article posted on March 16, available on: http://www.quackwatch.org/11Ind/eisen berg.html

Goldacre, B. 2007. Benefits and risks of homoeopathy. The Lancet, Amsterdam, NL: Elsevier Volume 370, No. 9600, pp. 1672–1673

Goodyear-Smith, F., and Buetow, S. 2001. *Power issues in the doctor-patient relationship*. Health Care Analysis 9: 449–462.

Groopman, J. 2007. *How doctors think*. New York: Houghton Mifflin.

Gungov, A.L. 2012. *Logic in Medicine: Approaches to Patient Safety*. Sofia, BG: Avangard.

Gungov, A.L. 2013. *Diagnostics in a Logical Perspective*, in Gungov, A.L., Kaneva V., and Kasabov, O. (eds). 2003. *Normativity: Contemporary Challenges*, Sofia, BG: St. Kliment Ohridski University Press.

Haas M., Spegman A., Peterson D., et al. 2010. *Dose response and efficacy of spinal manipulation for chronic cervicogenic headache: a pilot randomized controlled trial*. Spine Journal; 10(2): 117–128.

Hameroff, S.R. 2006. *The entwined mysteries of anesthesia and consciousness*. Anesthesiology 105 (2): 400–412. doi: 10.1097/00000542-200608000-00024. PMID 16871075.

Hampton, J.R. 2002. Evidence-based medicine, opinion-based medicine, and real-world medicine. *Perspectives in Biology and Medicine* 45: 549–68.

Hardin E.E., Robitschek, C., Flores, L.Y., Navarro, R.L., Ashton, M.W. 2014. *The Cultural Lens Approach to Evaluating Cultural Validity of Psychological Theory*. In *American Psychologist*. Vol. 69, Num. 7: 656–668 Washington, DC: APA, American Psychological Association

Hegel, G.W.F. *Phänomenologie des Geistes*, Suhrkamp Verlag Frankfurt am Main, I. Auflage (edition), 1986. For the English version, please refer to the translation by J. B. Baillie, Blackmask Online Edition, 2001.

Heintzelman, S.J., and King, L.A. 2014. *Life is Pretty Meaningful*. In *American Psychologist*. Vol. 69, Num. 6561–6574. Washington, DC: APA, American Psychological Association

Herman P.M., Szczurko O., Cooley K., et al. 2008. *Cost-effectiveness of naturopathic care for chronic low back pain*. Alternative Therapies in Health and Medicine; 14(2): 32–39..

Hill, A.B. 1965. The environment and disease: association or causation? *Proceedings of the Royal Society of Medicine* 58: 295–300.

Hollifield, M., Sinclair-Lian, N., Warner, T.D., and Hammerschlag, R. 2007. *Acupuncture for Posttraumatic Stress Disorder: A Randomized Controlled Pilot Trial*. The Journal of Nervous and Mental Disease.

Hofmann, E. 2003. *Progressive Muskelentspannung, ein Trainingsprogramm*. 2. Aufl. Göttingen, D: Hogrefe.

Holyoak, K., Morrison, R.G. 2012. *The Oxford Handbook of Thinking and Reasoning*. Oxford Library of Psychology. Oxford, UK: Oxford University Press

Hölzel B.K., Carmody J., Vangel M., et al. 2011. *Mindfulness practice leads to increases in regional brain gray matter density*. Psychiatry Research: Neuroimaging; 191(1): 36–43.

Hudziak JJ, Albaugh MD, et al. 2014. *Cortical thickness maturation and duration of music training: Health-promoting activities shape brain development*. JAACAP. 2014; 11: 1153–1161.

Illari, P.M., Russo, F., and Williamson, J., eds. 2011. *Causality in the sciences*. New York: Oxford University Press.

Illich, I. 1976. *Limits to Medicine; Medical Nemesis: The Expropriation of Health*. London, UK: Marion Boyars Publishers.

Jackson, M. 2005. *Existential Anthropology—Events, Exigencies, and Effects (Methodology and History in Anthropology)*, California: Berghahn Books.

Jansen, K.L.R. 1998. *The Ketamine Model of the Near Death Experience: A Central Role for the NMDA Receptor*. Journal Article, London, UK: The Maudsley Hospital, Denmark Hill.

Jedel S., Hoffman A., Merriman P., et al. 2014. *A randomized controlled trial of mindfulness-based stress reduction to prevent flare-up in patients with inactive ulcerative colitis*. Digestion. NIH PubMed; 89: 142–155

Jensen, M. P., Ehde, D. M., Gertz, K. J., Stoelb, B. L., Dillworth, T. M., Hirsh, A. T., .Kraft, G. H. 2011. *Effects of self-hypnosis training and cognitive restructuring on daily pain intensity and catastrophizing in individuals with multiple sclerosis and chronic pain*. International Journal of Clinical and Experimental Hypnosis, 59, 45–63.

Johansson, I., and Lynøe, N. 2008. *Medicine and philosophy: a twenty-first century introduction*. Frankfurt: Ontos Verlag.

Jonsen, A., Siegler, M., and Winslade, W. 2002. *Clinical ethics: a practical approach to ethical decisions in clinical medicine*. New York, NY: McGraw-Hill.

Joseph, G. M., & Patel, V. L. 1990. *Domain knowledge and hypothesis generation in diagnostic reasoning*. Medical Decision Making, 10(1), 31–46.

Jung, C.G. 1963 (1990 ed.), *Mysterium Coniunctionis. Untersuchungen über die Trennung und Zusammensetzung der seelischen Gegensätze in der Alchemie*, Olten und Freiburg im Breisgau: Walter-Verlag

Kaku, M. 2014. *The Future of the Mind: The Scientific Quest to Understand, Enhance, and Empower the Mind.* New York, NY: Doubleday

Kaptchuk, T.J. 2000. *The web that has no weaver: understanding Chinese medicine.* Chicago, IL: Contemporary Books.

Kaliman P., Álvarez-López M.J., Cosín-Tomás M., et al. 2014. *Rapid changes in histone deacetylases and inflammatory gene expression in expert meditators.* Psychoneuroendocrinology; 40: 96–107

Kearney, R. and Rainwater M. 1996. The Continental Philosophy Reader, London & New York: Routledge.

Kay, J. and Kay, R.L. 2003. *Ethnocultural Issues in psychotherapy*, in: Psychiatry: Therapeutics, Chapter 1: Individual Psychoanalytic Psychotherapy, II edition, Chichester, West Sussex, England: John Wiley & Sons

Kiecolt-Glaser, J.K., Graham J.E, Malarkey W.B., et al. 2008. *Olfactory influences on mood and autonomic, endocrine, and immune function. Psychoneuroendocrinology*; 33(3): 328–339.

Kiecolt-Glaser, J.K., Christian L., Preston H., et al. 2010. *Stress, inflammation, and yoga practice.* Psychosomatic Medicine; 72(2): 113–121.

Kienle, S.G., Kiene H. und Albonico H.-U. 2006. *Anthroposophische Medizin in der klinischen Forschung. Wirksamkeit, Nutzen, Wirtschaftlichkeit, Sicherheit.* Stuttgart, D: Schattauer

Kihlstrom J.F. 2002. *Mesmer, the Franklin Commission, and hypnosis: a counterfactual essay.* The International Journal of Clinical and Experimental Hypnosis 50 (4): 407–19

Klinger, B. 2015. *Non-Pharmacological Interventions to Chronic Pain. An evidence-based review of the use of integrative approaches including mind-body therapies and acupuncture to the management of chronic pain conditions.* University of Vermont College of Medicine / Laura Mann Integrative Healthcare Lecture Series, Burlington, VT.

Knight, J.A. 1982. The minister as healer, the healer as minister. *Journal of Religion and Health* 21: 100–114.

Kong J., Kaptchuk T.J., Polich G., et al. 2009. *Expectancy and treatment interactions: a dissociation between acupuncture analgesia and expectancy evoked placebo analgesia.* NeuroImage; 45(3): 940–949.

Kuipers, B., & Kassirer, J.P. 1984. *Causal reasoning in medicine: Analysis of a protocol.* Cognitive Science, 8(4), 363–385.

Kunstler, R., Greenblatt, F., & Moreno, N. 2004. *Aromatherapy and hand massage: Therapeutic recreation interventions for pain management*. Therapeutic Recreation Journal, 38, 133–147.

Lang, E.V., Berbaum, K.S., Faintuch, S. et al. 2006. *Adjunctive self-hypnotic relaxation for outpatient medical procedures: A prospective randomized trial with women undergoing large core breast biopsy*. Pain. PubMed.

Lee, M.S., Pittler, M.H., Ernst, E. 2008. *Effects of Reiki in clinical practice: a systematic review of randomized clinical trials*. International Journal of Clinical Practice 62 (6): 947–54

Lee, M.S., Oh, B., Ernst E. 2011. *Qigong for healthcare: an overview of systematic reviews*. JRSM Short Rep 2(2): 7.

Leurent, B., Nazareth, I., Bellón-Saameño, j., Geerlings, M.I., Maaroos, H., Saldivia, S., Švab, I., Torres-González, F., Xavier, M., and Kin, M. 2013. *Spiritual and religious beliefs as risk factors for the onset of major depression: an international cohort study*. Psychological Medicine. London, UK: Cambridge University Press.

Leung, L. 2012. *Neurophysiological basis of acupuncture-induced analgesia–an updated review*. Journal of acupuncture and meridian studies, 5 (6), 261–70.

Levinas, E. 1961. *Totality and Infinity. An Essay on Exteriority*. Pittsburg, PA: Duquesne University Press, 3rd ed. 1969.

Levinas, E. 1947. *Time and The Other*. Pittsburg, PA: Duquesne University Press, English Translation by Richard A, Cohen, 1987.

Licciardone J.C., Buchanan S., Hensel K.L., et al. 2010. *Osteopathic manipulative treatment of back pain and related symptoms during pregnancy: a randomized controlled trial*. American Journal of Obstetrics and Gynecology. 2010; 202(1): 43.e1–43.e8.

Lipton, P. 2004. *Inference to the best explanation*, 2nd edition. New York: Routledge.

Little, A.C., Jones, B.C., DeBruine, L.M. 2014. *Primacy in the Effects of Face Exposure: Perception Is Influenced More by Faces That Are Seen First*. Archives of Scientific Psychology, Washington, DC: APA, American Psychological Association, pp. 43–47

Loftus, S.F. 2006. *Language in clinical reasoning: using and learning the language of collective clinical decision making*. Sydney, AUS: Faculty of Health Sciences, School of Physiotherapy, University of Sydney

Lowen, A. 1975. *Bioenergetics*. New York, NY: Coward, McCarin & Geoghen.

Lutz A., Brefczynski-Lewis J., Johnstone T., et al. 2008. *Regulation of the neural circuitry of emotion by compassion meditation: effects of meditative expertise*. PLoS ONE. 2008; 3(3): e1897

Maier, B., and Shibles, W.A. 2010. *The philosophy and practice of medicine and bio-ethics: a naturalistic-humanistic approach*. New York: Springer.

Marcum, J.A. 2005. *Metaphysical presuppositions and scientific practices: reductionism and organicism in cancer research*. In: International Studies in the Philosophy of Science 19: 31–45.

Marcum, J.A. 2008. *An introductory philosophy of medicine: humanizing modern medicine*. New York: Springer.

Maslow, A.H. 1943. *A Theory of Human Motivation*. Originally published in *Psychological Review*, 1943, Vol. 50 #4, Washington, DC: APA, pp. 370–396

McDaniel, S.H., and deGruy III, F.V. 2014. *An Introduction to Primary Care and Psychology*. American Psychologist, Vol. 69, No. 4, 325–331. Washington, DC: American Psychological Association, p. 327

McKenzie, E. et al. 1998. *Healing Reiki*. Hamlyn Health & Well Being: Hamlyn

Miller, A. 2014. *Friends wanted. New research by psychologists uncovers the health risks of loneliness and the benefits of strong social connections*. Monitor on Psychology, Vol 45, No. 1 Washington, DC: American Psychological Association, pp. 54–58

Montgomery G.H., Bovbjerg D.H., Schnur J.B., David D., Goldfarb A., et al. 2007. *A Randomized Clinical Trial of a Brief Hypnosis Intervention to Control Side Effects in Breast Surgery Patients*. J National Cancer Institute; 99: 1304–1312

Montgomery, K. 2006. *How doctors think: clinical judgment and the practice of medicine*. New York, NY: Oxford University Press.

Moody, R. 1975. *Life After Life: the investigation of a phenomenon – survival of bodily death*, San Francisco, CA: Harper San Francisco

Murphy N., and Brown, W.S. 2007. *Did My Neurons Make Me Do It? : Philosophical and Neurobiological Perspectives on Moral Responsibility and Free Will*. Oxford, U.K.: Oxford University Press.

Napolitano J.G., Lankin D.C., Graf T.N., et al. 2013. *HiFSA fingerprinting applied to isomers with near-identical NMR spectra: the silybin/isosilybin case. Journal of Organic Chemistry*; 78(7): 2827–2839

Naylor, T.H., Willimon, W.H., Naylor, M.R. 1994. *The Search for Meaning*. Nashville, TN: Abigdon Press

Nestoriuc, Y., Martin, A., Rief, W., & Andrasik, F. 2008. *Biofeedback treatment for headache disorders: A comprehensive efficacy review*. Applied Psychophysiology and Biofeedback, 33, 125–140.

Nguyen H.T., Grzywacz J.G., Lang W., et al. 2010. *Effects of complementary therapy on health in a national U.S. sample of older adults*. Journal of Alternative and Complementary Medicine; 16(7): 701–706.

Nidich S.I., Rainforth M.V., Haaga D.A.F., et al. 2009. *A randomized controlled trial on effects of the Transcendental Meditation program on blood pressure, psychological distress, and coping in young adults.* American Journal of Hypertension. 2009; 22(12): 1326–1331

Norman, G.R., Brooks, L.R., Colle, C.L. and Hatala, R.M. 2010. *The Benefit of Diagnostic Hypotheses in Clinical Reasoning: Experimental Study of an Instructional Intervention for Forward and Backward Reasoning.* In: Cognition and Instruction, 17(4), 433–488, Hamilton, Ontario, CA: Lawrence Erlbaum Associates

Novotney, A. 2013. *Music as medicine. Researchers are exploring how music therapy can improve health outcomes among a variety of patient populations, including premature infants and people with depression and Parkinson's disease.* Monitor on Psychology, Vol. 44, N.10, Washington, DC: American Psychological Association, pp. 46–49.

Pagnini, A. (Ed.). 2010. *Filosofia della medicina. Epistemologia, ontologia, etica, diritto.* Roma, I: Carocci.

Pahal, J.S., and Li, H.Z. 2006. *The dynamics of resident-patient communication: Data from Canada.* In: Communication & Medicine, 3(2), pp. 161–170. New York, NY: Mouton de Gruyter.

Papakostas, Y.G., and Daras, M.D. 2001. *Placebos, placebo effects, and the response to the healing situation: the evolution of a concept.* Epilepsia 42: 1614–1625.

Patel, V. L., & Arocha, J. F. 2001. *The nature of constraints on collaborative decision making in health care settings.* In E. Salas & G. Klein (Eds.), *Linking expertise and naturalistic decision making.* pp. 383–405. Mahwah, NJ: Lawrence Erlbaum Associates.

Patel, V.L., Arocha, J.F., Zhang, J. 2004. *Thinking and reasoning in medicine.* In: Holyoak, K. 2004: *Cambridge Handbook of Thinking and Reasoning.* Cambridge, UK: Cambridge University Press.

Patel, V. L., Evans, D. A., & Kaufman, D. R. 1989. *Cognitive framework for doctor-patient communication.* In D. A. Evans & V. L. Patel (Eds.), *Cognitive science in medicine: Biomedical modeling,* pp. 257–312. Cambridge, MA, US: MIT Press.

Patel, V. L., & Kaufman, D. R. 1994. *Diagnostic reasoning and expertise.* Psychology of Learning and Motivation, 31, 137–252.

Patel, V. L., & Kaufman, D. R. 1995. *Clinical reasoning and biomedical knowledge: Implications for teaching.* In J. Higgs & M. Jones (Eds.), *Clinical reasoning in the health professions,* pp. 117–128. Oxford: Butterworth Heinemenn.

Patel, V.L., Arocha, J., Zhang, J. 2010. *Medical Reasoning and Thinking.* In K. Holyoak and Morrison (Eds.), Oxford Handbook of Thinking & Reasoning. New York, NY: Oxford University Press.

Penrose, R. 1989. *Shadows of the Mind: A Search for the Missing Science of Consciousness*. Oxford, UK: Oxford University Press.

Pinker, S. 2007. *The mystery of consciousness*. New York, NY: Time Magazine

Pinker, S. 2010. *Ethics and the Ethical Brain*. In: Reuter-Lorenz, P.A., Baynes, K., Mangun, G.R., and Phelps, A.E. 2010. *The Cognitive Neuroscience of Mind. A Tribute to Michael S. Gazzaniga*. Boston, MA: Massachusetts Institute of Technology

Pole, S. 2006. *Ayurvedic medicine: the principles of traditional practice*. Philadelphia, PA: Elsevier.

Plantinga A.C. and Dennet, D. 2010. *Science and Religion*. Oxford: Oxford University Press

Project of the ABIM Foundation, ACP-ASIM Foundation, and European Federation of Internal Medicine 2002. Medical professionalism in the new millennium: a physician charter. *Annals of Internal Medicine* 136: 243–246.

Relman, A.S. 2007. *A second opinion: rescuing America's healthcare*. New York: Perseus Books.

Rho, K., Han, S., Kim, K., & Lee, M. S. 2006. *Effects of aromatherapy massage on anxiety and self-esteem in Korean elderly women: A pilot study*. International Journal of Neuroscience, 116, 1447–1455.

Ritenbaugh C., Hammerschlag R., Dworkin S.F., et al. 2012. *Comparative effectiveness of traditional Chinese medicine and psychosocial care in the treatment of temporomandibular disorders-associated chronic facial pain*. Journal of Pain; 13(11): 1075–1089.

Rizzolatti G., and Sinigaglia C. 2006. *So quel che fai. Il cervello che agisce e i neuroni specchio*. Milan, I: Raffaello Cortina Editore.

Rizzolatti G., Sinigaglia C. 2010. *The functional role of the parieto-frontal mirror circuit: interpretations and misinterpretations*. Nature reviews neuroscience, 11(4) 264–274.

Robiner, W.N, Dixon, K.E., Miner, J.L., and Hong, B.A. *Psychologists in Medical Schools and Academic Medical Centers. Over 100 Years of Growth, Influence, and Partnership*. In: *American Psychologist*. Vol. 69, Num. 3: 217–315 Washington, DC: APA, American Psychological Association.

Safranski, R. 1999. *Martin Heidegger – Between Good and Evil*. Cambridge, MA: Harvard University Press.

Saper R.B., Phillips R.S., Sehgal A., et al. 2008. *Lead, mercury, and arsenic in U.S. and Indian-manufactured Ayurvedic medicines sold via the Internet*. Journal of the American Medical Association; 300(8): 915–923

Satel, S., Lilienfeld, S.O. 2013. *Brainwashed. The seductive appeal of Mindless Neuro-science*. New York, NY: Basic Books

Saunders J. 2000. *The practice of clinical medicine as an art and as a science*. Medical Humanities. 26: 18–22

Schaef, A.W. 1992. *Beyond Therapy, Beyond Science*. New York, NY: HarperCollins

Seifert, J. 2004. *The philosophical diseases of medicine and their cures: philosophy and ethics of medicine, vol. 1: foundations*. New York: Springer.

Senn, S. 2007. *Statistical issues in drug development*, 2nd edition. Hoboken, NJ: John Wiley & Sons.

Slagter, H.A., Lutz, A., Greischar, L.L., Francis, A.D., Nieuwenhuis, D., Davis, J.M., and Davidson, R.J. 2007. *Mental training affects distribution of limited brain resources*. PLOS Biology

Slayton, S.C., D'Archer, J., and Kaplan, F. 2010. *Outcome Studies on the Efficacy of Art Therapy: A Review of Findings*. Art Therapy: Journal of the American Art Therapy Association, 27(3) pp. 108–111

Spagnolo, A.G. 2008. *Quality of life and Ethical decisions in medical practice*. Journal of Medicine and The Person, vol.6, number 3: 118–122

Stefanelli, M., & Ramoni, M. F. 1992. *Epistemological constraints on medical knowledge-based systems*. In D. A. Evans & V. L. Patel (Eds.), *Advanced models of cognition for medical training and practice* Vol. 97, pp. 3–20. Heidelberg, D: Springer-Verlag.

Steger, M. F., Frazier, P., Oishi, S., & Kaler, M. 2006. *The Meaning in Life Questionnaire: Assessing the presence of and search for meaning in life*. Journal of Counseling Psychology, 53, 80–93

Steinhart, E.C. 2014. *Your Digital Afterlives: Computational Theories of Life after Death (Palgrave Frontiers in Philosophy of Religion)*. New York, NY: Palgrave McMillan

Stevenson, I. 1974 (2nd Ed.) *Twenty Cases Suggestive of Reincarnation*. Charlottesville, VA: University Press of Virginia.

Straus, S.E., and McAlister, F.A. 2000. *Evidence-based medicine: a commentary on common criticisms*. in *Canadian Medical Association Journal* 163: 837–840.

Tasman, A., Kay, J., Lieberman, J.A. 2003. *Psychiatry. Second Edition. Therapeutics*. Chichester, West Sussex, UK: John Wiley & Sons.

Tauber, A.I. 2005. *Patient autonomy and the ethics of responsibility*. Cambridge: MIT Press.

Teyber, E. 2000. *Interpersonal Process in Psychotherapy. A relational approach*. (4th Ed).Belmont, CA: Wadsworth/Thomson Learning.

Tillich, P.J. 1983. *Gesammelte Werke*, 14 Bände + 6 Ergänzungs- und Nachlassbände, 1958–1983, Hg. Renate Albrecht, Stuttgart, D: Evangelisches Verlagswerk, (new edition by Verlag Walter de Gruyter, Berlin)

Tjeltveit, A.C., and Gottlieb, M.C. 2012. *Avoiding ethical missteps. By drawing on the science of prevention, psychologists can develop skills, relationships and personal qualities to bolster ethical resilience and minimize risks related to unethical behavior*. Monitor on Psychology, Vol 43, No. 4. Washington, DC: American Psychological Association, Vol 44, No. 4, pp. 68–74.

Todorov, I., Kornell, N., Larsson Sundqvist, M., Jönsson, F.U. 2014. *Phrasing Questions in Terms of Current (Not Future) Knowledge Increases Preferences for Cue-Only Judgments of Learning*. Archives of Scientific Psychology, Washington, DC: APA, American Psychological Association, pp. 7–13

Tracey, J.G., Wampold, B.E., Lichtenberg, J.W., Goodyear, R.K. 2014. *Expertise in Psychotherapy. An Elusive Goal?* In: *American Psychologist*. Vol. 69, Num. 3: 217–315. Washington, DC: APA, American Psychological Association, pp. 225–226

Unschuld, P.U. 2010. *Medicine in China: a history of ideas*, 2nd edition. Berkeley, CA: University of California Press.

Van Dalen, D. 2012. *L.E.J. Brouwer – Topologist, Intuitionist, Philosopher: How Mathematics Is Rooted in Life*. London: Springer

Van der Steen, W.J., and Thung, P.J. 1988. *Faces of medicine: a philosophical study*. Dordrecht: Kluwer.

Verene, D.P. 1997. *Philosophy and the Return to Self-Knowledge*. New Haven, CT: Yale University Press.

Vickers A.J., Cronin A.M., Maschino A.C., Lewith G., MacPherson H., Foster N.E., Sherman K.J., Witt C.M., Linde K., & Acupuncture Trialists' Collaboration 2012. *Acupuncture for chronic pain: individual patient data meta-analysis*. Archives of internal medicine, 172 (19), 1444–1453

Vickers A.J., and Linde, K. 2014. *Acupuncture for chronic pain*. JAMA: the journal of the American Medical Association, 311 (9), 955–956

Vis, J., & Boynton, H. 2008. *Spirituality and transcendent meaning making: Possibilities for enhancing posttraumatic growth*. Journal of Religion & Spirituality in Social Work, 27, 69–86

Volk, S. 2011. *Fringe-ology: How I tried to Explain Away the Unexplainable—And Couldn't*, New York, NY: HarperCollins.

Vygotsky, L.S. 1962. *Thought and Language*. Cambridge, MA: MIT Press.

Vygotsky, L.S. 1978. *Mind in Society*. Cambridge, MA: Harvard.

Waterman, A.S. 2013. *The Humanistic Psychology-Positive Psychology Divide. Contrasts in Philosophical Foundations.* In *American Psychologist.* Vol. 68, Num. 3: 123–196 Washington, DC: APA

Weindling, P.J. 2004. *Nazi Medicine and the Nuremberg Trials. From Medical War Crimes to Informed Consent.* Houndmills, Basingstoke, Hampshire, UK: Palgrave Macmillan.

Weatherall, D. 1996. *Science and the quiet art: the role of medical research in health care.* New York: Norton.

Westen, D., and Weinberger, J. 2005. *In praise of clinical judgment: Meehl's forgotten legacy.* Journal of Clinical Psychology 61: 1257–1276.

Whitaker, R. 2001. *Mad In America: Bad Science, Bad Medicine, and The Enduring Mistreatment of the Mentally Ill,* New York, NY: Perseus Publishing

Whitaker, R. 2010. *Anatomy of an Epidemic: Magic Bullets, Psychiatric Drugs, and the Astonishing Rise of Mental Illness in America,* New York, NY: Crown

Witt C.M., Berling N.E.J., Rinpoche N.T., Cuomo M.; Willich S.N. 2009. *Evaluation of medicinal plants as part of Tibetan medicine prospective observational study in Sikkim and Nepal.* Journal of Alternative & Complementary Medicine, 2009-01-0115:1, 59(7)

Wittgenstein, L. 1958. *Preliminary Studies for the "Philosophical Investigations", Generally known as The Blue and Brown Books.* Hoboken, NJ: Blackwell Publishers

Wortman, J., Donnellan, M.B., and Lucas, R.E. 2014. *Can Physical Warmth (or Coldness) Predict Trait Loneliness? A Replication of Bargh and Shalev (2012).* Archives of Scientific Psychology, Washington, DC: APA, American Psychological Association, pp. 13–19

Wrathall, M. 2006. *How to Read Heidegger,* New York, NY: W. W. Norton, p. 100

Wulff, H.R., Pedesen, S.A., and Rosenberg, R. 1990. *Philosophy of medicine: an introduction,* 2nd edition. Oxford: Blackwell.

Yeh G.Y., McCarthy E.P., Wayne P.M., et al.. 2011. *Tai chi exercise in patients with chronic heart failure: a randomized controlled trial..* Archives of Internal Medicine; 171(8): 750–757; Wang C., Schmid C.H., Rones R., et al. 2010. *A randomized trial of tai chi for fibromyalgia.* New England Journal of Medicine; 363(8): 743–754..

Zaner, R.M. 1981. *The context of self: a phenomenological inquiry using medicine as a clue.* Athens, OH: Ohio University Press.

Zhang, J., Patel, V.L., Johnson, T.R., and Shortliffe, E.H. 2004. *A cognitive taxonomy of medical errors.* Journal of Biomedical Informatics 37 (2004) 193–204

Zürrer, R. 1989. *Reinkarnation. Die umfassende Wissenschaft der Seelenwanderung* (Reincarnation: the omni-comprehensive science of the migration of the body), IV. Aufl. 2000. Neuhausen, CH: Govinda-Verlag

Žižek, S., and Gunjević, B. 2012. *God in Pain: Inversions of Apocalypse*. New York, NY: Seven

3. Other Sources

- AA.VV. *CeSREM: Centro Studi San Raffaele Rischi Errori in Medicina*. http://www.sanraffaele.org/60316.html

- AA.VV. 2003. *20 Tips to Help Prevent Medical Errors*, http://www.ahrq.gov/Consumers & Patients/20 Tips to Help Prevent Medical Errors

- AA.VV. 2013. *10 common medical fallacies and how to avoid them*. First published in The Lawyers Weekly November 21, 2003, Vol. 23, No.28 http://www.medlit.info/lawweekly/2311medical_fallacies.htm

- AA.VV. 2014. *Sicurezza dei pazienti e gestione del rischio clinico: Manuale per la formazione degli operatori sanitari*. Ministero della Salute, Repubblica Italiana, Federazione Nazionale Ordine Medici Chirurghi ed Odontoiatri, Federazione Nazionale Collegi Infermieri.

- Barker, J. (Smith, M.W., review) 2013. Express Yourself: Your Mouth, Your Life. The Power of Positive Talking. New York, NY: WebMD. Available at: http://www.webmd.com/balance/express-yourself-13/positive-self-tal

- BioLogos Foundation, https://biologos.org/

- Borri, M. (Ed.) *Intervista ad Alessandro Pagnini*. In: Humanamente / Alessandro Pagnini, http://www.humanamente.eu/PDF/Intervista_Alessandro%20Pagnini_issue%209.pdf

- Consortium of Academic Health Centers for Integrative Medicine, http://www.imconsortium.org/

- Edzard Ernst official website: http://edzardernst.com/

- Gehirn und Geist, http://www.gehirn-und-geist.de/

- Atul Gawande, Being Mortal, on Frontline, http://www.pbs.org/wgbh/pages/frontline/being-mortal/

- Gemeinsamer Bibliotheksverbund / Illich: http://www.gbv.de/dms/faz-rez/771011_FAZ_0054_L22_0002.pdf

- Hall, H. 2008. *Death by Medicine. Science-Based Medicine. Exploring issues & controversies in science & medicine*. The complete discussion on the writing by Carolyn Dean, Gary Null, and others is available at http://www.sciencebasedmedicine.org/death-by-medicine/

- Kuhn, R.L. 2014. *Closer to Truth*, http://www.closertotruth.com/

- The Lancet, www.thelancet.com

- Loftus, S.F. 2006. *Language in clinical reasoning: using and learning the language of collective clinical decision making*, see in particular Chapter 2 -Clinical Reasoning in Medicine: Practice and Education, http://ses.library.usyd.edu.au/bit stream/2123/1165/3/03chapter2.pdf

- Meaning and Happiness, http://www.meaningandhappiness.com/

- Near Death Experience, Salon,

- Neue Medizin—http://neue-medizin.com/

- Open Sciences—http://www.opensciences.org/

- Quackwatch—www.quackwatch.org

- Rettew, D.C. 2014. *A Prescription for Music: Study Finds Musical Training Linked to Enhanced Brain Maturation in Children.* University of Vermont Medical Center Blog, December 17th, 2014,

- University of Vermont Medical Center Blog, https://medcenterblog.uvmhea lth.org/children-health/a-prescription-for-music-study-finds-musicaltraining-linked-to-enhanced-brain-maturation-in-children/

- Science-Based Medicine, http://www.sciencebasedmedicine.org/

- Journal of Translational Medicine, http://www.translational-medicine.com/

- University of Tartu's Blog, http://blog.ut.ee/religious-people-more-prone-to-dep ression/

- Wang, S. 2010. *Sartre's death-bed conversion?* In: Bridges and Tangents. Looking across the landscape of contemporary culture, https://bridgesandtangent s.wordpress.com/2010/07/31/sartres-death-bed-conversion/

ibidem-Verlag / *ibidem* Press
Melchiorstr. 15
70439 Stuttgart
Germany

ibidem@ibidem.eu
ibidem.eu